D1761084

30150 020861438

Beyond the Cognitive Map

Beyond the Cognitive Map
From Place Cells to Episodic Memory

A. David Redish

A Bradford Book
The MIT Press
Cambridge, Massachusetts
London, England

This book was set in Palatino by the author and was printed and
bound in the United States of America.

Library of Congress Cataloging-in-Publication Data

Redish, A. David.
     Beyond the cognitive map : from place cells to episodic memory
     A. David Redish.
          _____ p. _____ cm.
     "A Bradford book."
     Includes bibliographical references and index.
     ISBN 0-262-18194-0 (hc : alk. paper)
     1. Hippocampus (Brain). 2. Memory. 3. Animal navigation.
     4. Rodents as laboratory animals. 5. Space perceptions. I. Title.
     QP383.25.R43 1999
     573.8'6–dc21   98–41504
                                                                  CIP

For Laura,
for her faith and her patience

and for my parents,
for giving me the ambition
and the chutzpah to pull this off

Contents

Acknowledgements

I wish to thank first my doctoral advisor, David Touretzky, without whose high standards and support over the years, this book would not have been possible, and second the other members of my dissertation committee, Jay McClelland, Bruce McNaughton, and David Plaut, for helping make the book what it is. I am also grateful to Bruce McNaughton and Carol Barnes for their guidance and flexibility during my last year of work on the book.

I am deeply indebted to the many people who have given me critical comments (and some good arguments), and who have been so generous with their data, their comments, and their encouragement: Larry Abbott, Tad Blair, Neil Burgess, T. S. Collett, Howard Eichenbaum, Mark Fuhs, Kati Gothard, Michael Hasselmo, Jeremy Goodridge, Jim Knierim, Chip Levy, John Lisman, Etan Markus, Ali Minai, Bob Muller, Lynn Nadel, Doug Nitz, John O'Keefe, Gina Poe, Michael Recce, Lisa Saksida, Alexei Samsonovich, Pat Sharp, Bill Skaggs, Jiemin Shen, Rob Sutherland, Jeff Taube, Misha Tsodyks, Sid Wiener, Matt Wilson, Steve Wise, Brad Wyble, and Kechen Zhang, as well as the people at the Center for the Neural Basis of Cognition, the Computer Science Department at Carnegie Mellon University, and Arizona Research Laboratories, Division of Neural Systems, Memory and Aging, at the University of Arizona.

The work described in this book was partially funded by a National Science Foundation Graduate Fellowship (1991–1994) and a National Research Service Award from the National Institute of Aging (1997–1998). Additional support came from the Neural Processes in Cognition graduate training program, the Center for the Neural Basis of Cognition, the Department of Computer Science at Carnegie Mellon University, and a National Science Foundation grant awarded to David Touretzky. The views and conclusions contained herein are my own and should not be interpreted as representing those of Carnegie Mellon University, the University of Arizona, the National Science Foundation, the National Institute of Aging, the U.S. government, or anyone else. All mistakes are my own.

Last, but far from least, I have to thank my wife, Laura, for putting up with me for the year it took to write the book after surviving the year it took to write my dissertation.

Introduction

How do we remember the moments of our lives? In 1957, Scoville and Milner described a patient, H.M., who received bilateral lesions of his temporal lobes (including the hippocampus, a distinctive structure in the back of the temporal lobe) to alleviate intractable epilepsy. After the surgery, H.M. no longer had epileptic seizures but had developed a profound anterograde amnesia — he could not remember the things that happened to him after the surgery. Although he could remember a number, for example, if he concentrated, as soon as he was distracted, he forgot what the number was and even that he had been given a number to remember (Milner, 1970). It was subsequently discovered that H.M. could learn new skills, such as how to read mirror writing, although he could not remember having been taught them (Corkin, 1968). Even decades later, he still cannot remember the names of his caregivers (Cohen and Eichenbaum, 1993). Cohen and Squire (1980; see also Cohen and Eichenbaum, 1993) suggested that there were two kinds of memory: (1) *declarative* or *episodic* memory (memories of events, moments, episodes, such as where you left your car keys last night); and (2) *procedural* memory (skills, habits, abilities that take practice, such as how to throw a baseball).[1] Cohen and colleagues suggested that H.M. had a problem with storing new episodic memories.

The declarative/procedural distinction is a taxonomy of memory, but it is not a computational theory. It says nothing about how the brain stores memories, nor what the anatomy of memory is, which makes it very hard to build computational models of episodic memory that can be compared (even qualitatively) to real tasks. Almost all published simulations of episodic memory demonstrate the storage and retrieval of random binary vectors (for example, Marr, 1970; Alvarez and Squire, 1994; McClelland, McNaughton, and O'Reilly, 1995). The only two papers that make comparisons between simulations and specific experiments or that model specific cases of episodic memory do so in a navigation domain (Shen and McNaughton, 1996; Redish and Touretzky, 1998a).

The hippocampus has been strongly implicated in navigation (O'Keefe and Nadel, 1978). Models reproducing the navigation roles of hippocampus are detailed and computational; they address very specific changes in cellular firing rates after complex environmental manipulations (e.g., Zipser, 1985; McNaughton and Morris, 1987; Hetherington and Shapiro, 1993; Burgess, Recce, and O'Keefe, 1994; Touretzky and Redish, 1996; Samsonovich and McNaughton, 1997, to list a few; see also chapter 8 for more). Perhaps if we understood the role of the hippocampus in navigation, we could also begin to model episodic memory in a computational, quantitative manner.

The domains of navigation and space have a long history. The earliest navigators developed concepts that allowed them to cross vast distances of open water. Humans have been studying the geometry of space for thousands of years, going back to the ancient Greeks (Euclid, Pythagoras, Archimedes, etc.), and continuing through Newton, Descartes, Leibniz, and others. (For reviews of the history of ideas about space, see Collinder, 1955; Jammer, 1969; Cotter, 1968; Lanczos, 1970; O'Keefe and Nadel, 1978; and Gallistel, 1990). Understanding the mathematics of space, in particular how to represent two- and three-dimensional spatial extents, allows us to address the navigation domain with theories that make explicit predictions about specific experiments.

I begin the book by framing the hippocampus debate, after which I synthesize (in the Hegelian sense of "pulling ideas together") a theory of navigation in the rodent. Then I return to episodic memory to ask, computationally, what is the role of the hippocampus? In pulling together a navigation theory, this book can also serve as an introduction and review of navigation in the rodent. Researchers interested in navigation (for example, roboticists and those studying animats) will find chapters 2–11 and appendix B a useful introduction to the neurophysiology and neuroanatomy of rodent navigation, as well as a valuable source of references.

NEUROSCIENCE AND COMPUTATION

The brain can be understood on many levels. At an abstract level, we can ask what information has to be represented and how that information might be processed. For example, animals have the ability to take a circuitous path, and then, using no external information, return directly to the starting point of that path (see chapter 6). This is called *path integration* or *dead reckoning*. Because the path they take includes both direction and distance, animals must be representing a two-dimensional spatial vector. Although, mathematically, we generally represent such vectors using either Cartesian coordinates (x, y) or polar coordinates (r, ϕ), algorithms designed to handle Cartesian or polar coordinates may not be well suited for the representations actually used by rodents.

To understand how path integration occurs in the rodent brain, we need to ask how the information is represented by populations of neurons. Location in space is represented by *place cells* in the hippocampal formation (see chapter 8 and appendix B). Each of these cells has a high probability of firing when the animal is in a small, circumscribed portion of the environment. The population of these cells represents the location of the animal in the environment. Algorithms appropriate for these kinds of representations are very different from those intended for Cartesian or polar coordinates.

To understand the computation required to accomplish a task, we need to define the *functional structure* of the task, which in turn will divide the task into *subsystems*. On the other hand, there is not necessarily a one-to-one correspondence between a subsystem and an anatomical structure. Each subsystem is realized by an interaction between different brain structures, and each brain structure plays roles in multiple subsystems.

Any book purporting to address the relation between function and neurophysiology has to be careful not to fall into the trap of trying to answer the question *what does structure x do?* I take it as axiomatic that each brain structure works as one component in a network, and that each structure plays multiple roles in different networks. Having said this, we must not push too far in the other direction. Different structures are constructed differently, receiving different inputs, having different internal properties, and playing different roles.

This division into abstract functionality and detailed implementation is analogous to Marr's three levels of "understanding complex information-processing systems": (1) computational theory, (2) representation and algorithm, and (3) hardware implementation (Marr, 1982). *Computational theory* asks what computation the system must be performing, which in the path integration example, corresponds to the recognition that animals must maintain a representation of the vector home. *Representation and algorithm* asks how the information is represented by the system and how that information gets processed, which corresponds to the recognition that place cells represent a location in a coordinate system, mathematically equivalent to a two-dimensional vector. (See chapter 6 for discussions about how that representation is maintained and updated.) *Hardware implementation* asks how the representation and algorithm are realized physically, which concerns questions of neuronal connections, neurotransmitters, and so on. Although Marr assumed that the levels were separable, so that questions about computation could be addressed without addressing representation or algorithm, and questions about representation and algorithm could be addressed without addressing the actual implementation, I will not make this assumption.

An example of the inseparability of levels is the self-localization process described in chapter 9. This process allows an animal to resolve ambiguous local view inputs and reset the path integrator representation to a value consistent with the local view. Although an abstract computation of this process would select between possible candidate locations (e.g. Collett, Cartwright, and Smith, 1986; Touretzky and Redish, 1996), the actual process probably occurs by a pseudo-winner-take-all (pWTA) network settling to a stable state (chapter 9), a process that averages nearby candidate locations, but selects between candidate locations more distant from each other (appendix A). The pWTA process can only be understood by examining the neurophysiology (hardware implementation level), because it changes the computation. The computation as understood abstractly and neurophysiologically have different behavioral effects.

Because the levels are interrelated, theory cannot address only one level. It is not enough to say that to accomplish path integration there must be a representation of a vector home; we must also ask how that vector is represented and address any data available about the representation and implementation. The key to creating a theory that addresses multiple levels is to address multiple data levels as well.

Data about the brain comes in many forms. Behavioral data gives clues to what is represented and what is not, neurophysiological data is be the key to understanding representations, and anatomical data is crucial to understanding how the data flow occurs and how representations are processed. In addition, there is neuropharmacological data, which is very useful to help get at Marr's hardware implementation level, although there are cases in which the neuropharmacological data informs even the computational level (e.g. the role of acetylcholine, chapter 9).

Finally, there is lesion data, in which one or more brain structures are destroyed. Lesion data tells little about what a brain structure does, only what the brain can do without that structure. The fact that an animal can perform a task without part of its brain does not mean that that part of the brain is not involved in the task during normal operation. An animal may even be using a different technique to solve the specific problem. Similarly, that an animal cannot perform a task after a lesion does not imply that the brain structure was critically involved in the computation. For example, the brain structure may provide necessary tonic input into another brain structure that does not provide any informational content but is necessary for the second structure to perform its computations. When interpreting lesion data, it is important to be clear about what roles the structure may play in the task. I will primarily use lesion data for two purposes: to establish that certain brain structures are critically involved in a task and to confirm theories built on the foundations from other data paradigms. That is, once the theory has been built based on data from other paradigms, it will predict lesion effects that the lesion data must corroborate, but the lesion data will not generally be used to drive the specifics of the theory.

Data from all of these levels are useful constraints on a theory. In a sense, theoretical neuroscience can be thought of as a constraint satisfaction problem. On the other hand, we have to be careful about what data to include. While more constraints limit the range of candidate theories and make us more confident of our predictions, too many unrelated constraints confuse the issue.

The key to answering this problem is the concept of a *domain*, a set of experiments that a theory can be reasonably expected to address. The limits of the domain should be unrelated to the actual theory itself. A single domain is explicable by a variety of theories. Requiring all theories to address the same set of experiments allows the rejection of theories that do not fit the experimental data.

A domain should be broad enough to encompass data from multiple levels and relate them, but not so broad as to be unwieldy. The main purpose of defining a domain is to allow other people beyond the originator of the theory to decide whether an experiment is addressable by a theory. This book will address the twin domains of hippocampal function and rodent navigation.

WHAT THIS BOOK IS NOT

This book is not a replacement for O'Keefe and Nadel's 1978 book *The Hippocampus as a Cognitive Map*. I have tried, instead, to build on the foundation they laid out. In the last twenty years, hundreds of experiments have been done to test their hypotheses, measuring the effects of hippocampal lesions on spatial tasks and measuring the effects of environmental and other manipulations on hippocampal place cells. Although the experimental literature has generally supported the original hypothesis that the rodent hippocampus plays a role in locale (map-based) navigation, the theory is still not accepted by everyone (Eichenbaum, Otto, and Cohen, 1992; Eichenbaum, 1996a; see also Nadel, 1991). There are still a number of competing theories of hippocampal function. But none of these theories deny that the hippocampus is involved in navigation.

Nor is this book an answer to Cohen and Eichenbaum's 1993 book, *Memory, Amnesia, and the Hippocampal System*. This book addresses the same questions, but from a different starting point, trying to be more explicitly computational and beginning from the rodent navigation domain. But in the end, the conclusions are remarkably similar (chapter 13).

This book starts from the hypothesis that the rodent hippocampus is involved in navigation, but may also be involved in memory or other processes. It builds a theory of rodent navigation that is consistent with the anatomical, neuropharmacological, neurophysiological, and behavioral experimental literature. Although the theory draws heavily from the theoretical and experimental work done by other researchers over the last century, some specific aspects of the overall theory are novel. Once I have identified a role for the hippocampus in navigation, I return to the other theories. The role hypothesized for the hippocampus in navigation in rodents may open a new window on its role in memory in primates. This book represents only a snapshot of the state of the field of hippocampal research and rodent navigation as of January 1998. Many questions are still open and many issues still unresolved.

OUTLINE OF THE BOOK

Chapter 1 reviews the hippocampus debate, identifying key results and the two major competing theories of hippocampal function: episodic memory (Cohen and Eichenbaum, 1993) and the cognitive map (O'Keefe and Nadel, 1978). Chapters 2–7 detail a comprehensive theory of navigation and explore aspects of navigation that occur outside the hippocampus. Chapters 8–12 focus on the role of the hippocampus in navigation, arguing that it allows the animals (1) to reset their internal coordinate systems from external input (chapter 9), and (2) to store and replay recently traveled routes (chapters 11–12). Chapter 13 returns to hippocampal function, generally, while chapter 14 addresses the role of the hippocampus in primates and asks whether it is conserved across species.

Beyond the Cognitive Map

1 The Hippocampus Debate

Over the last hundred years, the hippocampus has been one of the brain's most studied structures; Ramón y Cajal (1968) dates his studies as beginning in 1888 and cites Schaffer's studies in 1892 as a key starting point. Anatomically laid out in straightforward layers, the hippocampus is clearly identifiable as different from cortex (Ramón y Cajal, 1968; Lorento do Nó, 1933, 1934; Witter et al., 1989; see figure 1.1). In the rat, the hippocampus is located just under the parietal cortex, which makes the dorsal aspect of it easily accessible to electrode probes. Because its internal structure is so regular, the hippocampus was the first place that long-term potentiation (LTP)[1] was identified in the mammalian brain (for reviews, see Racine, Milgram, and Hafner, 1983; Bliss and Lynch, 1988; Bear and Kirkwood, 1993; McNaughton, 1993).

Two key experimental effects have driven hippocampal studies:

1. *In the rodent.* Although the hippocampus is far removed from sensory stimuli, in the freely moving rodent, hippocampal pyramidal cells show a remarkable correlation to the location of the animal (O'Keefe and Dostrovsky, 1971; see appendix B for a review). Each *place cell* only shows activity in a limited portion of the environment. Hundreds, if not thousands, of experiments have examined the effects of various manipulations on place cells. Much of the theory in this book is driven by an attempt to explain these diverse effects within a single model.

2. *In the primate.* Lesions of the hippocampus (and adjacent cortical areas) in primates (particularly humans) cause a profound anterograde amnesia (Scoville and Milner, 1957; see Cohen and Eichenbaum, 1993, for a review). Lesioned subjects cannot remember facts from one day to the next. More

CA1

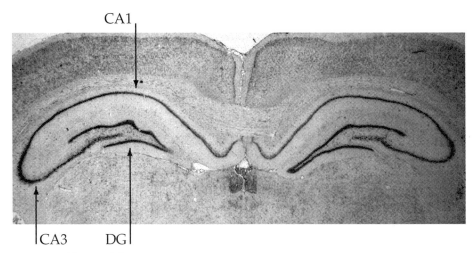

CA3   DG

Figure 1.1
Cresyl violet stain of a coronal slice of rat brain, showing the two interlocking Cs of the dentate gyrus (DG) and the hippocampus proper (CA3, CA1) on each side of the brain. (Picture courtesy C. Barnes.)

than forty years after receiving a temporal lobe lesion (including much of hippocampus, Scoville and Milner, 1957), H.M. still cannot recall the names of the doctors and nurses he sees every day (Cohen and Eichenbaum, 1993). However, he could learn some tasks. For example, he still has a very good vocabulary and can do complex crossword puzzles, although he forgets that he had done them soon afterward (Scoville, 1968). Many theories have been put forward to attempt to reconcile the complexities of this amnesia with the neural correlates found in rodents. I will address these issues in depth in chapters 12 and 14.

Each of these two effects has driven a major hippocampal theory: (1) that the hippocampus stores a *cognitive map* for navigation (O'Keefe and Nadel, 1978), and (2) that the hippocampus stores memories of events (*episodes*) temporarily for eventual storage in cortex (Marr, 1970; Squire, 1992; Cohen and Eichenbaum, 1993; McClelland, McNaughton, and O'Reilly, 1995).

Although these two theories are the most popular theories today, other theories have proposed that the hippocampus serves as an emotional center (Papez, 1937; Isaacson, 1974), that it serves as a predictive comparator (Gray, 1982a), that it stores configural associations (associations between stimuli; Sutherland and Rudy, 1989), that it is critical for working memory (within-task information; Olton and Samuelson, 1976), that it supplies context for contextual retrieval (Hirsh, 1974), that it is necessary for spanning temporal discontiguities (Rawlins, 1985), that it is necessary for recognition of novelty (Gaffan, 1972), and that it stores and replays sequences (Levy, 1989; Skaggs and McNaughton, 1996).

That the rodent hippocampus plays a role in navigation is well evidenced by lesion, EEG, and single-cell neurophysiological data. No one denies that the rodent hippocampus is involved in spatial navigation, although some believe that space is only one aspect of a more general system (e.g., Eichenbaum, Otto, and Cohen, 1992; Eichenbaum, 1996a; Rolls, 1996).

Let us therefore assume that the hippocampus is involved in spatial navigation and also that its role is conserved across spatial and nonspatial tasks. If these assumptions are correct, then we may find we can simplify the issue by concentrating on the role of the hippocampus in spatial tasks. Therefore, I will start from the question: *What is the role of the rodent hippocampus in spatial navigation?*

Because many of the spatial theories proposed to address place cell reactions to experimental manipulations are explicitly computational, they can address specific experiments, both quantitatively and qualitatively. Many of the alternate theories are not particularly computational, in part because many of the alternate domains do not have their component concepts as explicitly worked out as spatial navigation. For example, it is not yet understood how episodes are represented in the brain. We understand the mathematics of space, we know the difference between two- and three-dimensions, what it takes to represent position in space. But we have no comparable mathematics for the representation of episodes. This makes it very difficult to build explicit models of episodic memory in real tasks. There are almost no models of hippocampal function in spe-

cific episodic memory tasks. Published models of declarative
memory that include simulations or computational analyses generally address storage and retrieval of random binary vectors
(Marr, 1971; McNaughton and Morris, 1987; McNaughton, 1989;
Rolls, 1989; Alvarez and Squire, 1994; Hasselmo and Schnell, 1994;
O'Reilly and McClelland, 1994; McClelland, McNaughton, and
O'Reilly, 1995; Levy, 1996; McClelland and Goddard, 1996;
Rolls, 1996). Although these models can address general principles involved in memory, they cannot address the role of the
hippocampus in specific tasks. This makes it difficult to compare
their results with real experiments or to generate testable predictions. The two exceptions are Shen and McNaughton (1996)
and Redish and Touretzky (1998a), models of episodic memory
in navigation tasks, that show storage and retrieval of recently
experienced environments, locations, and routes.

Hippocampal studies have been performed on rodents, rabbits, and both human and nonhuman primates. However, it is not
necessarily true that the hippocampus plays the same role across
diverse species. To be sure we can construct a consistent theory
from the data, I begin by discussing only rodents. Although I
return to the question of the primate hippocampus in Chapter 14,
arguing there that the role is mostly conserved across species, I
do not want to begin from that assumption.

2 Navigation Overview

Let us begin our discussion of navigation with a canonical task, the water maze, first introduced by Morris (1981). Although it is very straightforward, it allows a relatively clean separation of navigational subsystems. The water maze consists of a large pool of water mixed with milk, chalk, or paint so as to make the water opaque. Somewhere in the pool, there is a platform on which the rodent can stand and be out of the water (see figure 2.1). Sometimes the platform is submerged just below the surface; this is called the *hidden platform water maze*. Other times, the platform sticks out above the surface; this is called the *visible platform water maze*. Sometimes the location of the platform is indicated by a colocalized cue (such as a lightbulb hanging directly over the platform), which indicates the location of the platform. This version is called the *cued water maze* and is similar to the visible platform water maze.

Because of its simplicity, the Morris water maze is one of the most used navigational tasks. It has been used to examine effects of lesions (Morris et al., 1982; Sutherland, Whishaw, and Kolb, 1983; Schenk and Morris, 1985; Kolb and Walkey, 1987; Sutherland, Whishaw, and Kolb, 1988; DiMattia and Kesner, 1988; Annett, McGregor, and Robbins, 1989; Dean, 1990; Eichenbaum, Stewart, and Morris, 1990; Morris et al., 1990; Sutherland and Rodriguez, 1990; Packard and McGaugh, 1992; Taube, Klesslak, and Cotman, 1992; McDonald and White, 1993; Sutherland and Hoesing, 1993; McDonald and White, 1994; Nagahara, Otto, and Gallagher, 1995; Whishaw, Cassel, and Jarrard, 1995; Whishaw and Jarrard, 1996; Schallert et al., 1996), neuropharmacological manipulations (Schallert, De Ryck, and Teitelbaum, 1980; Sutherland, Whishaw, and Regehr, 1982; DeVietti et al., 1985; Whishaw, 1985; Packard and White, 1991; Day and Schallert, 1996), grafts (Nilsson et al., 1987; Bjorklund,

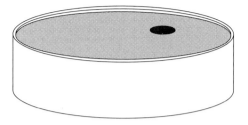

Figure 2.1
Water maze. Black circle indicates location of the platform. In the
hidden platform version, the platform is beneath the water surface and
thus not visible to the animal. Typical tank diameters are 1–2 m.

Nilsson, and Kalen, 1990), and genetic mutants (Silva et al., 1992;
Tsien, Huerta, and Tonegawa, 1996; Wilson and Tonegawa, 1997),
as well as aging effects (Gallagher and Burwell, 1989; Gallagher, Burwell, and Burchinal, 1993; Gallagher and Nicole, 1993;
Gallagher and Colombo, 1995; Gallagher, Nagahara, and Burwell,
1995; Barnes et al., 1997; Barnes, 1998).

There are five strategies an animal can take to find the platform
(O'Keefe and Nadel, 1978; Sutherland, Whishaw, and Kolb, 1983;
Whishaw and Mittleman, 1986; Gerstner and Abbott, 1997):

- *Random navigation.* If the animal has no information about
  the location of the platform, it must search randomly for it.

- *Taxon navigation.* The animal can find a cue toward which it
  can always swim. For example, if the platform is visible, it
  can simply "swim toward the platform."

- *Praxic navigation.* The animal can execute a constant motor
  program. For example, if the animal always starts at the
  same location, in the same orientation, and the platform
  is never moved, it can use praxic navigation to reach the
  platform.

- *Route navigation.* The animal can learn to associate a direction with each sensory view. In more complex mazes, this entails planning a sequence of subgoals. For example, many early navigation tasks used complex mazes that consisted of sequences of T-junctions. Route navigation can be thought of as chaining sequences of taxon and praxic substrategies.

- *Locale navigation.* The animal can learn the location of the platform relative to a constellation of cues. It can learn a map on which the location of the platform is known. If it knows both its own location and the location of the platform in the same coordinate system, then it can plan a path from one to the other.

These five strategies make up the taxonomy of rodent navigation.

Other taxonomies have been proposed (O'Keefe and Nadel, 1978; Gallistel, 1990; Kuipers et al., 1993; Trullier et al., 1997). O'Keefe and Nadel (1978) separate out route and locale navigation but separate out orientations and guidances under the rubric of route navigation. *Orientations* are beaconings to a landmark and *guidances* are landmark based responses such as following along a wall.

Gallistel (1990) divides navigation into two components that allow an animal to determine its position on a cognitive map: piloting and dead reckoning. *Piloting* is a process by which a navigator determines its position from landmarks, while *dead reckoning* is a mechanism to update that representation of position from internal cues identifying the navigator's direction of motion and speed. These two components correspond to the influence of local view and path integration on the place code (see chapters 3, 6, and 8, respectively).

The local view subsystem represents the animal's relationship to landmarks. These cues can be differentiated from, say, vestibular cues, which can only tell the animal how quickly it is turning or accelerating. Cues can be categorized as being either external or internal.[1] *External* cues allow an animal to calculate its position given general knowledge about the environment, but require no prior knowledge about the position; *internal cues* allow the animal to calculate its position at time t given a known position at $t - t$, but require no knowledge of the environment.

Kuipers et al. (1993) suggest a three-level hierarchy of (1) control strategies; (2) topological representations; and (3) geometric representations. *Control strategies* consist of simple stimulus-response abilities (such as wall-following), equivalent to the taxon and praxic strategies here. *Topological representations* consist of places linked by paths, which allow navigation in complex environments, but do not allow shortcuts across open spaces. I will not dwell on them because data is lacking on the neurophysiology underpinning topological navigation. Finally, Kuipers et al.'s hierarchy includes *geometric representations*, which include metric properties. Again, data is lacking from the rodent, but this corresponds to path planning and what data is available will be discussed in the context of the *goal memory* in chapter 7.

Trullier et al. (1997) have reviewed animat models (robotics and simulated-life models), characterizing navigation in a five-stage hierarchy: (1) target-approaching, (2) guidances, (3) place navigation, (4) topological navigation, and (5) metric navigation. *Target approaching* simply consists of beaconing to a landmark (taxon navigation here). *Guidances* are stimulus responses to a complex array. Target approaching and guidances together correspond to Kuipers et al.'s control strategies (1993), and are discussed in chapter 4. *Place navigation* corresponds to locale navigation here — it requires a mechanism for self-localization (chapter 9) and goal finding (chapter 7). *Topological* and *metric navigation* in Trullier et al.'s hierarchy are equivalent to topological and geometric navigation in Kuipers et al.'s taxonomy.

In addition, there are navigation taxonomies that divide out different kinds of taxes (Fraenkel and Gunn, 1961; Tinbergen, 1969; Schöne, 1984), such as chemotaxis (orientation to chemical odors) and phototaxis (orientation to light), which I have categorized under the rubric of taxon navigation.

One should note as well the relation between this taxonomy and the procedural/declarative distinction made in the episodic memory theory (Cohen and Squire, 1980; Squire, 1987; Mishkin and Appenzeller, 1987; Squire and Zola-Morgan, 1988;

Cohen and Eichenbaum, 1993). Declarative memory stores facts, names, and such, while procedural memory stores skills. This distinction is usually framed in terms of general memory properties, whereas in the navigation domain, locale navigation would be declarative while taxon and route navigation would be procedural. Although there are other navigation taxonomies, I will stick to the five strategy taxonomy described at the begining of this chapter because it is the easiest with which to understand the neurophysiology. Most of the navigation section of this book is devoted to locale navigation because, as originally hypothesized by O'Keefe and Nadel (1978), it is locale navigation that requires the hippocampus.

RANDOM NAVIGATION

When first put into the hidden platform water maze, an animal has no information about the location of the platform and must search for it randomly. When an animal first sees a novel environment, it spends a significant amount of time exploring that environment; indeed, many animals will explore rather than look for food reward in novel environments (for reviews, see Archer and Birke, 1983; Renner, 1990).

In addition to novel environments, there is one other case in which an animal must fall back on random navigation: when it cannot determine any information about where it is. If the animal does not always start from the same location relative to the platform, then it cannot use a praxic strategy. Taxon, route, and locale strategies all require information from the external world — without this *local view* information, the animal would be reduced to using a random search strategy.

TAXON NAVIGATION

The term *taxon navigation* comes from the word *taxis*, used in ethology to mean "a drawing towards," or "to approach," as in phototaxis, an orientation toward the light. It refers to a strategy of moving directly toward a landmark. Because they entail orienting to a landmark and using it as a beacon, taxon strategies are sometimes called *orienting* or *beaconing* strategies. They are essentially stimulus-response strategies.

The suggestion that rodents use taxon strategies go back to the very earliest navigation models (e.g. Hull, 1943, 1952; Fraenkel and Gunn, 1961; Tinbergen, 1969; for reviews, see Schöne, 1984, and Gallistel, 1990). Taxon strategies have been most extensivly studied in insects and other primitive organisms (Fraenkel and Gunn, 1961; Tinbergen, 1969; Schöne, 1984). In the water maze, only the cued and visible platform versions can be solved using taxon strategies.

Taxon strategies have the computational advantage that they are very simple and so can be learned using straightforward Pavlovian stimulus-response mechanisms. On the other hand, they are limited in their flexibility. If the animal has learned to approach a single landmark and then that landmark is moved or if it disappears entirely, the animal is out of luck and cannot find the goal.

Anatomically, there is evidence that taxon strategies are based in phylogenetically old structures, such as the superior colliculus (Drager and Hubel, 1975, 1976; Goodale, Foreman, and Milner, 1978; Ellard and Goodale, 1988; Goodale, 1983) and the basal ganglia (Potegal, 1982; Packard and McGaugh, 1992; Wiener, 1993; McDonald and White, 1994; Mizumori and Cooper, 1995).

Animals with superior collicular lesions cannot orient toward stimuli (Goodale, Foreman, and Milner, 1978; Ellard and Goodale, 1988; Goodale, 1983; Dean and Redgrave, 1984a). Cells in the superior colliculus respond to input from multiple modalities (Drager and Hubel, 1975, 1976; Stein and Meredith, 1993); electrical stimulation of the superior colliculus produces orientation motions (Dean and Redgrave, 1984a; Stein and Meredith, 1993). Because the cells in the superior colliculus are laid out in a highly regular format (Drager and Hubel, 1975, 1976; Sparks, 1986; Sparks and Nelson, 1987; Stein and Meredith, 1993), stimulation of a single point in the superior colliculus fires a population of neurons encoding a single orientation direction.

In addition, the caudate nucleus seems to be involved in taxon navigation. Lesions of the caudate nucleus disrupt navigation to cued platforms, such as visible platforms or platforms with a large black card marking the quadrant containing the goal, but not to hidden platforms (McDonald and White, 1994; Packard and McGaugh, 1992). Wiener (1993) and Mizumori and Cooper (1995) have both recorded from neurons in caudate nucleus and found cells related to taxon strategies. (All of these results will be discussed in depth in chapter 4.)

Parietal cortex is also involved in taxon strategies. In the hidden platform water maze, parietal lesions produce random search (DiMattia and Kesner, 1988). Even when a visible cue is available, animals with parietal lesions reverted to circling at the appropriate distance from the wall, a praxic strategy (Kolb and Walkey, 1987; Kolb, 1990b). Parietal cortex may be involved in the representation of the local view, which represents spatial aspects of local and distal landmarks (see chapter 3 for discussion and references). Obviously, in order for an animal to use taxon strategies (say, approach to a landmark), the animal must be able to represent spatial parameters such as the egocentric bearing to the landmark.[2]

Taxon strategies can be understood using simple stimulus-response models. Given a single stimulus, the animal simply orients toward it and proceeds. Models of taxon strategies have been extensively studied. (Some of these models and other issues relating to taxon navigation will be discussed in greater depth in chapter 4.)

PRAXIC NAVIGATION

Taxon navigation consists of a simple response to a stimulus; praxic strategies consist of complex responses, but usually to very simple stimuli. In the water maze, an animal can use praxic strategies to find the platform if it is always started at a specific point in the environment. For example, if the animal always starts facing the east wall at the easternmost point of the environment and the platform is always along the northernmost part of the wall, then the animal only needs to learn to turn left and then proceed to the platform (Eichenbaum, Stewart, and Morris, 1990; Moghaddam and Bures, 1994; Save and Moghaddam, 1996). This is a praxic strategy.

Praxic strategies are sometimes called *kinetic strategies*, referring to internally guided movements (from the Greek *kinein*, "to move," American Heritage, 1969). The term *praxic* comes from the Greek word *praxis*, meaning "doing," "action," as in the English word *practice* (American Heritage, 1969). Praxic strategies generally consist of stereotyped movements independent of starting position. They are thus only useful if an animal's spatial relationship to the goal does not change from trial to trial. However, the term *praxic strategy* is also sometimes used to refer to a strategy completely guided by internal cues (for example, dead reckoning or path integration).

Early experiments on rodents used very complex mazes made up of many elevated tracks all of the same length, joined at T-junctions (Watson, 1907; Carr and Watson, 1908; Carr, 1917; Dennis, 1932; Honzik, 1936; Hull, 1943; Tolman, 1948; Hull, 1952). See figure 2.2.

Some of the important results to come out of these early experiments seem to imply that animals were using praxic strategies (Watson, 1907; Carr and Watson, 1908; Carr, 1917; Dennis, 1932; Honzik, 1936; see also Gallistel, 1990, for review.) For example, well-trained rats can navigate complex mazes under extreme sensory deprivation (Watson, 1907; Carr and Watson, 1908; Carr, 1917; Honzik, 1936). Honzik (1936) found that rats could navigate his 14-junction maze (figure 2.2c) even after being blinded or made anosmic. Watson (1907) found that animals could navigate a Hampton-Court maze (figure 2.2a) without ever touching the walls, even when made simultaneously blind, deaf, anosmic, and lacking vibrissae. If animals are using internally driven, praxic strategies, they could navigate these mazes by knowing how much they turn and how many steps they take. Chapters 5 and 6 review evidence that rodents can do both.

Another demonstration that animals may use praxic strategies is that well-trained rats run into walls when the lengths of the

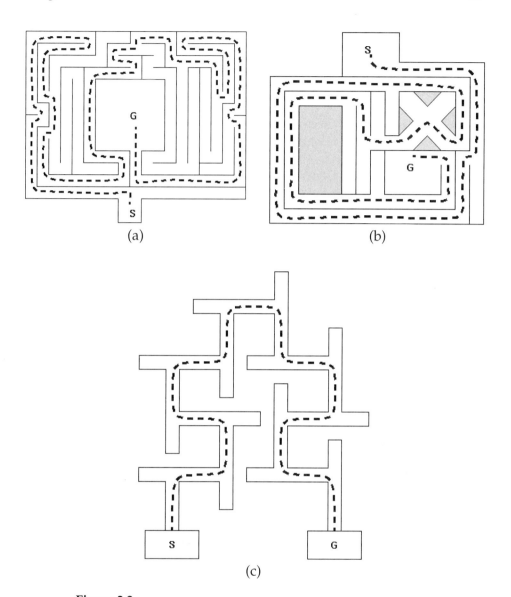

Figure 2.2
Complex mazes used in the early rodent navigation literature. S indicates the start and G indicates the goal. Dashed line indicates successful path. (a) Hampton-court maze used by Watson (1907). (b) Maze used by Carr and Watson (1908). (c) Fourteen–dead end maze used by Honzik (1936).

corridors are shortened (Carr and Watson, 1908; Dennis, 1932). Carr and Watson (Watson, 1907; Carr and Watson, 1908; Carr, 1917) report that well-trained rats run a maze very fast and "with confidence." They note that the rats do not seem to be using external sensory cues to guide them. When placed in the maze at a point along the route (i.e. not the start), the rats seem confused at first but then once they "get their cues," they run at top speed to the goal (Carr and Watson, 1908). Unfortunately, this means that if a corridor is shortened or lengthened, the rats run full tilt into the wall (Carr and Watson, 1908). Analogously, Dennis (1932) reports that when dead ends on an elevated maze are changed, rats run right off the edge, sometimes barely catching themselves with their hind claws

Although I have separated taxon and praxic strategies in the navigation taxonomy here, it is not absolutely clear that they are separable. For example, in the hidden platform water maze task, rodents with hippocampal lesions learn to circle the tank at the correct distance from the wall (Morris et al., 1982; Eichenbaum, Stewart, and Morris, 1990). This is neither a true taxon strategy, in that it is a complex response to the cue, but nor is it a true praxic strategy, in that it is cue-driven.

Path Integration

A special case of a praxic strategy, *path integration* is the ability to take a circuitous path, and, using only internal cues, plan a journey home, that is, to the begining of that path (Barlow, 1964; Gallistel, 1990; Maurer and Seguinot, 1995). Path integration has been demonstrated in a variety of species, ranging from gerbils (Mittelstaedt and Mittelstaedt, 1980) to humans (Beritashvili, 1965).

One possible explanation of some recent findings that rats are capable of remembering the location of a visible platform is that the water maze can be solved by path integration if an animal is not disoriented between trials (Alyan, Touretzky, and Taube, 1995). Animals with hippocampal lesions were trained to find a visible platform; when the visible platform was removed, they searched at the location of the missing platform (Whishaw, Cassel, and Jarrard, 1995; Whishaw and Jarrard, 1996). Because the animals were not disoriented between trials, they might have been able to path integrate and remember the direction and distance that they had to travel to reach the platform. Another explanation of these findings will be discussed in the next section. (Issues of whether the hippocampus is necessary for path integration will be discussed in chapter 6.)

Like other praxic strategies, path integration requires a mechanism for tracking both the angles turned and the distance traveled. (A mechanism by which rodents track angles turned will be discussed in chapter 5 and the complete path integration system will be discussed in chapter 6.)

ROUTE NAVIGATION

Taxon and praxic navigation are both special cases of a more general navigation strategy: that of route navigation. They thus have often been referred to as *route strategies* (e.g., O'Keefe and Nadel, 1978). Route navigation can be understood as the sequencing of taxon and praxic strategies dependent on sensory input.

There are two major types of route navigation: complex routes such as those used to solve the mazes shown in figure 2.2, and associations of direction to travel with the view available from each location (the local view, see chapter 3). Complex routes are more applicable to corridor and T-junction mazes like Honzik's fourteen-junction maze (Honzik, 1936), while the association is most applicable to open arenas (such as the water maze), but both are examples of route strategies. They are essentially chains of taxon and praxic strategies.

In ethology, a difference is often made between a stimulus that *releases* an action and a stimulus that *directs* one (Tinbergen, 1969; Schöne, 1984). Taxon strategies consist of approaching toward directing (or *orienting*) stimuli, while praxic strategies consist of stereotyped motor actions. Both taxon and praxic strategies can be released by stimuli. For example, an animal always placed in the same point of a water maze can learn to reach an immobile platform by swimming in a certain direction for a certain distance (Eichenbaum, Stewart, and Morris, 1990; Moghaddam and Bures, 1994; Save and Moghaddam, 1996). This is a praxic strategy released by the stimulus of being placed into the water maze. Route strategies can be thought of as chaining taxon and praxic strategies by sequences of releasing stimuli.

A number of robotics and artificial intelligence algorithms have been proposed to solve these sequencing problems (see Trullier et al., 1997, for a review). They usually consist of sequences of symbolic links. For example, Kuipers and colleagues (Kuipers, 1977, 1978; Kuipers et al., 1993) define each corner as a *place*; Levitt and colleagues (Levitt et al., 1987; Kuipers and Levitt, 1988) define areas by changes in landmark perceptual order (i.e., which landmark is to the left of which other landmarks); Schölkopf and Mallot (1993) and Poucet (1993) define places as areas in which the local view does not change. Once these authors have defined symbolic areas, connected by topological edges, algorithms such as graph search (Bondy and Murty, 1976; Cormen, Leiserson, and Rivest, 1990) can be used to identify routes to goals. None of these algorithms allow simple neural implementations; they all require complex symbolic computations. The mechanism by which this occurs in rodents is still not known, although McNaughton (1989) and Poucet (1993) have suggested that the hippocampus serves to chain together places and to learn how to make transitions from one to another. We will see that place cells are not well suited for this purpose, but are for determining where the animal is (chapter 8); other systems probably subserve path planning (chapter 7).

In contrast, there are a number of plausible models that associate a representation of the external world with direction in which to travel to reach a goal (McNaughton, 1989; Leonard and McNaughton, 1990; Brown et al., 1991; Brown and Sharp, 1995; Blum and Abbott, 1996; Gerstner and Abbott, 1997; Redish and Touretzky, 1998a). In some of these models, the hippocampus serves as the route storage mechanism ((McNaughton, 1989; Leonard and McNaughton, 1990; Blum and Abbott, 1996; Gerstner and Abbott, 1997); in other models, the hippocampus serves as the input to a route system (Brown et al., 1991; Burgess, O'Keefe, and Recce, 1993, 1994; Brown and Sharp, 1995). In Redish and Touretzky (1998a), the hippocampus is used to train the association in *long-term memory*.

If there were a way to show the animal the route to the goal, it might be possible to train the route system even without a hippocampus. For example, Schallert et al. (1996) showed that animals could learn to solve the water maze even with hippocampal lesions if they were trained with a certain paradigm. Schallert et al. used animals with hippocampal lesions (created with injections of both colchicine and kainate, which destroy the DG and CA3/CA1 fields, respectively). The animals were first trained with a large hidden platform that filled almost the entire maze. Once the animals could reach that platform reliably, it was shrunk trial by trial until it was the size of a typical platform in a water maze task. These animals learned to solve the water maze without a hippocampus. One way to explain these results is that nonhippocampal processes are being used to train the route system. In the Schallert et al. (1996) experiments, the route system may be being explicitly trained by their experimental methodology.

Redish and Touretzky (1998a) have suggested similar explanations for Whishaw and colleagues' experiments, in which animals with fimbria-fornix (Whishaw, Cassel, and Jarrard, 1995) or hippocampal (Whishaw and Jarrard, 1996) lesions can remember the location of a previously visible platform, but McDonald and White (1994) tried to train animals with fimbria-fornix lesions to find hidden platforms in locations previously occupied by visible platforms. They were unable to train rats with fimbria-fornix lesions to find the hidden platform. The difference between these two experiments is that Whishaw and colleagues did not disorient the animals between trials, and therefore path integration might have been a factor (Alyan, Touretzky, and Taube, 1995) while McDonald and White (1994) gave the visible and hidden trials on different days, thereby precluding praxic strategies.

Route navigation as defined here has the advantage of being simple to compute once it has been trained. The animal simply moves in a certain direction when it sees a certain (possibly complex) local view.

The main disadvantage of route navigation is that it takes a long time to train; it cannot be trained in a single trial. Each position needs to be associated with a direction. This means that enough time has to be spent in each location learning the association. The methodological paradigm used by Schallert et al. (1996) may have given the animal enough time to learn the necessary association.

Alternatively, route navigation could be trained off-line, for example, during sleep (Levy, 1996; Levy and Wu, 1996; Skaggs and McNaughton, 1996; Redish and Touretzky, 1998a). This issue relates very strongly to that of consolidation (Marr, 1970; Buzsáki, 1989; Squire, 1992; Cohen and Eichenbaum, 1993; McClelland, McNaughton, and O'Reilly, 1995), and will be discussed in detail in chapters 11 and 12.

Unfortunately, if route navigation is defined as an association between positions and vectors (directions of intended motion), then the only way an animal can plan a shortcut is either to recognize a position farther along the chain or to interpolate the vectors. Animals can take shortcuts along areas beyond the reach of interpolation (Tolman, Ritchie, and Kalish, 1946a; Tolman, 1948; Matthews et al., 1995). Planning a path from an unexplored area by vector interpolation requires that the unexplored areas be in the convex hull of the explored areas.

Sutherland et al. (1987) trained rats to find a hidden platform in half the water maze (with a barrier blocking the other half) and then removed the barrier and started the animals on the unexplored side. Although the rats spent a longer time finding the platform than previously, Matthews et al. (1995) argued that the animals may have been spending their time exploring where the barrier had been. Matthews et al. (1995) also trained rats in a water maze with a barrier closing off half of the maze, but they then moved the barrier slightly, exposing more of the maze with each trial. At first, the animals spent time exploring near the moved barrier, but eventually, they began to ignore the barrier. At this point, Matthews et al. (1995) removed the barrier and started the animals in the unexplored area of the water maze, which had previously been beyond the barrier. The rats swam directly to the platform, showing that they could indeed plan paths from unexplored areas. Such behavior requires a more complex strategy: locale navigation.

LOCALE NAVIGATION

In contrast with the other four strategies, locale navigation requires the construction of a *cognitive map*, as originally proposed by Tolman (1948) as an explanation for shortcut abilities and for latent learning, where prior experience in an environment makes tasks easier to learn in that environment (Blodget, 1921; Tolman, 1948). For example, on a Y-maze, Tolman (1948) tested animals with a food reward at the end of one arm of the Y and a water reward at the other. Animals who were neither hungry nor thirsty were allowed to explore this environment. Half of the animals were then made hungry and the other half thirsty. The hungry animals immediately ran to the food source and thirsty animals to the water source (Tolman, 1948). This demonstrates that animals do not have to be strongly rewarded for them to learn goal locations. Latent learning is also seen in the ability of animals to learn navigation tasks faster in an environment if they have had a chance to explore the environment beforehand (Blodget, 1921).

One of the key points that separates locale navigation from route strategies is that locale navigation should be an all-or-none phenomenon (O'Keefe and Nadel, 1978). The animal either knows where it is on the map or doesn't. In a beautiful demonstration of this, Barnes et al. (1997) looked back over hundreds of trials of old and young animals in the water maze. They found that histograms of path length[3] were strongly bimodal. On any trial, animals either traveled a very short path to the goal or took a long, roundabout route searching for the goal. With increased training, the samples shift from the long-path mode to the shorter-path mode.

On the basis of EEG, lesion, and extracellular recording results, O'Keefe and Nadel (1978) proposed that the hippocampus
is the anatomical locus of the cognitive map. A tremendous corpus of data has been added to the literature over the last twenty
years, most of it confirming their hypothesis (see Jarrard, 1993;
Redish and Touretzky, 1997a; Redish, 1997; and appendix B). I
will argue that the role of the hippocampus is to localize the
animal on the cognitive map, and that it works through a host
of other anatomical and functional structures to perform locale
navigation.

A rodent's ability to perform locale navigation tasks such as
the hidden platform water maze depends on an interaction between five different spatial representations:

1. *Local view*: a representation of the animal's relationship to
   landmarks in its environment.

2. *Path integrator coordinates*: a metric representation of position
   that accommodates vector arithmetic.

3. *Head direction*: a representation of orientation in space.

4. *Place code*: a distributed representation of position that ties
   local views to path integrator coordinates.

5. *Goal memory*: a representation that associates motivational
   and spatial inputs and that accommodates trajectory planning.

These abstract subsystems should not be expected to be anatomically localized; their functions will be distributed across several
brain structures.

Chapters 3–8 address the five subsystems. None of the subsystems work independently of each other, but I have tried to order
them in the most straightforward way, with the fewest forward
dependencies. Because it is the least dependent on other systems
yet is involved in all of the other systems, we will begin with the
local view (chapter 3). Next, we turn to taxon, praxic, and route
navigation (chapter 4), and then address the major components of

locale navigation: the head direction system (chapter 5), the path integration system (chapter 6), and the goal memory (chapter 7). Finally, we will consider the place code and the hippocampus proper in chapter 8. The remaining navigation chapters (chapters 9–11) address processes involving the place code.

3 Local View

The local view subsystem represents the sensory aspects of landmarks; it should at a minimum include representations of spatial aspects of the various landmarks (such as distance and bearing). Although the term *local view* was first introduced to mean what can be seen from a particular viewing position (McNaughton, 1989, see Leonard and McNaughton, 1990, for a review), even the earliest theories of local view did not require the landmarks to be solely visual (e.g., Leonard and McNaughton, 1990). Rodents can navigate based on any number of nonvisual cues, such as auditory, olfactory, and somatosensory cues (Schöne, 1984; Goodale and Carey, 1990; Kelly, 1990; Stein and Meredith, 1993), and rats with severe sensory deficits can still navigate accurately using external cues (Watson, 1907; Carr and Watson, 1908; Carr, 1917; Dennis, 1932; Honzik, 1936; Zoladek and Roberts, 1978; Hill and Best, 1981; Save et al., 1998).

Of course, rodents are generally nocturnal and their visual acuity is much less than ours, but they are sensitive to distal cues that are only detectable visually. For example, their search patterns on the radial maze follow rotations of distal cues (Suzuki, Augerinos, and Black, 1980), and their place fields also follow rotations of distal cues around the room, Muller and Kubie, 1987; O'Keefe and Speakman, 1987; McNaughton, Knierim, and Wilson, 1994; Knierim, Kudrimoti, and McNaughton, 1995). For our purposes, I will accept that rodent vision is poor but useful, and assume that *local view*, irrespective of its name, includes nonvisual cues as well as visual.

Thus local view consists of the sensory input available from a particular viewing position and orientation in a specific environment. With a sufficiently rich set of cues and no pathological symmetries in the environment, local views describe unique

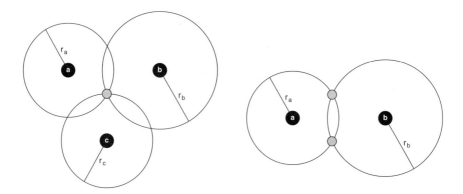

Figure 3.1
Knowing the distances to three unique, noncolinear landmarks allows localization to a single point (*left*), but knowing distances to only two does not (*right*). (From Redish, 1997.)

places. However, in the real world, some cues move from time to time, and others appear and disappear. I will argue that animals handle these ambiguities in the place code in the hippocampus (see chapter 8).

SPATIAL ASPECTS

Because the point of the local view system is to allow the animal to determine its position from external cues, we can make some computational claims about the spatial aspects included in the local view. The local view must include enough spatial cues to uniquely define a point. For example, three distance measurements are sufficient, but two are not. As can be seen in figure 3.1, having only two distance measurements leaves an ambiguity of two points. The actual representation of landmark spatial aspects is likely to be noisy, so the local view can be expected to overdetermine position in order to compensate.

Distance

Distance to landmarks is correlated with aspects such as size on the retina and position relative to the horizon. Both of these aspects vary regularly with respect to the distance an object is from the animal. Thus a cell tuned to these aspects will appear to be tuned to distance.

Primates have forward-facing eyes, which allow them to use stereo vision to determine distance. Rodents are prey animals and in general do not have forward-facing eyes, but the overlap of the visual fields of the nasal retinas does allow about 50° to 80° of binocularity (Goodale and Carey, 1990). Both Goodale and Carey (1990) and Dean (1990) suggest that head movements seen during rearing in discrimination-learning tasks may be designed to bring discriminants into the temporal retinas so that they can be viewed stereoscopically. Gallistel (1990) suggests that the purpose of these movements is to produce parallax, which could also provide distance information.

Egocentric and Allocentric Bearing

In addition to distance, orientation to landmarks must be a key component of local view. Orientation can be encoded egocentrically or allocentrically. *Egocentric bearing* measures the angle between the landmark and the animal's heading (θ_j in figure 3.2), while *allocentric bearing* measures the angle between the landmark and a reference direction (ϕ_j in figure 3.2). Allocentric bearing can be calculated from egocentric bearing given the angle between the animal's heading and the reference direction (H in figure 3.2).

$$\phi_j = \theta_j + H \tag{3.1}$$

Allocentric bearings have the advantage that they are independent of the animal's orientation, but they require a representation of the animal's heading relative to the reference direction (H in equation 3.1), which is exactly what is provided by the representation of head direction (see chapter 5).

Taxon navigation is generally based on egocentric bearing: orient to a stimulus and approach it. Evidence that animals can

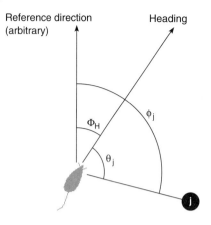

Figure 3.2
Ego- and allocentric bearings. $_H$: angle between head direction and reference orientation; θ_j: egocentric bearing to landmark j; ϕ_j: allocentric bearing to landmark j. (From Redish, 1997.)

use egocentric bearing for navigation is extensively reviewed by Schöne (1984). (Taxon navigation, and the particular role of the superior colliculus in orientation, is discussed in chapter 4.)

Evidence that rodents have access to allocentric bearing is more subtle. Animals have been trained to find food at a constant bearing and distance to a single landmark; they do not search at an annulus around the landmark (Collett, Cartwright, and Smith, 1986). Collett and colleagues attempted to control the available external directional cues. They used a circularly symmetric landmark and a black curtain around the walls of the room. The search distribution they observed can be explained by access to allocentric bearing. When they disoriented their animals before each trial, Biegler and Morris (personal communication) had difficulties training an animal to search at a single point relative to a circularly symmetric landmark. If the allocentric bearing computation is dependent on the representation of head direction, then the disorientation used by Biegler and Morris would be like putting the food at a different orientation from the landmark with each trial. This issue has also been examined by Knierim, Kudrimoti, and McNaughton (1995), who found that when animals were disoriented prior to each experience, the tuning curves of head direction cells no longer followed a distal cue (a cue card, placed along one wall of the arena). As they noted, if the internal representation of head direction is primary, then the effect of disorientation is like putting the cue card at a different location with every trial.

CUE TYPES

Point Landmarks

Although there are many examples of rodents navigating based on small objects (e.g., the cylinders in Collett, Cartwright, and Smith, 1986), whether these are seen as single objects by the rodents is an open question. Most models treat landmarks as *points* in space. This gives the distinct advantage that distance and bearing are easily defined. Of course, even though no object is a true point (i.e., all objects have extent), whether one considers navigation to an object or a point on an object is irrelevant. What matters is that rodents can measure spatial parameters of pointlike landmarks.

Surface Landmarks

Rodents with hippocampal damage solve the water maze by swimming at a set distance from the wall (Morris et al., 1982; Whishaw and Mittleman, 1986; Eichenbaum, Stewart, and Morris, 1990), strongly implying they have a representation of their relation to the wall, which can then be used in taxon navigation. An important question is how far away from the surface an animal can detect the surface orientation. If rodents used their vibrissae to detect local surface orientation, they would only be able to use the wall as a sensory cue when close.

Another indication that the local view might include some representation of local surface orientation is that changes in the local surface orientation produce changes in place fields (Muller and Kubie, 1987; Muller, Kubie, and Ranck, 1987).

Muller and Kubie (1987) found that when a barrier was added to a cylinder, the firing rates of 9 out of 10 cells whose fields intersected the barrier diminished. The remaining cell increased its firing rate. Substituting a transparent barrier did not affect the results. The effect only occurred if the barrier interfered with the rat's motion. They also experimented with a small heavy object that did not interfere with travel (the base of the barrier). If only this base was put into the place field, there was no effect on firing rate. Barriers outside the place field also had no effect.

Muller, Kubie, and Ranck (1987) reported cells with place fields along the wall of a cylindrical arena. The interior edges of these fields are concave (i.e., the fields "hug" the arena wall), which implies that the cells must be sensitive to the arena wall.[1] That these cells have only been seen near the wall may imply that the detection range of surface orientation might be very local. That only barriers intersecting a cell's place field changed the field (Muller and Kubie, 1987) also supports the hypothesis that the detection range of surface orientation might be local.

Compass Points

If a landmark is very distant to the environment, the egocentric bearing to it will change very little as the animal moves around an arena. In addition, accurate distances would be hard to determine (beyond that it is very far). These cues are sometimes called *compass points*, because they can be used to inform the head direction system directly. An association between the egocentric bearing to a distal cue and a head direction is valid no matter where an animal is in the environment. Like the North Star, the distal cue can serve as a direct orienting cue.

Whether local view preferentially includes information from distal or local cues has been measured behaviorally by examining whether rodents follow intramaze or extramaze cues (e.g., Watson, 1907; Dennis, 1932; Honzik, 1936; Olton and Samuelson, 1976; Suzuki, Augerinos, and Black, 1980). Early experiments (e.g., Dennis, 1932; Honzik, 1936) tested this by training rats to solve complex mazes made of elevated tracks and then interchanging or replacing the tracks without changing the basic shape of the maze. Presumably, the distinctive features of the tracks (such as odor or texture) would then conflict with the extramaze cues. They found that generally this manipulation had little or no effect, suggesting that animals followed distal cues.

Other attempts at this question rotated or translated the maze (Watson, 1907; Carr and Watson, 1908; Honzik, 1936). Unfortunately, rotating the maze has the unintended consequence of changing the allocentric bearing of intramaze cues as well as the relation to extramaze cues. Watson (1907) found that rotating the maze produced severe deficits while translating the maze did not.

More modern behavioral attempts to get at this question have looked at the radial maze (e.g., Suzuki, Augerinos, and Black, 1980). By rotating the radial maze, internal and external cues are in conflict. Again, animals generally follow extramaze cues, but can be trained to follow the internal cues.

Whether the local view preferentially incorporates information from distal or local cues has also been tested by measuring whether place cells prefer to follow distal or local cues. Many early experiments used T, plus, or radial mazes with cues available on the walls of the surrounding room (e.g. O'Keefe and Conway, 1978; Miller and Best, 1980; O'Keefe and Speakman, 1987; Shapiro et al., 1989; Young, Fox, and Eichenbaum, 1994). Sometimes there were differing textures on each arm of the maze, but even if without differing textures, one would expect some sort of local intramaze cues. The local and distal cues can then be separated by rotating the maze. Place cells generally follow the distal cues (Miller and Best, 1980; Shapiro et al., 1989). Similar results have been found by Cressant, Muller, and Poucet (1997), who found that inside a small circular arena place fields only follow the rotated cues if the landmarks were pushed all the way against the wall, that is, if they were *orienting* or *distal* stimuli.

On the other hand, animals can be trained to perform tasks based on local cues, such as searching for food at a position relative to an array of local landmarks (Collett, Cartwright, and Smith, 1986; Biegler and Morris, 1993; Saksida et al., 1995; Biegler and Morris, 1996; Gothard, Skaggs, and McNaughton, 1996, 1996; Redish, 1997). However, training can take a long time. This implies that rodents may be initially sensitive to distal landmarks, but can learn to attend to local landmarks if they are stable relative to the animal's internal representations and provide spatially constant clues to reward location.

NONSPATIAL ASPECTS

Traditionally, the term *local view* has been used to refer to spatial parameters of landmarks (both local and distal); most place cell models allow each landmark to have a unique identity T (see, for example, Sharp, 1991; Hetherington and Shapiro, 1993; Touretzky and Redish, 1996). Although these labels do not have to be unique for each landmark (in many models they are), they are assumed to identify landmarks perfectly. That is, each landmark is associated with a type and these types are not confusable. For example, if there are three white cylinders in an environment and an arena wall, the three cylinders might have a type $T_1 = T_2 = T_3 = A$, while the arena wall might have type $T_4 = B$.

Rodents are also sensitive to non-spatial aspects of the environment, such as luminosity of a cue (Bostock, Muller, and Kubie, 1991). Although it is still unknown how these aspects inform the local view, they should probably be included in the concept.

ANATOMY

In the primate, there is strong evidence that there are two representational pathways (or *streams*) for the local view: the dorsal stream representing spatial aspects (passing through parietal cortex) and the ventral stream representing identity aspects (passing through inferotemporal cortex). For reviews of the extensive evidence supporting this distinction in the primate see Mishkin, Ungerleider, and Macko (1983); Ungerleider and Haxby (1994); and Goodale et al. (1994).

There is evidence that this same distinction occurs in rodents (Kolb, 1990a; Kolb et al., 1994). The discussion of the two streams generally occurs in the visual mode (discussing how visual information is processed). It should be remembered, however, that the local view is not solely visual. Neurons in posterior parietal cortex (PPC) of the rodent are multimodal (Chen, 1989, 1991; Chen et al., 1994b; McNaughton et al., 1994), as they are in the primate (Hyvarinen, 1982; Colby and Duhamel, 1991). Although there are no recordings of neurons in rodent inferotemporal cortex (Te2), in the primate inferotemporal cortex neurons are primarily visual (Desimone et al., 1985; Tanaka et al., 1991). This suggests that while spatial parameters may be encoded in a supramodal representation, object identity might not be.

Evidence that the spatial aspects of local view are represented in posterior parietal cortex comes from anatomical, lesion, and neurophysiological data. More extensive neurophysiological work on parietal cortex has been done in the monkey (for reviews, see Andersen et al., 1993; Colby, Duhamel, and Goldberg, 1995) and extensive neurological work has been done in humans with parietal lesions (for reviews, see Bisiach and Vallar, 1988; Ungerleider and Haxby, 1994). In both the human and nonhuman primate, parietal cortex seems to be critically involved in representing nearby space (Stein, 1991, 1992). There is extensive cytoarchitectonic and neurophysiological evidence that primate parietal cortex consists of a variety of subareas (Andersen, 1988; Colby and Duhamel, 1991); rodent parietal cortex is also likely to consist of a variety of subareas, but more work needs to be done to decode what these areas are and the roles they play in representing the local view. Zilles (1990) identifies four parietal areas and three secondary visual areas, the latter corresponding to Krieg's area 7, which Krieg (1946) suggests as the homologue of primate parietal cortex. Zilles notes that even these areas are not necessarily cytoarchitectonically homogeneous and may need to be subdivided even further in the course of additional anatomical studies. For now, I will continue to treat posterior parietal cortex as a single unified brain structure, keeping in mind the caveat that it is actually quite diverse.

Posterior parietal cortex in the rat receives input from the lateral dorsal and lateral posterior thalamic nuclei (LDN and LPN, respectively), as well as from primary visual cortex (Kolb and Walkey, 1987; Chandler et al., 1992). The superior colliculus sends information to the posterior parietal cortex via the LPN (Dean, 1990). I suspect that parietal cortex also receives input from auditory representations (as evidenced in the primate by auditory responses of parietal neurons; Stricanne, Andersen, and Mazzoni, 1996), but have found no data supporting or refuting this hypothesis. Parietal cortex sends output to the posterior cingulate cortex (Chandler et al., 1992), the postsubiculum (van Groen and Wyss, 1990), the superior colliculus (Kolb, 1990a), and to the postrhinal cortex, which sends robust efferents to the entorhinal cortex (Burwell, Witter, and Amaral, 1995). Some cells in parietal cortex show directional and behavioral correlations that may indicate they play a role in local view processes (Chen, 1989; McNaughton, Chen, and Markus, 1991; Chen, 1991; Chen et al., 1994a, 1994b; McNaughton et al., 1994). LDN cells also show directional correlates but are dependent on intial availability of light (Mizumori, Ward, and Lavoie, 1992) indicating that they too may play a role in local view processes.

Parietal cortex lesions impair performance on a dry version of the water maze: finding food in one hole of 177 in an open field (Kesner, Farnsworth, and DiMattia, 1989). Animals with posterior parietal lesions can learn to navigate to hidden platforms with enough training, but their trajectories include strong amounts of looping and they do not swim directly to the platform (Kolb and Walkey, 1987). Although animals with posterior parietal cortex lesions can learn to navigate directly to a visible platform, they cannot learn to navigate to a platform indicated by a colocalized cue (Kolb and Walkey, 1987). Therefore parietal cortex cannot be the only local view pathway. (In chapter 4, evidence will be reviewed that the superior colliculus can also drive orientation to a landmark.) In the rodent, superior colliculus receives direct retinal input and projects directly to brainstem motor structures (for reviews, see Dean and Redgrave, 1984a, 1984b, 1984c).

In contrast to posterior parietal lesions, Te2-lesioned rats are poor at visual pattern discriminations, although not at spatial orientation discriminations (Kolb, 1990a). They are unable to learn to perform a visual match-to-sample task, even with no delay (Kolb, 1990a). But they can learn the hidden platform water maze normally. While I know of no recordings from Te2 neurons in rats, in the primate, temporal cortex neurons are sensitive to visual patterns and to object identities (Desimone et al., 1985; Tanaka et al., 1991).

Rodent inferotemporal and parietal cortices project to the perirhinal and postrhinal cortices, respectively, which both project to entorhinal cortex (EC), but perirhinal cortex receives stronger input from inferotemporal regions while postrhinal cortex receives its primary input from parietal cortex (Burwell, Witter, and Amaral, 1995). The perirhinal and postrhinal cortices receive direct afferents from a host of other cortical and subcortical sources, including (among others) the somatosensory, auditory, and medial prefrontal cortices as well as the anterior and posterior cingulate cortices, amygdala, nucleus accumbens, and caudate nucleus (Burwell, Witter, and Amaral, 1995). Te2 also sends direct projections to the lateral EC (Staubli, Ivy, and Lynch, 1984; Myrher, 1991). Both medial and lateral EC send projections into the hippocampus via the perforant path.

Data from Burwell and Eichenbaum (1997) may provide preliminary evidence that the dorsal/ventral (space/object) separation may continue into the perirhinal and postrhinal cortices. They recorded from perirhinal cells on a plus maze and did not find any spatial correlations. In contrast, Young et al. (1997) did find firing correlated with odor in a delayed nonmatch-to-sample task.

Otto et al. (1996) even report data suggesting that the dorsal/ventral separation is maintained into lateral/medial entorhinal cortex. They found that in a task that paired an odor with a location (given a specific odor, go to a specific location), lateral entorhinal lesions produced occasional odor discrimination errors (animal went to the location indicated by the wrong odor). When the lesions encroached on medial EC, the animals also occasionally made spatial errors (animal went to a location not associated with any odor). As we will see in the discussion of *multiple maps* (chapter 10), while one entorhinal input pathway may inform the hippocampus of the animal's location, the other may inform it of the environment (map/chart/reference frame) it is in.

The local view is necessary for all the navigation strategies (except, perhaps, random navigation). Taxon navigation requires representations of cues to orient towards; even praxic navigation requires some sensory input if only as releasing stimuli. Its main role, however, is to provide input to the locale navigation system.

4 Route Navigation: Taxon and Praxic Strategies

The taxonomy of navigation developed in chapter 2 separated three non-locale-based strategies: taxon strategies, praxic strategies, and route strategies. Because all three strategies can be understood as components of stimulus-response-based navigation in which each stimulus produces a specific and rigid response, all three strategies will be reviewed together. There is also some preliminary evidence that both taxon and praxic strategies use similar neurophysiological structures.

OVERVIEW

Taxon Strategies

Although taxon navigation strategies have been studied for more than fifty years (see Schöne, 1984, for a review), most of the work has been behavioral (Fraenkel and Gunn, 1961; Tinbergen, 1969) and most of the models kybernetic[1] (Schöne, 1984). While there are no large-scale neural models of the rodent taxon navigation system comparable to those of the locale system (e.g, O'Keefe and Nadel, 1978; McNaughton et al., 1996; or Touretzky and Redish, 1996), there is evidence that at least three key specific anatomical structures are involved: (1) the posterior parietal cortex, (2) the superior colliculus, and (3) the caudate nucleus. Because we lack the neurophysiological data to pull together a taxon navigation theory, I will review the evidence for the involvement of each of these three key structures and attempt to synthesize some hypotheses about their role in taxon navigation.

Praxic Strategies

Praxic strategies can be subdivided into spinal reflexes/patterns
and central sequencing strategies. What makes both of these
praxic strategies is that they require complex sequences of responses, but that once each sequence begins, it completes to the
end without external input. We can say that it is ballistic.

Surprisingly complex reaction sequences have been studied in
the spinal cord, particularly in lower vertebrates, in the ganglia of
insects, and in other invertebrates such as the swimming lamprey
(Wilson, 1966; Herman et al., 1975; Pearson, 1976; Brooks, 1986;
Gallistel, 1980; Bizzi, Mussa-Ivaldi, and Giszter, 1991). As with
taxon navigation, however, there is not enough neurophysiological data to construct a systems-level praxic navigation theory for
rodents, although some specific neural structures can definitely
be said to be involved (see below).

NEUROPHYSIOLOGY

Parietal Cortex

Extensive neurophysiological data suggests that the posterior parietal cortex in primates plays a major role in orienting movements, particularly visually cued orientations (Andersen, Essick, and Siegel, 1985; Bisiach and Vallar, 1988;
Colby and Duhamel, 1991; Stein, 1991, 1992; Andersen et al., 1993;
Ungerleider and Haxby, 1994; Colby, Duhamel, and Goldberg,
1995). But also in auditory (Stricanne, Andersen, and Mazzoni,
1996). Tactile cues have not been tested. In the rodent, the homologous areas are Krieg's area 7 (Krieg, 1946).

In chapter 3, we reviewed data implying that the parietal
cortex in rodents plays a role in representing distal cues. Parietal
cortex does not, however, seem to be involved in praxic strategies.
Animals with parietal cortex lesions can learn to make a single
turn, according to Kesner, Farnsworth, and DiMattia (1989), who
trained animals to find food on an eight-arm maze adjacent to the
entry arm (i.e., the animals were placed on an arm and the two
adjacent arms were baited) — this is a praxic strategy. Certain

authors (e.g., Save and Moghaddam, 1996) have suggested an influence of the parietal cortex in what seems to be a praxic task, the hidden platform water maze with a constant start. However, Moghaddam and Bures (1994) found that normal animals trained to do this task increase their latency to the platform after a 90° rotation of the environment. This means that the animals could not have been using a purely praxic strategy; otherwise, the rotation of the environment would have had no effect. Moghaddam and Bures also found that subsequent rotations did not increase the latency, implying that the animals may have learned to ignore the rotation and to use a purer praxic strategy. Because Save and Moghaddam (1996) did not rotate the environment, it is unlikely that normals were using a purely praxic strategy. Therefore, finding that posterior parietal lesions impair this task relative to normals does not imply that posterior parietal cortex is involved in praxic strategies.

Obviously, if an animal is to use a taxon navigation strategy to reach a stimulus, a representation of distal cues would be a necessary input component. Because animals with parietal lesions can learn to navigate directly to a visible platform (Kolb and Walkey, 1987), there must be taxon mechanisms that sidestep the parietal cortex. Evidence suggests that the superior colliculus may be one of those structures.

Superior Colliculus

In the rodent, the superior colliculus receives a strong direct retinal projection (Dean and Redgrave, 1984a; Goodale and Carey, 1990; Stein and Meredith, 1993). Although there is a large literature implicating the superior colliculus of primates in oculomotor abilities (e.g., Robinson, 1973; Sparks, 1986; Sparks and Nelson, 1987; Colby and Duhamel, 1991), in these experiments the animal's head is bolted to the apparatus. When the head is allowed to move freely, stimulation of the superior colliculus in rodents and felines produces general orienting movements of the eyes, ears, and head toward a stimulus (for reviews, see Dean and Redgrave, 1984c; Stein and Meredith, 1993). In the bat, stimulation of the superior colliculus evokes echolocating vocalization movements as well as head and ear pinnae movements (Valentine, Iannucci, and Moss, 1994; Valentine and Moss, 1997). The superior colliculi are laid out topologically, with the left colliculus covering the right side of space and the right colliculus the left side (Stein and Meredith, 1993). The midline of the colliculi represent the midline of the animal.

Drager and Hubel (1975, 1976) found that superior collicular cells in the mouse were sensitive to tactile and auditory as well as visual stimuli and that the receptive fields for all these modalities overlapped. Stein and Meredith (1993) have examined this issue in detail and found a remarkable overlap between tactile, auditory, and visual receptive fields in the feline colliculus; they review data suggesting that the rodent also shows these overlaps. Stein and Meredith also report that there is a nonlinearity in the summation of the different sensory cues. If simultaneous sensory cues from multiple modalities are consistent in their external location (i.e., if they overlap), then the neuron representing that location shows a rate more than twice as strong compared to the case when only one sensory modality informs the animal of the cue. Rodents with superior colliculus lesions show visual neglect of the external world contralateral to the lesioned side of the colliculus (Dean and Redgrave, 1984a). Animals with bilateral lesions show severe orienting impairments (Goodale, Foreman, and Milner, 1978; Ellard and Goodale, 1988).

Goodale (1983) trained gerbils to run to an escape hole in a semicircular environment. They found that gerbils with collicular lesions could only run to the hole if it was within about 40° of their initial orientation. They identified the problem as an inability to orient the head appropriately in the initial entry into the environment. Goodale and Murison (1975), on the other hand, showed that gerbils with superior colliculus lesions could approach visual stimuli. The term *orientation* is used for (1) detection by and turning of sensory organs toward a stimulus and (2) actual locomotion toward a stimulus. These two aspects were distinguished in the early ethological work (Fraenkel and Gunn, 1961; Tinbergen, 1969; Schöne, 1984). As the study of navigation has grown to accommodate more complex strategies, the two aspects have merged into one term. The superior colliculus seems to be strongly involved in sensory orientation, but not in locomotion toward a stimulus. Gerbils with superior colliculus lesions could still go to an open door on the opposite side of the arena from their entry as long as the cue was less than 40° off midline, but they ignored novel stimuli in their peripheral vision, stimuli that were investigated by normal animals.

Milner and Lines (1983) explicitly hypothesized that superior colliculus was involved in goal-directed orientation movments. In one of their experiments, they tested animals with superior colliculus lesions in the water maze. SC-lesioned animals were severely impaired in both the hidden platform and visible platform versions.

The rodent superior colliculus has also been identified as being involved in identifying threats and producing antitaxon behavior such as freezing and flight (Dean and Redgrave, 1984a, 1984b, 1984c; Ellard and Goodale, 1988; Dean, Redgrave, and Westby, 1989). Because this issue is beyond the scope of this book, we will leave the superior colliculus having noted that it plays a role in orientation and taxon navigation even if that is not its only role.

Cingulate Cortex

There is also some evidence that the cingulate cortex may play a role in navigation (Chen, 1991; Chen et al., 1994a, 1994b; Sutherland and Hoesing, 1993). It receives strong input from the anterior thalamic nuclei (Bentivoglio, Kultas-Ilinsky, and Illinsky, 1993; van Groen, Vogt, and Wyss, 1993), which are likely to play a role in the head direction system (chapter 5). Although a few cells in the cingulate cortex show head direction correlates (Chen, 1991; Chen et al., 1994a, 1994b), extensive recordings from posterior cingulate cortex cells have not been done during spatial tasks.

Lesions of the posterior cingulate cortex impair learning the hidden platform water maze, even if the lesions are done long after training (Sutherland, Whishaw, and Kolb, 1988; Sutherland and Hoesing, 1993). However, Neave and colleagues (Neave et al., 1994; Neave, Nagle, and Aggleton, 1997) have suggested that these lesions impaired the animals' navigation abilities because the cingulum bundle was damaged. The cingulum bundle connects the anterior thalamus and the postsubiculum (components of the head direction system; chapter 5).

It is important to distinguish posterior cingulate cortex from anterior cingulate cortex which seems to play a role in visceral control, emotion, pain, affect and reward (Neafsey et al., 1993; Vogt, Sikes, and Vogt, 1993; Bussey, Everitt, and Robbins, 1997; Bussey et al., 1997). For example, lesions of the anterior cingulate cortex do not affect the hidden platform water maze (Sutherland, Whishaw, and Kolb, 1988; Sutherland and Hoesing, 1993; Neave et al., 1994, 1997) or other spatial tasks (Bussey, Everitt, and Robbins, 1997; Bussey et al., 1997). The specific role played by posterior cingulate cortex has not been resolved. Redish and Touretzky (1998a) has suggested that it may play a role in storing long term routes, while McNaughton et al. (Chen, 1991; McNaughton, Chen, and Markus, 1991) have suggested that it might play a role in associating head directions with external and internal coordinate systems.

Caudate Nucleus

A part of the *basal ganglia*, the caudate nucleus, together with the putamen and the nucleus accumbens, forms the *striatum*, and is thus sometimes referred to as *dorsal striatum*. In the rodent, the putamen is not anatomically separable from the caudate nucleus, and is thus sometimes referred to as the *caudatoputamen*. (For in-depth reviews of the complex anatomy and structure of the basal ganglia, see White, 1989; Graybiel, 1990; Smith and Bolam, 1990; Afifi, 1994; Groves et al., 1995; Houk, Adams, and Barto, 1995; Beiser, Hua, and Houk, 1997; White, 1997.)

The caudate nucleus receives a convergence of input from much of the cortex (Parent, 1990; Afifi, 1994; Finch, 1996), although recently questions have been raised about whether the input is truly convergent or remains separated into specific cortical loops through the basal ganglia (Alexander and Crutcher, 1990; Beiser, Hua, and Houk, 1997). However, Finch (1996) reports converging influence from a variety of sources onto caudate neurons.

The basal ganglia have in general been associated with stimulus-reward associations (Mishkin and Appenzeller, 1987; Saint-Cyr, Taylor, and Lang, 1988; White, 1989; Barto, 1995; Gabrieli, 1995; Houk, Adams, and Barto, 1995; Schultz et al., 1995a, 1995b; Wickens and Kotter, 1995; Schultz, 1997; White, 1997), as well as with the sequencing of action (Berridge and Whishaw, 1992; Pellis et al., 1993; Barto, 1995; Houk, Adams, and Barto, 1995; Cromwell and Berridge, 1996; Aldridge and Berridge, 1998). Often the dorsal and ventral striatum have been contrasted in terms of stereotyped movements and locomotor movements, respectively (see, for example, Whishaw and Mittleman, 1991).

Chapter 7 will review data and theories suggesting that the nucleus accumbens (the ventral striatum) associates location information (from the place code in the hippocampus) with reward and emotional information (from the ventral tegmental area and the amygdala, respectively). If the caudate nucleus takes as input local view information directly (for example via the parietal or cingulate cortices) and associates that local view information with reward and emotional information, then it could be a key connection in taxon navigation.

If the nucleus accumbens is a major component of goal finding (see chapter 7), then it would need to sequence actions based on the input location information. Similarly, if the caudate nucleus sequences actions, it could be a key component to praxic navigation as well, released by simple stimuli and transmitted via direct connections between local view representations and the caudate nucleus itself.

Any discussion of the role of the caudate nucleus in taxon navigation must start from the dissociation papers of McDonald,

McGaugh, Packard, and White (Packard, Hirsh, and White, 1989; Packard and McGaugh, 1992; McDonald and White, 1994; Packard, 1994; Packard and McGaugh, 1996). These authors have examined caudate lesions and hippocampal lesions in four important tasks: the radial maze, the plus maze, and the cued and hidden platform water maze.

On the water maze, hippocampal lesions impair navigation to hidden platforms (Morris et al., 1982; Sutherland, Whishaw, and Kolb, 1983; Eichenbaum, Stewart, and Morris, 1990; Morris et al., 1990; Sutherland and Rodriguez, 1990; Packard and McGaugh, 1992), while caudate lesions impair navigation to cued platforms (Packard and McGaugh, 1992; McDonald and White, 1994). Packard and McGaugh (1992) compared caudate and fornix lesions[2] on a water maze with two platforms, one stable, one unstable. If the animal tried to climb up on the unstable platform, it fell back into the water. Both platforms were hidden. Packard and McGaugh ran two versions of the experiment: In the first version, the stable platform was always in one quadrant, while the other was always in the opposite, so that the location of the platform denoted its stability; in the second version, the platforms alternated quadrants randomly from trial to trial, but a visual cue demarcated which of the two was stable. They found that fornix lesions impaired acquisition of the location-stable platform, while caudate lesions did not affect performance. On the other hand, caudate lesions impaired acquisition of the cue-stable platform, while fornix lesions did not affect performance.

In another experiment, Packard (1994) found that amphetamine injections into caudate enhanced memory of the cued water maze, while injections into hippocampus enhanced memory of the hidden platform water maze.[3]

McDonald and White (1994) trained rats to find a visible platform for three days and then gave them a fourth day of training to find a hidden platform. They repeated this sequence three times (twelve days). After which, they tested the animals with a visible platform moved to another location. They found that both rats with dorsal caudate lesions and rats with fimbria-fornix lesions could find the visible platform, but rats with fimbria-fornix lesions could not find the hidden platform even though it was in the same position. Most significantly, when McDonald and White (1994) moved the visible platform, animals with dorsal caudate lesions ignored the visible cue and searched where the platform had been. By lesioning the caudate nucleus, McDonald and White uncovered a locale navigation strategy.

Packard and McGaugh (1996) tested rats on a plus maze: rats were always started on the south arm and trained to turn left (to the west arm). As noted by Tolman, Ritchie, and Kalish (1946b), animals learn place strategies (locale strategies) first, and only later (if at all) develop response strategies (taxon and praxic strategies). In Packard and McGaugh's experiment, the animals were given seven days of four trials per day. On the eighth day, they were placed on the north arm. They all turned right (to the west arm), demonstrating a locale strategy. The animals were then trained for seven more days to turn left from the south arm to the west arm. On the sixteenth day, they were again placed on the north arm. They all turned left (to the east arm), demonstrating a response (presumably praxic) strategy. We should note that they might have been using a taxon strategy: there might have been a texture difference on the floor or some cue they learned to approach. Packard and McGaugh then inactivated caudate (with lidocaine) and tested the animals on the north arm. They all turned right, indicating the locale strategy again.

Finally, the caudate nucleus has been implicated in cued-response tasks on the radial arm maze. In a variant of the standard radial arm task, Packard, Hirsh, and White (1989) trained animals to find food on four of the eight arms with lights at the ends of each arm. This makes the task into a *win-stay* task, as compared to the standard *win-shift* task usually associated with the radial arm maze (Olton and Samuelson, 1976; see also appendix B, for a review of the radial arm maze task). Packard, Hirsh, and White (1989) found that caudate lesions impaired the cued task, but not the standard radial arm maze task, and vice versa for fimbria-fornix lesions. This result has been replicated by McDonald and White (1993). Posttraining injections of dopamine agonists into caudate enhanced the win-stay task, while posttraining injections into hippocampus enhanced the win-shift task (Packard and White, 1991).

There are only three reports of recordings from the rodent caudate nucleus in spatial tasks (Wiener, 1993; Mizumori and Cooper, 1995; Mizumori, Unick, and Cooper, 1996) and the two most recent are preliminary reports available only in abstract form. While Wiener (1993) stresses cells correlated with head direction, in the small rectangular arena used, a number of other factors such as approach to a corner are also correlated with head direction. Any of these factors could produce head direction sensitivity. Wiener reports that the directional preferences of these cells rotated with rotation of the arena and were independent of extramaze room cues and a light which did not rotate with the arena. Wiener also reports that a few units showed location and task effect (such as rotation of the arena) correlations.

When Mizumori and Cooper (1995) recorded from caudate cells on the radial maze, they found that most cells were tuned to single directions along pairs of arms, but also found that some cells changed their preferred directions suddenly and drastically within a single trial. Others were tuned, not to direction, but to a path along a pair of arms. Mizumori, Lavoie, and Kalyani (1996) report correlations to direction and location as well as egocentric rotations (for example, at the ends of the arms). They also report reward related activity similar to that found in nucleus accumbens cells (Lavoie and Mizumori, 1994, see also chapter 7).

The caudate nucleus has been hypothesized to form the key to a procedural or habit-based memory system (Mishkin and Appenzeller, 1987; Cook and Kesner, 1988; White, 1989). Models of how this stimulus-response memory system might work for general conditioning rather than for spatial taxon navigation strategies have been proposed (Barto, 1995; Houk, Adams, and Barto, 1995).

SYNTHESIS

Although we have not reached a large-scale coherent model of taxon or praxic navigation strategies, we have identified structures which must play specific roles: the parietal cortex as playing a role in the local view system (see chapter 3); the superior colliculus as critical to orienting towards a peripheral cue, though not locomoting to it; but the key seems to be the caudate nucleus. A number of authors have associated the basal ganglia with stimulus-response abilities (Mishkin and Appenzeller, 1987; Saint-Cyr, Taylor, and Lang, 1988; White, 1989; Barto, 1995; Gabrieli, 1995; Houk, Adams, and Barto, 1995; Schultz et al., 1995a, 1995b; Wickens and Kotter, 1995; Schultz, 1997; White, 1997), as well as with the sequencing of action (Berridge and Whishaw, 1992; Pellis et al., 1993; Barto, 1995; Houk, Adams, and Barto, 1995; Cromwell and Berridge, 1996; Aldridge and Berridge, 1998). As will be reviewed in chapter 7, the nucleus accumbens seems to be involved in generating directions of movement, given inputs representing location (from the hippocampus) and motivation (from the amygdala). If this is true, then we can follow Mogenson and Nielsen (1984), Mogenson (1984), and Whishaw and Mittleman (1991) in hypothesizing similar computational functions for the caudate nucleus (dorsal striatum) and nucleus accumbens (ventral striatum). Both structures associate their inputs with motor actions, but the caudate nucleus associates sensory inputs, whereas the nucleus accumbens associates location inputs.

5 Head Direction

Cells with firing rates reflecting head direction have been discovered in a number of structures in the rodent brain: postsubiculum (PoS; Ranck, 1984; Taube, Muller, and Ranck, 1990a, 1990b), the anterior thalamic nuclei (ATN; Blair and Sharp, 1995; Knierim, Kudrimoti, and McNaughton, 1995; Taube, 1995a), the lateral mammillary nuclei (LMN; Leonhard, Stackman, and Taube, 1996), the lateral dorsal nucleus of the thalamus (LDN; Mizumori and Williams, 1993), and to a lesser extent the posterior parietal and cingulate cortices (PPC and PCC; Chen et al., 1994a, 1994b; McNaughton et al., 1994).

Head direction cells have a single *preferred direction* at which they fire maximally, and their firing rates decrease monotonically as the animals' orientation moves progressively farther away from the preferred direction (see figure 5.1). The firing rates of these cells are not correlated with the angle between the head and the body, but with the orientation of the head relative to the surrounding environment. Because a cell's preferred direction does not change over the space of an environment (Taube, Muller, and Ranck, 1990a, 1990b), the cell cannot be encoding egocentric bearing to a landmark; it must be encoding allocentric bearing to a *reference direction*.

Many of the areas that contain head direction cells are tightly linked anatomically: The anterior dorsal (AD) nucleus of the thalamus and the postsubiculum are directly interconnected (van Groen and Wyss, 1990; Witter, Ostendorf, and Groenwegen, 1990); postsubiculum sends a strong projection to the lateral mammillary nucleus (van Groen and Wyss, 1990; Witter, Ostendorf, and Groenwegen, 1990), which in turn sends a strong projection to the AD nucleus (Bentivoglio, Kultas-Ilinsky, and Illinsky, 1993). The lateral dorsal nucleus of the thalamus is also interconnected with the postsubiculum (van Groen and

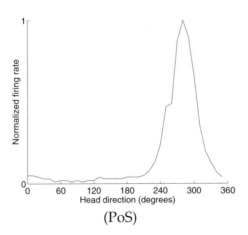

(PoS)

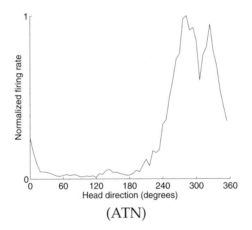

(ATN)

Figure 5.1
Sample head direction tuning curves from postsubiculum (PoS) and
anterior thalamic nuclei (ATN). (Data courtesy T. Blair and P. Sharp.)

Wyss, 1990). The posterior parietal cortex receives input from LDN and sends efferents to PoS, as well as to the cingulate cortex (van Groen and Wyss, 1990; Kolb, 1990a), while posterior cingulate is interconnected with both the anterior thalamus and the postsubiculum directly (van Groen and Wyss, 1990; Wyss and van Groen, 1992; Bentivoglio, Kultas-Ilinsky, and Illinsky, 1993). There are differences between these areas that can be used to narrow down the possible roles each structure might play in the head direction system.

Most *head direction cells* are recorded from a small cylinder (less than a meter in diameter) with a cue card subtending about 90°, although a few of the recordings were done in other environments (such as the eight-arm maze or a small rectangular arena). In complex environments, *beaconing cells* can be confused with head direction cells (in chapter 4, I argued that the striatal head direction cells reported in Wiener, 1993, are really beaconing cells). Because the preferred orientation of head direction cells is constant over the entire environment, they are unlikely to be beaconing cells.

Head direction cells are generally sensitive to rotation of distal cues (Taube, Muller, and Ranck, 1990b; Taube, 1995a; Goodridge and Taube, 1995; Knierim, Kudrimoti, and McNaughton, 1995; Leonhard, Stackman, and Taube, 1996), and when two head direction cells have been simultaneously recorded, their tuning curves have always rotated synchronously (Taube, Muller, and Ranck, 1990b; Goodridge and Taube, 1995; Taube et al., 1996). Cells in the lateral dorsal thalamus, in parietal and cingulate cortex, and in striatum do not always show such a clean tuning to directional cues (Mizumori and Williams, 1993; Wiener, 1993; Chen et al., 1994a, 1994b; Mizumori and Cooper, 1995).

Head direction cells in lateral dorsal thalamus are not sensitive to the movement of single cues, although they are sensitive to movement of the entire visual world (Mizumori and Williams, 1993). They are also dependent on the presence of visual input, unlike anterior thalamic and postsubicular head direction cells, which show normal activity in the dark, even when the animal is first placed into the environment in the dark (see Taube et al., 1996, for a review).

Similarly, cells in parietal and cingulate cortices are sensitive to behavioral cues as well as directional cues (Chen, 1989, 1991; McNaughton et al., 1994; Chen et al., 1994a, 1994b), such as whether the animal is turning left or right or moving straight, or whether the animal is proceeding inward or outward on a radial maze (McNaughton et al., 1994). Chen et al. (1994a) found that approximately 5–10% of the cells were sensitive to direction on the radial arm maze, and that of those, half required a cue in order to show a directional tuning. These cells only fired if the cue was present. But if the cue was present and then removed, some of the cells continued to show a tuning to direction, as if the cell remembered the direction the cue had been. They tended to show a broader tuning to direction than postsubicular head direction cells (Chen et al., 1994a). They also did not show the clean sensitivity to distal cues reported for anterior thalamic and postsubicular head direction cells. Some cells showed bimodal head direction tuning curves during cue manipulation trials (Chen, 1991; Chen et al., 1994b), something never seen in anterior thalamic or postsubicular recordings. Lateral dorsal thalamus and parietal cortex may be better understood as part of the local view subsystem (chapter 3) than the head direction subsystem, while cingulate may be part of the goal memory (chapter 7) or route navigation (chapter 4) systems.

When multiple head direction cells have been recorded from anterior thalamus, postsubiculum, or the lateral mammillary nucleus, the difference between their preferred directions is a constant across all environments (Taube, Muller, and Ranck, 1990b; Goodridge and Taube, 1995; Taube et al., 1996). If the population of head direction cells were imagined as a one-dimensional ring with each cell placed in a position on that ring corresponding to its preferred direction (figure 5.2), then at any time the population would always encode a single direction. One can therefore talk about the *precession of the head direction representation as a whole*.

One way of interpreting the activity of these cells is as a distributed representation of the rat's current head direction. A pop-

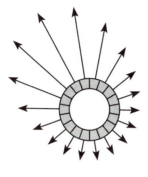

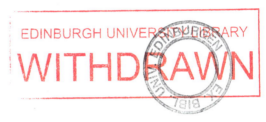

Figure 5.2
Head direction population as a ring. Each shaded segment corresponds to a cell with a preferred direction pointing away from the center. Lengths of the arrows are proportional to firing rate. This figure does not show simulation or experiment, it is meant to be explanatory only. (After a figure from Skaggs et al., 1995.)

ulation of head direction cells with preferred directions ϕ_i evenly distributed through 360° represents the direction of the weighted vector sum $\sum_i F_i \cdot \vec{v}_i$, where F_i is the normalized firing rate of cell i and $\vec{v}_i$ is a unit vector pointing in direction ϕ_i. This is the weighted circular mean (Mardia, 1972), and is also known as a *population vector encoding* (Georgopoulos et al., 1983). Of course, real head direction cells are not necessarily evenly distributed, but as long as the cells are distributed approximately evenly, this interpretation is still valid (Georgopoulos, Kettner, and Schwartz, 1988; Redish and Touretzky, 1994).

Early reports (Blair and Sharp, 1995; Knierim, Kudrimoti, and McNaughton, 1995; Taube, 1995a) suggested that anterior thalamic cells showed tuning curves very similar to those of postsubicular cells, but more recent reports have suggested differences. While postsubicular head direction cells are best correlated with current head direction, anterior thalamic head direction cell activity is best correlated with head direction approximately 20–40 ms in the future (Blair and Sharp, 1995; Taube and Muller, 1995; Blair, Lipscomb, and Sharp, 1997).[1]

Leonhard, Stackman, and Taube (1996) also report that lateral mammillary cells are correlated with future direction (by as much as 83 ms), at least in one direction, but it is not yet clear whether this anticipation occurs for both clockwise and counterclockwise turns. Because lateral mammillary activity is also correlated with angular velocity (see below), it might seem to anticipate future head direction when the animal is turning in one direction but not the other.

Another important difference between anterior thalamic and postsubiculum head direction cells is that even when the animal is not turning, AD head direction cells show multiple peaks in the tuning curve (Blair, Lipscomb, and Sharp, 1997). Because these cells anticipate head direction, the tuning curves shift to one side with clockwise turns and to the other with counterclockwise turns (see figure 5.3). However, Blair, Lipscomb, and Sharp (1997) showed that this "shift" is not really a shift at all. Both peaks are present when the animal is not turning, and when the animal turns, one peak of the tuning curve rises while the other falls. This confirmed a prediction (first made in Redish, Elga, and Touretzky, 1996) of the attractor network model (see below). Because AD head direction cells are hypothesized to receive offset connections, the theory predicts (1) that there will be two peaks, even when the animal is not turning, each peak a consequence of one set of those offset connections; and (2) that the width between the two peaks seen when the animal is not turning will correlate with the *anticipatory time interval*, the future time to which the tuning curve is best correlated. Both predictions have been confirmed (Blair, Lipscomb, and Sharp, 1997). For example, a cell that is best tuned to head direction 40 ms in the future has a large separation between the two peaks, but a cell that is best tuned to head direction only 20 ms in the future has a small

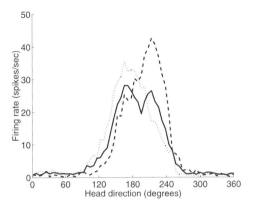

Figure 5.3
Tuning curves for a single anterior thalamic head direction cell at three different angular velocities. Note the two peaks during nonrotations (black line). With clockwise rotations (dotted gray line), the left peak rises (the cell is anticipating its preferred head direction when the animal is not yet at that direction). Likewise, with counterclockwise rotations (dashed gray line), the right peak increases. (Data courtesy T. Blair and P. Sharp.)

separation. Figure 5.3 shows a cell with a large anticipatory time interval; the two peaks are clearly visible even when the animal is not turning.

Cells in other areas also show more complicated correlations than the simple orientation correlations that the term *head direction cell* implies. For example, lateral mammillary cell activity is strongly correlated with angular velocity as well as direction (Leonhard, Stackman, and Taube, 1996). In other words, although they show normal head direction tuning curves correlated with the orientation of the animal, the overall firing rate is modulated by the angular velocity as well. Some cells in parietal cortex are also correlated with both head direction and angular velocity (McNaughton, Chen, and Markus, 1991), as are some postsubicular cells (Taube, Muller, and Ranck, 1990b; Sharp, 1996). These cells are also accounted for by the standard model (see below) and were in fact predicted by an early model of the head direction system (called $\mathcal{HH}'$ *cells*, McNaughton, Chen, and Markus, 1991).

THEORETICAL ISSUES

Tracking head direction accurately requires three components: a means of maintaining a stable representation (Skaggs et al., 1995; Redish, Elga, and Touretzky, 1996; Zhang, 1996), a means of updating the representation from vestibular input (McNaughton, Chen, and Markus, 1991; Skaggs et al., 1995; Redish, Elga, and Touretzky, 1996; Zhang, 1996), and a means of updating the representation from local view input (McNaughton, Chen, and Markus, 1991; Knierim, Kudrimoti, and McNaughton, 1995). The key to understanding these three components lies in properties of *attractor networks*, reviewed (with example code) in appendix A. The key properties of these networks are

1. A coherent representation of head direction is a stable state;

2. Slightly offset excitatory input forces the representation to precess; and

3. Strong, distally offset excitatory input forces the representation to reset to match the offset input.

Shift Register Models of the Head Direction System

McNaughton, Chen, and Markus (1991)

In this associative mapping model for updating head direction based on angular velocity, a head direction cell population $\mathcal{H}$ and an angular velocity population $\mathcal{H}'$ jointly produce activity in a direction velocity population $\mathcal{HH}'$. Each $\mathcal{HH}'$ cell is tuned to both a specific direction and a specific angular velocity. Thus, given the representation in the $\mathcal{HH}'$ population, the representation of head direction in the $\mathcal{H}$ population can be updated by a linear associative memory. Various anatomical areas, such as parietal and retrosplenial cortex, are discussed as sources of the $\mathcal{H}$ and $\mathcal{H}'$ signals, and postsubiculum is suggested as a possible site for the $\mathcal{H}\mathcal{H}'$ population. In this state shift model, a new representation of head direction is generated at each time step from the representation of the head direction $\times$ angular velocity state. Although McNaughton, Chen, and Markus (1991) presented the first model that explained how head direction could be maintained from vestibular and reset by extrinsic cues, they reported no simulations.

Blair (1996)

In this somewhat different shift register model, angular velocity–modulated head direction cells (AVHD cells) in the reticular thalamic nucleus selectively inhibit cells in ATN that are offset from the corresponding AVHD cells. Th model suggests that the activity of anterior thalamic nuclei (ATN) cells is also governed by a modulatory input from angular speed cells hypothesized to exist in the mammillary bodies. This modulatory input varies the rate of shifting because the ATN cells provide input that helps drive the AVHD cells; ATN also drives HD cells in postsubiculum and retrosplenial cortex. While Blair (1996) was the first to propose a model in which the ATN representation leads the postsubiculum (PoS) representation, there is no evidence for the necessary cell types in the reticular thalamus or the mammillary bodies. Moreover, the model did not produce realistic tuning curves, and Blair did not report tracking performance on realistic data sets, and did not examine rotations at multiple angular velocities, although he did show that his simulations could track a single turn.

Attractor Network Models of the Head Direction System

Skaggs et al. (1995)

This model of the head direction system accounts for both the shape of the head direction tuning curves and provides a means of updating the representation as the animal moves through space. A population of head direction cells forms an *attractor network* in which *coherent representations*[2] *of head direction* are stable states of the network. Head direction cells project to corresponding left and right *rotation cells*, whose activity is controlled by *vestibular cells* that fire when the animal is making a left or right turn. The rotation cells play a role similar to the $\mathcal{H}\mathcal{H}'$ cells of McNaughton, Chen, and Markus (1991) and project back to either the left or right neighbors of the head direction cell that drives them. Thus, during a turn, the hill of activity over the head direction cell population gradually shifts. Although Skaggs et al. (1995) did not include simulation results, it formed the basis for the subsequent simulations by a number of authors (e.g., Redish, Elga, and Touretzky, 1996; Zhang, 1996).

Zhang (1996)

Zhang (1996) presented the first simulation results of a pure attractor model of the head direction system. He defined a Gaussian-shaped hill of activation and derived weights and an activation function that produce self-sustaining activity patterns of this form, then derived another weight function to dynamically translate the activity pattern to the left or right. He did not separate the roles of ATN and PoS, however, nor did he measure tracking ability on realistic data sets.

Redish, Elga, and Touretzky (1996)

This model included two populations, one representing current head direction and the other future head direction, identified with PoS and ATN respectively. As in the Skaggs et al. (1995) and Zhang (1996) models, offset connections drove the update function, but here the offset connections were hypothesized to exist between PoS and ATN. Both PoS and ATN were assumed to maintain representations by attractor networks but Redish, Elga, and Touretzky (1996) noted that anatomical evidence for the necessary inhibition structure required to make the ATN an attractor network was lacking. Redish, Elga, and Touretzky (1996) predicted that if the ATN was not an attractor network, then there should be specific deformations in the ATN head direction tuning curves during rotations. These deformations have been found (Blair, Lipscomb, and Sharp, 1997). A new version of this model has recently been developed (Goodridge et al., 1997). This model is shown in figure 5.4 and will be detailed in the rest of this chapter.

Synthesis

The attractor network models can be understood as a combination of two different weight matrices: (1) during periods of nonrotation, the weight matrix among the head direction cells has a local excitation and global inhibition structure; and (2) during rotations, the offset cells become active and input extra activity into the system that effectively makes the weight matrix asymmetric in the direction of rotation. This kind of local excitation/global inhibition network has been well studied, both with symmetric weight matrices (when the weight matrix is symmetric, a *hill* of activation is a stable state in the network; Wilson and Cowan, 1973; Amari, 1977; Ermentrout and Cowan, 1979; Kishimoto and Amari, 1979; Kohonen, 1982, 1984; Murray, 1989), as well as asymmetric (in which traveling waves can form Wilson and Cowan, 1973; Ermentrout and Cowan, 1979; Murray, 1989). Fundamentally similar models have also been proposed as explanations of saccade generation by the superior colliculus (Droulez and Berthoz, 1991; Munoz, Pélisson, and Guitton, 1991; Lefévre and Galiana, 1992; van Opstal and Kappen, 1993; Arai, Keller, and Edelman, 1994). Attractor networks and their properties are reviewed in appendix A, including sample code for anyone who wants to experiment with them.

Maintaining a Stable Representation

Skaggs et al. (1995) were the first to suggest that a stable representation of head direction could be maintained by an attractor network; Zhang (1996) the first to simulate it; and Redish, Elga, and Touretzky (1996) the first to propose the postsubiculum as a likely candidate. It is not known whether the real head direc-

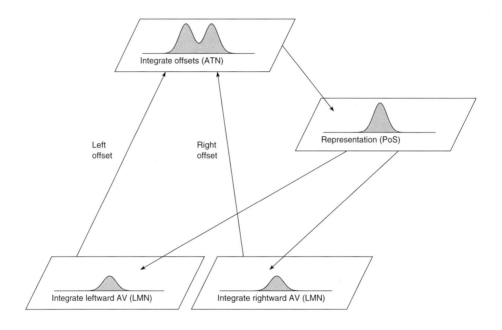

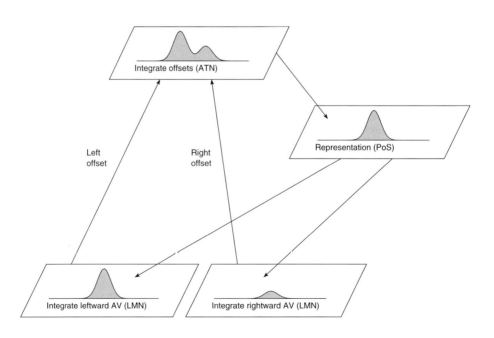

tion system actually includes an attractor network — this is a hypothesis.

The attractor nature of the system could be demonstrated with multiunit recordings. If one were to record from multiple head direction cells simultaneously (say 20 cells), then the population encoding (see figure 5.2) could be observed directly. If noise were injected into the system by microstimulation, the representation should be transiently disrupted. Even in darkness, without external or self-motion cues, the population's firing rates should return to a well-formed representation of head direction.

Resetting Head Direction from Local View

Within any environment, the head direction system must represent a consistent orientation — if a cell's preferred direction corresponds to, say, northwest at one point in the environment, it should always correspond to northwest when the animal experiences that environment, even though it may correspond to a totally different direction in another environment. This requirement implies that the head direction representation must not drift during a single session, and that it must be reset upon re-entry into the environment. That both these conditions can occur can be seen from evidence that (1) the head direction system can drift in animals trained with disorientation (Knierim, Kudrimoti, and McNaughton, 1995)

Figure 5.4
Attractor network model of the head direction system. The plots in each box show populations of cells at a single moment in time, with the activity of each cell plotted at its preferred direction (thus when the representation is *coherent*, only cells with similar directions are active and the population diagram shows a single hill of activity). Plots are diagramatic only. When the animal is not turning, the offset connections are balanced (top). When the animal is turning (in this case, turning left), the offset connections become unbalanced and the system precesses leftward (bottom).

and (2) in the absence of an orienting cue card, the head direction system does not reset to the same orientation on re-entry into a familiar environment (Goodridge and Taube, 1995; Taube and Burton, 1995). One possible solution is an association between local view inputs and head direction orientations (McNaughton, Chen, and Markus, 1991).

Postsubiculum is interconnected with both parietal cortex and LDN, structures that appear to support the local view subsystem (chapter 3). Through correlational long-term potentiation (LTP) occurring between representations of head direction based purely on distal cues (θ_i in figure 3.2) and head direction cells, external information about head direction can be associated with actual head direction (McNaughton, Chen, and Markus, 1991; Knierim, Kudrimoti, and McNaughton, 1995; Skaggs et al., 1995).

External orientation cues are associated with internal (idiothetic) cues, and not the other way around. Knierim, Kudrimoti, and McNaughton (1995) disoriented rats by carrying them from their home cage to the arena in an enclosed box that rotated slowly. Behaviorally, rats that are disoriented like this cannot learn to find one arm on a plus maze (Martin et al., 1995), nor can they learn to decide between opposite corners of a rectangle (Cheng, 1986; Margules and Gallistel, 1988; Gallistel, 1990), or to find food relative to a single landmark (Biegler and Morris, 1993), even when distal cues are available. All of these tasks are easy to learn without disorientation.

Knierim, Kudrimoti, and McNaughton found that head direction cells in rats with disorientation training did not follow the cue card as well as they did in control rats, and that even in control rats, after a number of probes with rotated cues, the head direction representations did not follow the cues as well as they had previously. As they pointed out, their findings imply that the internal cues are primary and the external cues are associated with them. If the external cues were primary and head direction representations were associated with them, one would expect to see head direction representations following the cue card in both disoriented and control rats. This is the opposite of what Knierim, Kudrimoti, and McNaughton found. The most parsimonious explanation for their data is that external cues are associated with head direction representations. Knierim, Kudrimoti, and McNaughton (1995) suggested that to the disoriented rats, the cue card was an unstable cue (because the rats' reference orientation changed from trial to trial, the cue card's orientation seemed to change from trial to trial). Because stable cues are associated with the same directions but unstable cues are not, only stable cues can reset head direction representations. The mechanism by which this reset can occur was first suggested by McNaughton, Chen, and Markus (1991), clarified by Skaggs et al. (1995), and simulated by Zhang (1996).

As shown in figures A.2 and A.4 (appendix A), sufficiently strong tonic excitatory input added into an attractor network will either slowly rotate the representation until it matches the tonic input or will shift it suddenly. Which of these two processes occurs depends on the angular difference between the current representation and the input direction. Note that, according to this theory, the input into postsubiculum from local view is not the orientation of the distal cue but rather the head direction in the environment as informed by the distal cue.

An important question immediately arises as to what happens when an animal enters a cue conflict situation. Animals exposed to a conflict between internal and external representations sometimes reset head direction on entry into the new environment and sometimes do not (Taube and Burton, 1995). Sometimes, they shift partway toward the reset, but not all the way (Taube and Burton, 1995). Note that whenever more than one cell was recorded simultaneously, the representation shifted by the same amount. Thus the reference direction shifted, but the system still maintained a coherent representation of head direction.

Updating the Representation

From the earliest recordings of head direction cells, researchers believed that internal cues (i.e., vestibular and self-motion cues) were being used to update the head direction representation (Ranck, 1984; Taube, Muller, and Ranck, 1990a, 1990b). The first hypothesis for how this could happen was suggested by McNaughton, Chen, and Markus (1991), clarified by Skaggs et al. (1995), and simulated by Zhang (1996); it was understood anatomically and shown to be able to track accurately by Redish, Elga, and Touretzky (1996; see figure 5.5).

The first key hypothesis is that there is a population of cells that receives input from both the head direction representation and vestibular input and that represents the product of angular velocity and head direction (McNaughton, Chen, and Markus, 1991). Following Blair (1996), I refer to these as *AV × HD cells*. (They were called $\mathcal{HH}'$ *cells* by McNaughton, Chen, and Markus, 1991.) The second key hypothesis is that these AV × HD cells project to cells in the head direction representation with slightly offset connections, where the effective strength is dependent on the preferred angular velocity (clockwise or counterclockwise) (Skaggs et al., 1995; see also Redish, Elga, and Touretzky, 1996; Zhang, 1996; Goodridge et al., 1997).

Given the recent data from Leonhard, Stackman, and Taube (1996) that lateral mammillary cells are correlated with both head direction and angular velocity, the most parsimonious explanation is that the AV × HD cells are in two head direction populations in lateral mammillary nuclei (LMN), differentiated by whether they increase their firing with left rotations or with right rotations. A *left-offset* cell with preferred direction ϕ_i would send projections to ATN cells with preferred direction counterclockwise to ϕ_i, while a *right-offset* cell with preferred direction ϕ_i would send projections to ATN cells with preferred direction clockwise to ϕ_i.

This architecture entails that the locations of the represented directions in all three structures (postsubiculum, PoS; anterior dorsal thalamic nucleus, AD or ATN; and lateral mammillary nuclei, LMN) will be synchronized during periods of no rotation, but during rotations ATN will lead PoS (Redish, Elga, and Touretzky, 1996). Furthermore, the amount of lead in ATN will depend on the angular velocity of the rotation (Redish, Elga, and Touretzky, 1996) as well as other complex factors such as the magnitude of

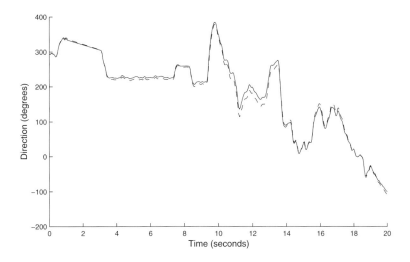

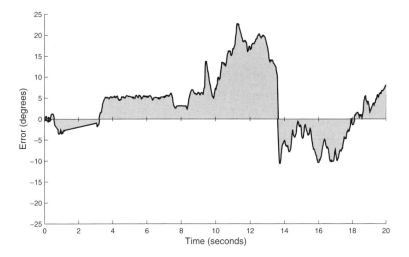

Figure 5.5
Tracking ability of the standard model. Top panel: Solid line indicates
sequence of head orientations recorded by T. Blair and P. Sharp. Dashed
line indicates head direction represented by excitatory pool of simulated
postsubiculum. Direction has been unrolled for clarity. Bottom panel:
Cumulative tracking error, namely angular difference between actual
and simulated head directions. These results actually show one vari-
ation of the standard model, from Redish, Elga, and Touretzky (1996).
Similar results have been shown for the full model (Goodridge et al.,
1997).

the asymmetry produced by the offset connections (Goodridge et al., 1997).

A prediction of this model, originally made by in Redish, Elga, and Touretzky (1996), is that the tuning curves of ATN cells will change with angular velocity. As reviewed above (see figure 5.3), this prediction has been recently confirmed by Blair, Lipscomb, and Sharp (1997), who found that during nonrotations, ATN cells show two peaks, and during left and right rotations, one of those peaks grows; they hypothesized that the two peaks seen in the nonrotation condition are indicative of the left- and right-offset connections. Figure 5.6 shows the ability of the standard model to account for this effect.

Relation to the Lesion Data

Lesions to the anterior thalamus cause a disruption of directional selectivity in the postsubiculum head direction population (Goodridge and Taube, 1994). The theory argued for here is compatible with this result because without the offset connections, the representation of head direction in PoS can not be updated.

Stackman and Taube (1997) have shown that with vestibular lesions, the ATN head direction cells are no longer correlated with head direction. However, it is not clear whether the ATN head direction population still shows a coherent representation of head direction that has been decoupled from the real world, or whether the representation itself is disrupted. Multiunit recordings could differentiate these two possibilities. According to this theory, as long as PoS and LMN were still intact, the ATN population should still contain a coherent representation of head direction, but the representation should be decoupled from rotations made by the animal.

Golob and Taube (1994) examined lesions of the lateral dorsal thalamus (LDN) and found that they did not affect the directional selectivity of PoS head direction cells. One possibility is that although LDN is interconnected with PoS (van Groen and Wyss, 1990), the local view information can also enter the system via parietal cortex which receives input from primary visual cortex,

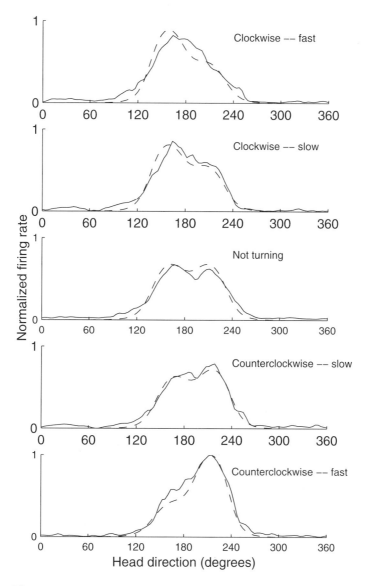

Figure 5.6
Model of an anterior thalamic (ATN) cell showing the two-peak effect.
Solid lines indicate data recorded by T. Blair and P. Sharp. Dashed
lines indicate computer simulation by J. Goodridge, A.D. Redish, and
D. Touretzky. Each panel shows the match between simulation and
data at a different angular velocity. Data has been normalized over all
conditions.

LDN, LPN, and superior colliculus. This means that a combined LDN/parietal lesion may be necessary to affect PoS sensitivity to visual cues.

There is no published data on LMN lesions, on how LDN lesions affect ATN cells, or on how parietal or cingulate lesions affect the head direction system.

Unfortunately, postsubiculum lesions do not seem to disrupt the directional selectivity of anterior thalamic cells (Goodridge and Taube, 1994; Taube et al., 1996). This result is incompatible with the attractor network model. There are three possible explanations that can make the theory and data compatible again:

1. *The postsubiculum may be only part of a larger structure, such as the presubiculum* (Taube, Muller, and Ranck, 1990a), at which point the lesions made by Goodridge and Taube were incomplete. The anatomical connections of the ventral presubiculum are slightly different from those of the postsubiculum (van Groen and Wyss, 1990) suggesting that the two structures may really play different roles. Because no one has yet recorded from the ventral presubiculum, we do not know whether we will find head direction cells there.

2. *Another brain structure can play the role normally played by the postsubiculum.* The cingulate cortex also sends projections to the ATN (Bentivoglio, Kultas-Ilinsky, and Illinsky, 1993; van Groen, Vogt, and Wyss, 1993). Chen et al. (1994a) have found head direction cells in cingulate cortex; perhaps the cingulate cortex can take over the role normally played by postsubiculum.

3. *The theory may be wrong or incomplete.* For example, the head direction signal may be generated by deeper subcortical structures projecting through LMN to ATN and thence to PoS (Taube et al., 1996). While this is always a possibility, the anatomical instantiations of the attractor network theory laid out in this chapter are compatible with all available data except for Goodridge and Taube (1994; see also Taube et al., 1996). I hesitate to suggest abandoning the theory without at least exploring the two other possibilities.

SYNTHESIS

The head direction subsystem provides the animal with an effective *internal compass*, which can define a *reference orientation*, allowing the system to measure allocentric bearings (see chapter 3) and to perform path integration (see chapter 6).

The head direction system is a crucial part of the navigation system. Without it, an animal should be unable to perform any locale navigation task. Lesions of the anterior thalamus and of the postsubiculum do disrupt the ability to perform the water maze (Sutherland and Rodriguez, 1990; Taube, Klesslak, and Cotman, 1992). Although an animal should be able to perform taxon navigation, many praxic navigation strategies will also be unavailable, particularly those which rely on updating internal directional coordinates, such as path integration.

An important consideration is that because the fornix carries fibers from the postsubiculum to the anterior thalamus (Witter, Ostendorf, and Groenwegen, 1990), fornix lesions are likely to severely impair the head direction system. Many experiments have included fornix lesions instead of hippocampal lesions (e.g., Eichenbaum, Stewart, and Morris, 1990; Sutherland and Rodriguez, 1990; Packard and McGaugh, 1992; Whishaw, Cassel, and Jarrard, 1995) and some have even argued that the inability of an animal with fornix lesions to return from foraging implies that the hippocampus is the key to path integration (e.g. Whishaw and Maaswinkel, 1997). The issue of the hippocampus and path integration will be discussed in the next chapter, but we should note here that because fornix lesions should disrupt the head direction system, they should also severely impair the path integration system independent of the role played by the hippocampus.

6 Path Integration

Path integration is the ability to return directly to a starting point (sometimes called a *home base* or *reference point*) from any location in an environment, even in the dark or after a long circuitous route (Barlow, 1964; Gallistel, 1990; Maurer and Seguinot, 1995). Sometimes called *dead reckoning*, this ability has been shown in gerbils (Mittelstaedt and Mittelstaedt, 1980; Mittelstaedt and Glasauer, 1991), hamsters (Etienne, 1987, 1992; Chapuis and Scardigli, 1993), house mice (Alyan and Jander, 1994), rats (Tolman, 1948; Alyan et al., 1997; Whishaw and Maaswinkel, 1997), birds (Mittelstaedt and Mittelstaedt, 1982; von Saint Paul, 1982), and even insects (Wehner and Srinivasan, 1981) and arthropods (Mittelstaedt, 1983), as well as dogs, cats, and humans (Beritashvili, 1965).

Path integration in animals has been the subject of argument for more than a century, including a notable debate in 1873 between Alfred Wallace and Charles Darwin in which Wallace suggested that animals find their way back via sequences of smells and Darwin argued that animals must be using dead reckoning (see Wallace, 1873a, 1873b; Darwin, 1873a, 1873b; *Nature*, 1873; Forde, 1873; Murphy, 1873). The carefully controlled experiments of Mittelstaedt and Mittelstaedt (1980) and Etienne (1987) have demonstrated conclusively that this ability is a consequence of integrating internal cues from vestibular signals and motor efferent copy.

Mittelstaedt and Mittelstaedt (1980) showed that a female gerbil searching for a missing pup via an apparent random walk could execute a straight-line return to the nest once the pup was found. The experiment was performed in the dark to rule out visual homing. Displacement of the animal during its search at

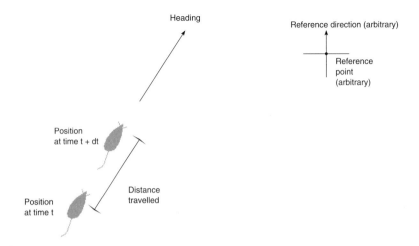

Figure 6.1
Path integration. Given a representation of its position at time t, $\langle x_t, y_t \rangle$, and representations of its speed and heading, an animal can calculate its position at time $t + t$, $\langle x_{t+t} = x_t + x_t,\ y_{t+t} = y_t + y_t \rangle$. (From Redish, 1997.)

speeds below the vestibular detection threshold caused the return path to be offset by a comparable amount, eliminating the possibility that auditory or olfactory cues guided the trajectory.

Etienne (1987) showed similarly that golden hamsters trained to find food at the center of a circular arena used path integration to return to the nest. When the environment was rotated 90° or 180° while the animal was at the center of the arena, the animal returned to where the nest had been originally, ignoring the rotation of the arena (Etienne et al., 1986; Etienne, 1987; Etienne, Maurer, and Saucy, 1988). The fact that animals always went to the center of the arena only implies angular integration; linear integration is not necessary if the animals always go to the center (B. McNaughton, personal communication). However, Etienne does note that the hamsters could return accurately from locations other than the center (cited as "unpub. res." in Etienne, 1987), but does not present the data in detail.

The basic idea of path integration is shown in figure 6.1: if one knows one's location at time t as well as one's speed and direction at time t, then position at time $t + t$ can be calculated. The main problem with path integration is that if your measurements of speed and direction are wrong, your representation of position will be increasingly inaccurate.

Path integration has been used in shipboard navigation for thousands of years. Polynesian navigators used path integration techniques to cross the Pacific Ocean over distances of thousands of miles with no land in sight (Gladwin, 1970; Oatley, 1974). Even as late as the eighteenth century, European navigators were still using dead reckoning to determine longitude (Encyclopædia Britannica, 1994, "Navigation"), often with disastrous results (Sobel, 1995). While latitude can be determined by azimuth of the North Star in the Northern Hemisphere and by azimuth of known southern stars in the Southern Hemisphere, determining longitude on the open sea requires accurate comparisons between time at a known longitude and local time. Although local time can be deterined by comparing stellar observations and the calendar date, keeping track of time at a known longitude requires accurate timepieces, which were not invented until the 1760s (Sobel, 1995). With modern technology, however, submarines can navigate under the polar ice cap using dead reckoning with errors of less than a mile per week (Encyclopædia Britannica, 1994, "Navigation").

Because errors in the path integrator can be corrected from local view information, there may be some systematic error in the path integrator that is corrected by external cues. When Müller and Wehner (1988) examined path integration in desert ants (*Cataglyphis fortis*), they found systematic errors. Testing hamsters on simple one- to five-stage paths and measuring the direction they took on their journey home, Seguinot, Maurer, and Etienne (1993) also found systematic errors depending on specifics of the path taken. Other species make similar errors (see Maurer and Seguinot, 1995, for review). However, a path integrator that drifts too much will be useless.

A number of models of path integration have been introduced (Jander, 1957; Mittelstaedt, 1962, 1985; Müller and Wehner, 1988; McNaughton and Nadel, 1990; Touretzky, Redish, and Wan, 1993; McNaughton, Knierim, and Wilson, 1994; McNaughton et al., 1996; Redish, 1997; Samsonovich and McNaughton, 1997; Samsonovich, 1997). The following sections present a review and summary of the major models of path integration. These models fall into two categories: (1) *kybernetic* models, which endeavor to describe the abilities and errors but do not insist on a neural understanding; and (2) *connectionist* models, which emphasize an understanding of the underlying neural mechanism.

After reviewing the models, we will turn to the current debate about the anatomical instantiation of the path integrator, which has concentrated on whether the hippocampus is directly involved or not. McNaughton et al. (1996) and Samsonovich and McNaughton (1997) have suggested that it is, while Sharp (1997) has suggested that the key anatomical structure is the subiculum, and Redish and Touretzky (1997a) have suggested a three-stage loop of subiculum, parasubiculum, and superficial entorhinal cortex. These theories make predictions about the results of lesion experiments. McNaughton and colleagues' models (McNaughton et al., 1996; Samsonovich and McNaughton, 1997; Samsonovich, 1997) predict that animals should be unable to path integrate after any hippocampal lesion. In contrast, Redish and Touretzky (1997a) predicted that ibotenic lesions of the hippocampus should not produce path integration deficits, while fornix lesions should. Two recent experiments (Alyan et al., 1997; Whishaw and Maaswinkel, 1997) explicitly tested these predictions. After reviewing the models and the anatomical debate, we will return to these two experiments and discuss their implications in depth.

MODELS OF PATH INTEGRATION

Kybernetic Models

Early models of path integration addressed issues of the computational components of path integration, attempting to account for the animals' behavior, but generally not addressing the anatomy or neurophysiology (e.g. Jander, 1957; Mittelstaedt, 1962, 1983, 1985; Müller and Wehner, 1988; for reviews, see Gallistel, 1990; Maurer and Seguinot, 1995). Many of the kybernetic models address path integration in insects, which is not to suggest that path integration in insects and rodents necessarily occurs by the same mechanism.

Jander (1957)

In this model, a representation of the animal's *angle of return* α_r (the angle home) is maintained by calculating the integral

$$\alpha_r = \frac{1}{t_Z - t_N} \int_{t_N}^{t_Z} \alpha_t dt \tag{6.1}$$

where the journey lasts from t_N to t_Z, and α_t is the angle turned at time t. Note that Jander's model does not include a representation of the distance necessary to return home, only the direction. As pointed out by Maurer and Seguinot (1995), although this equation works for specific cases, it does not match either perfect path integration or the actual abilities of insects.[1]

Mittelstaedt (1962)

Here, the Cartesian coordinates of the animal's path home are explicitly represented, so that after a step of distance d at angle ϕ, the animal changes its representation of position by

$$\begin{aligned} x(t+t) &= x(t) + d(t) \cdot \cos(\phi(t)) \\ y(t+t) &= y(t) + d(t) \cdot \sin(\phi(t)) \end{aligned} \tag{6.2}$$

which corresponds to the mathematically ideal path integration. Noise in the system produces scatter in the position returned to

(Benhamou, Sauve, and Bovet, 1990), which can produce non-systematic errors. However, as pointed out by Maurer and Seguinot (1995), because this model corresponds to the mathematical ideal path integration mechanism, it cannot explain systematic errors.

Fujita et al. (1990) examined a linearization of the mathematically accurate path integrator model but they found it a very poor fit to the path integration abilities of ants. (It made errors in the opposite directions from the actual ants.)

Müller and Wehner (1988)

Keeping track of the animal's mean direction home by weighted averages of distance traveled along each direction, this model replicates inaccuracies seen in ants. The representation of the direction home is updated at each step by:

$$\phi_{n+1} = \phi_n + k\frac{(180° + \delta)(180° - \delta)}{l_n} \tag{6.3}$$

where δ is the angle turned in step n, k is a constant (empirically determined to be $4.009 \times 10^{-5} \deg^{-2}$ for *Cataglyphis fortis* ants), and l_n is a measure of the distance from the home base and is updated by

$$l_{n+1} = l_n + 1 - \frac{\delta}{90°} \tag{6.4}$$

Although this model is does not perfectly track the vector home, it does fit the path integration abilities of ants remarkably well (Müller and Wehner, 1988). Seguinot, Maurer, and Etienne (1993) show that it also reasonable approximates the path integration abilities of hamsters on short journeys consisting of 1–5 straight segments.

Connectionist Models

While the kybernetic models do not address the neurophysiology of path integration, there have been three connectionist models of path integration in rodents that do.

Associative Memory Models

McNaughton and colleagues (McNaughton, 1989; McNaughton and Nadel, 1990; McNaughton, Chen, and Markus, 1991; McNaughton, Knierim, and Wilson, 1994) suggested in their early models that path integration could be accomplished by an associative memory in which a representation of position was associated with a representation of spatial displacement. The association produces a representation of the new position. The discrete form of this is a table lookup model and the continuous version can be described by a linear associator. McNaughton and colleagues reported no simulations of these proposals.

These models use self-motion information to regenerate local views, requiring that an animal explore an environment before it can show path integration in that environment. Because animals can path integrate from a first experience in an environment (Beritashvili, 1965; Mittelstaedt and Mittelstaedt, 1980; Wehner and Srinivasan, 1981; von Saint Paul, 1982; Alyan and Jander, 1994), these associative memory models are insufficient to fully describe path integration.

Sinusoidal Arrays

Touretzky, Redish, and Wan (1993) described a representation of two-dimensional vectors they called the *sinusoidal array* that accommodates several vector arithmetic operations including addition, in which the error grows linearly. This representation can thus be used to implementat the vector addition theory of Mittelstaedt (1962).

The representation consists of a population of cells in which each cell fires at a rate

$$F_i = b_i + k_i \cdot r \cos(\phi - \phi_i) \tag{6.5}$$

where b_i is a baseline firing rate, k_i is a gain parameter, and ϕ_i is a preferred direction, analogous to that of head direction cells. This representation is one possible extension of the head direction representation shown in chapter 5 and appendix A, as well as an extension of a represention found in primary motor cortex and first described by Georgopoulos et al. (1983). Redish and Touretzky (1994) have shown that some motor control results can be explained by it. Although head direction cells have been found in the rodent (see chapter 5), directionally tuned cells with a linear relation to speed have not yet been found.

Because error grows linearly in this model, the effect of noise will be similar to that seen by Benhamou, Sauve, and Bovet (1990). Although no one has tested whether combining this model with realistic neuronal time courses can reproduce the systematic errors seen in hamsters (Seguinot, Maurer, and Etienne, 1993), Wittmann and Schwegler (1995) have shown how this encoding could be used to model path integration in ants.

Two-dimensional attractor networks

Another extension of the head direction representation is for each cell to have a *preferred spatial coordinate* (in two dimensions) and to fire at a rate proportional to a Gaussian of the distance between the represented coordinates and its preferred coordinates, analogous to preferred directions in the head direction representation. This representation was suggested as a substrate for path integration by McNaughton and colleagues (McNaughton et al., 1996; Samsonovich and McNaughton, 1997; Samsonovich, 1997) and by Zhang (1996).

An appropriately formulated connection matrix will produce a two-dimensional attractor network analogous to a one-dimensional attractor network (Kohonen, 1982, 1984; Droulez and Berthoz, 1991; Munoz, Pélisson, and Guitton, 1991; Arai, Keller, and Edelman, 1994; McNaughton et al., 1996; Zhang, 1996; Samsonovich and McNaughton, 1997; Samsonovich, 1997; Redish, 1997; Redish and Touretzky, 1998a). Offset connections can move the two-dimensional representation around just as they can the one-dimensional representation in chapter 5 (Droulez and Berthoz, 1991; Munoz, Pélisson, and Guitton, 1991; Arai, Keller, and Edelman, 1994; McNaughton et al., 1996; Zhang, 1996; Samsonovich and McNaughton, 1997; Samsonovich, 1997; Redish and Touretzky, 1998a).

The basic theory is a straightforward extension of the head direction system (chapter 5). Samsonovich and McNaughton (1997) suggest that the system works in two stages: a $\mathcal{P}$-stage, which represents the position (analogous to the role assigned to post-subiculum in chapter 5) and an $\mathcal{I}$-stage, which represents position $\times$ velocity (analogous to the role assigned to lateral mammillary nuclei in chapter 5). One can also imagine a third stage (which I call $\mathcal{R}$ for *reintegration*, with a role analogous to that assigned to anterior thalamus in chapter 5). This third stage was not separated from the $\mathcal{P}$-stage by Samsonovich and McNaughton (1997). All three stages were incorporated into a single population by Zhang (1996).

ANATOMY

Computational Requirements

Having reviewed the connectionist models of path integration, we can now ask *What brain structures are directly involved in path integration?* These structures must meet the following five criteria:

1. *They must collectively be able to represent the position of the animal.* That is, the cells must show activity patterns correlated with the position of the animal.

2. *They must receive input from the head direction system.* To update the representation of position, the path integration system must know the direction the animal is moving.[2]

3. *They must receive information about self-motion from the motor and vestibular systems.* In addition to direction of motion, path integration requires information about the speed of the animal.

4. *They must update the representation as the animal moves around the environment.* In other words, the path integration system must be able to perform the equivalent of the vector addition shown in figure 6.1, at least for small vectors along the direction of motion.

5. *They must send output to the area associated with the place code.* If hippocampal place cell activity in the dark or in the absence of cues is a consequence of path integrator input (O'Keefe, 1976; O'Keefe and Speakman, 1987; McNaughton, Leonard, and Chen, 1989; Leonard and McNaughton, 1990; Kubie and Muller, 1991; Markus et al., 1994; Wan, Touretzky, and Redish, 1994b, 1994c; McNaughton et al., 1996; Touretzky and Redish, 1996; Redish and Touretzky, 1997a; Samsonovich and McNaughton, 1997; see chapter 8 and Appendix B for reviews of this phenomenon), then the hippocampus must either be directly involved in path integration, or the cells must receive input from the path integrator.

Hypotheses

Hippocampus

McNaughton and colleagues (McNaughton and Nadel, 1990; McNaughton et al., 1996; Samsonovich and McNaughton, 1997; Samsonovich, 1997) suggested that the key to a rodent's ability to path integrate lies in the hippocampus. The place cell representation can represent the position of the animal, thus it meets criterion 1.

Each place cell can be modeled as a Gaussian representation of position. Because the set of Gaussians covering all positions forms a basis set representation of position, the population of place cells can be viewed as a basis set.[3] And because any mathematical function of the inputs to a basis set can be approximated by a linear combination of the activities of the set's elements, any function of position can be calculated by a linear transformation applied to the representation of position in the place code. This includes the position update function necessary for path integration.

Animals can return to their starting point even in novel environments (Eilam and Golani, 1989; Leonard and McNaughton, 1990; Golani, Benjamini, and Eilam, 1993; Touretzky, Gaulin, and Redish, 1996). This means that the mechanism subserving path integration must be already wired up before the animal enters an environment. However, the topology of place fields changes from environment to environment (O'Keefe and Conway, 1978; Kubie and Ranck, 1983; Thompson and Best, 1989), which means that the update function allowing the vector arithmetic (criterion 4) would have to be prewired in the hippocampus for each separate environment. Samsonovich and McNaughton (1997) have suggested exactly this, calling each prewired coordinate system a *chart*.

Updating the two-dimensional attractor network requires a very complex interaction between the head direction system and the representation of location in the path integrator. There must either be an interpretation function that transforms an environment-sensitive representation of location (the P-stage, identified with hippocampus) into an environment-independent representation of location $\times$ velocity (the I-stage), or there must be multiplicative connections between the P-stage and the I-stage that are correctly matched with head direction input. Samsonovich and McNaughton (1997; see also Samsonovich, 1997) have argued that this complex connection matrix may be trained up early in life and that a limited number of environment-dependent maps (called *charts* by Samsonovich and McNaughton) make the theory plausible, but they have not given any method (nor shown any simulations) by which this connection structure could be trained. I find the identification of the P-stage with the hippocampus implausible and unnecessarily complex. A strong prediction of this hypothesis is that hippocampal lesions should devastate path integration in rodents. There are alternative hypotheses that do not require the complex prewiring required by this instantiation.

Subiculum

Because subicular cells show similar place fields across different environments, Sharp (1997) proposed the subiculum as the locus of the path integrator. Because there are place cells in subiculum (Sharp and Green, 1994; Sharp, 1997), it can represent the current position of the animal (thus meeting criterion 1), and subicular cells do show a (weak) directional signal (Sharp and Green, 1994), which means it can also meet criterion 2. Because each environment is represented by the same subset of place cells (Sharp, 1997), only one update function needs to be learned. This means that it can be learned once early in life, or even prewired genetically. However, the subiculum does not send output directly to the place code; it sends output to the postsubiculum, to the parasubiculum, to layer IV of the entorhinal cortex, and to a variety of other structures via the fornix, but not to the hippocampus (Kohler, 1986, 1988; Witter et al., 1989, 1990). Thus the subiculum acting alone does not meet criterion 5.

Subiculum – Parasubiculum – Superficial Entorhinal Cortex

Redish and Touretzky (1997a; see also Redish, 1997) proposed that the path integrator is a two-dimensional attractor, as suggested by Samsonovich and McNaughton (1997) and Zhang (1996), reviewed above, but that, anatomically, path integration occurs via the subiculum (Sub), the parasubiculum (PaS), and the superficial layers of entorhinal cortex (ECs).

These three structures are connected in a loop (Kohler, 1986, 1988; Witter et al., 1989, 1990; van Groen and Wyss, 1990; Wyss and van Groen, 1992). Parasubiculum receives input from the postsubiculum (van Groen and Wyss, 1990), which is a key component of the head direction system (see chapter 5), and parasubiculum is interconnected with posterior cingulate cortex (Wyss and van Groen, 1992), which includes directional and behavioral representations (Chen et al., 1994b) that could supply self-motion information. This proposed loop meets the five criteria listed above:

1. Because each of these areas show place cells, each of the three can represent the position of the animal (Quirk et al., 1992; Sharp and Green, 1994; Taube, 1995b).

2. The parasubiculum receives input from the postsubiculum (van Groen and Wyss, 1990), which represents the head direction of the animal (see chapter 5).

3. The parasubiculum is interconnected with parietal and cingulate cortex (Wyss and van Groen, 1992), which includes directional and behavioral representations (Chen et al., 1994b).

4. Even though there is no data showing that the update mechanism described above occurs in the Sub-PaS-ECs loop, it is nevertheless plausible because only one complex connection structure would have to be learned. Thus a mechanism that produced such a structure early in life (e.g., from exploration in an early-experienced environment) could be used in any subsequent environment.

5. As required, this path integrator proposal includes direct projections into the hippocampus (from ECs, a proposed component of the path integrator.)

LESIONS

The anatomical hypotheses make very strong predictions about the effect of hippocampal and hippocampal formation lesions. Specifically, the hippocampal theory (McNaughton et al., 1996; Samsonovich and McNaughton, 1997) predicts that any lesion affecting the hippocampus should impair path integration. In contrast, the other theories (subiculum: Sharp, 1997; three-stage loop of subiculum, parasubiculum, and superficial entorhinal cortex: Redish and Touretzky, 1997a; Redish, 1997) predict that cytotoxic lesions of the hippocampus (destroying cell bodies but not fibers of passage) should not impair path integration. Although evidence that the hippocampus is not involved in path integration tasks such as return from passive transport goes back to 1979 (Abraham and Potegal, 1979; Abraham, Potegal, and Miller, 1983), these early experiments did not do the controls necessary to explicitly test path integration. These predictions were explicitly tested by two recent experiments (Alyan et al., 1997; Whishaw and Maaswinkel, 1997).

In Alyan et al. (1997), rats had to perform two tasks. In the first, the animals were lured via a circuitous route to a location in the arena, from which they were allowed to return back to the nest. They went directly to the nest. In probe trials, animals were lured to the center. A rotation of the arena (with no corresponding rotation of the animal) ruled out intramaze cues driving the return journey.[4] In the second task, the rats were trained to take an L-shaped path and then the path was blocked, forcing them to try another route back. They started back along the shortest path, turning directly toward the other end of the L. Both tasks were performed in the dark to rule out visual homing. In both cases, there were no significant differences between normals and lesioned animals, implying that even the lesioned animals had intact path integrative abilities.

In Whishaw and Maaswinkel (1997), rats were tested on a large platform: they had to leave a hole, find a food pellet, and return to a specific hole. There were also distractor holes that did not lead to exit paths. After training, blinders were placed on some rats and they were released from a different hole. The rats without blinders found the food and then returned to the original hole they had been trained from (indicating that they were using some sort of visually guided navigation). The rats with blinders returned to the new hole (indicating that they were using some sort of path integration). When the fornix of some rats was lesioned, those without blinders returned to the hole they were trained from, but those with blinders were totally lost, returning to a random hole. Whishaw and Maaswinkel interpret a fornix lesion as equivalent to a hippocampal lesion, but it is not. In addition to affecting the neuromodulatory input into the hippocampus, lesioning the fornix disconnects the subiculum from the nucleus accumbens and the postsubiculum from the thalamus (Witter, Ostendorf, and Groenwegen, 1990). As discussed in the previous chapter, the postsubiculum and the anterior thalamus are involved in the head direction system. Without a working head direction system, an animal cannot path integrate.

These two experiments strongly support the subiculum and three-stage loop (Sub-PaS-ECs) hypotheses over the hippocampal hypothesis. They show that animals can path integrate when hippocampus is lesioned, but cannot when the subicular output (fornix) is. Although they support the nonhippocampal hypotheses, it needs to be noted that the fornix lesions should devastate the head direction system (chapter 5). Thus Whishaw and Maaswinkel (1997) cannot be taken as proof that the subiculum is involved in path integration.

Although the Alyan et al. (1997) results are incompatible with the hypothesis that hippocampus is the key to behavioral path integration, it does not disprove the hypothesis that hippocampal place cells are updated by path integration mechanisms occurring within hippocampus. Given the existence of an extrahippocampal path integrator, however, the complex intrahippocampal mechanism is unnecessary (Redish and Touretzky, 1997a; Redish, 1997; Redish and Touretzky, 1998b).

EDGE EFFECTS

The attractor network model of path integration has a problem at the edges of its representations. What happens when the animal *falls off the edge of the map*? There are three possible mechanisms that might allow the system to handle problems at the edges of its representations:

- *The map might be toroidal*, which would mean that there are no edges. Representations that fall off the top appear at the bottom while representations that fall off the left edge appear on the right and vice versa. This would lead to an intriguing prediction: when exposed to a large enough environment, the place fields recorded from the path integrator components should repeat after a certain distance traveled.

- *The map might be scalable*, so that when faced with a large environment, the place fields of the path integrator components would scale appropriately. Even so, there is a limit to how large an environment can be accommodated by scaling. As fields get larger, the representational accuracy decreases, because, as the fields enlarge, a distance x is distinguished by smaller and smaller changes in firing rates. In addition, if an animal misjudged the size of an environment, the scale of the place fields would be incorrect and some recovery mechanism would have to exist.

- *The system might shift centers when it approaches the edge of the representation.* This would ensure that the system always had a valid representation of its position in some coordinate frame. However, for the animal is to be able to path integrate back across that *reference frame shift*, there must be a representation of how the two reference frames are associated. (Evidence supporting this third possibility will be discussed in chapter 10.)

PATH INTEGRATION AND PREDICTION

There is an interesting relationship between the concept of path integration and prediction in sensory systems. Path integration can be thought of as a means of predicting one's position from knowledge about one's previous position and idiothetic cues. There is evidence that under certain conditions, sensory systems can predict the stimulus using motor efferent copy.

Two examples from the primate are in parietal area 5 in a reaching task (Kalaska et al., 1990; Kalaska and Crammond, 1992) and in the lateral intraparietal area (LIP) in a double-step saccade task (Colby, Duhamel, and Goldberg, 1993, 1995). In area 5, neurons encoding the position of the arm during a reach begin to fire before the action (Kalaska et al., 1990); this is likely to be driven by motor efferent copy (Kalaska and Crammond, 1992).

Colby, Duhamel, and Goldberg (1993) found predicting neurons in a double-step saccade task. In this task, monkeys were trained to look at two dots in sequence, but the dots appeared and disappeared so fast that they had already disappeared before the animal began its first saccade. Colby, Duhamel, and Goldberg recorded from neurons in the lateral intraparietal area (LIP) and found that the visual receptive fields of these neurons shifted 70 ms before the saccade began. Effectively, the neurons were *predicting* the location of the stimulus based on the planned eye movements. Psychophysical studies by Dassonville and colleagues (Dassonville, Boline, and Georgopoulos, 1993; Dassonville, Schlag, and Schlag-Rey, 1994) show that humans use motor efferent copy to predict the location of the eye or the arm during ballistic movements. The time courses of Dassonville and colleagues' results match the time courses found neurophysiologically in the reaching domain by Kalaska et al. (1990) and in the oculomotor domain by Colby, Duhamel, and Goldberg (1993) These results are from primates, but there is no reason to suspect that rodents could not also predict ballistic movements similarly. We should note that while these results only demonstrate prediction of ballistic movements by motor efferent copy, and thus are not equivalent to path integration, they do show that animals can predict sensory stimuli from idiothetic cues.

Recce and Harris (1996) have suggested that because of this, path integration may be ubiquitous throughout the cortex. In their model, each landmark representation is updated from motor efferent copy. This, however, has the problem that without a mechanism to keep these updated representations synchronized, errors will accumulate and the representations will drift apart. One possibility is that it is the role of the place code to correct these errors.

Having a unique path integration mechanism that tracks one's home base does not suffer from this problem. Only one system needs to correct its errors. However, it is plausible that prediction based on idiothetic cues is ubiquitous but that one system is tracking the home base. That system then would be identified as the path integrator.

7   Goal Memory

It is not enough for an animal to be able to return to a starting point, it must also be able to reach a goal from that starting point. For example, many of the demonstrations that animals can navigate in natural settings come from cache behavior (Vander Wall, 1990; Sherry and Duff, 1996), and controlled experiments suggest that animals use locale navigation to find their caches (Jacobs and Liman, 1991; Jacobs, 1992). If the locale navigation system represents the location of the animal within some coordinate system,[1] this information will not help the animal find its cache without a representation of the location of the cache in that same coordinate system. This is the role played by the *goal memory*.

COMPUTATION

For each task, in each environment, goal memory must (1) represent the location of the goal within the coordinate system the animal uses for that task; and (2) compute the path from the current location of the animal to the goal.

There are two possible computational means by which this can be accomplished. Either the animal can compute the path each time or it can learn to associate a direction with representations of location and task. It is not clear what the anatomy of path planning is, but I will argue that the association of direction with representations of location and task is maintained by the nucleus accumbens.

One important role of the goal memory is to plan a trajectory from the animal's current position to a goal. If there are obstacles in the way or if the animal must take a complex path to reach the goal, the goal memory system should be able to plan these kinds of complex trajectories. Rodents can learn extremely complex trajectories such as the mazes in figure 2.2. It is not currently known how obstacles are represented in the rodent brain or how the planning is done to avoid them. A number of robotics algorithms have been developed to avoid obstacles or plan complex paths: *potential field navigation* (Khatib, 1986; Connolly, Burns, and Weiss, 1990; Tarassenko and Blake, 1991; Connolly and Grupen, 1992), *occupancy grids* (Moravec, 1988), *sinusoidal transforms* (Pratt, 1991a, 1991b); and *graph search* (Kuipers and Levitt, 1988; Muller, Kubie, and Saypoff, 1991, 1996). See also Trullier et al. (1997) for a review of some additional proposals. But because they do not lend themselves easily to neural implementations, and it is unclear what brain structures subserve these roles, strategies for planning complex trajectories will not be reviewed here.

We can, however, identify some computational requirements that the two components of the goal memory must meet. The role of the goal memory is to plan a route to a goal, given information about the position of the animal and the current needs and desires. The structures subserving the goal memory can thus be expected to meet the following four criteria:

1. They must receive input from the place code or path integrator, probably both.

2. They must be *motor areas*, that is, manipulations to them should affect locomotion, or they should send projections to motor areas.

3. They must be able to represent intended actions and directions of motion.

4. They must play an essential role in navigation, that is, lesions of the area should cause impairments in navigation tasks.

ANATOMY

Posterior Cingulate Cortex

As noted in the discussion of praxic navigation (chapter 4), there is evidence that the cingulate cortex may play a role in navigation

(Chen, 1991; Chen et al., 1994a, 1994b; Sutherland and Hoesing, 1993; but see Neave et al., 1994; Neave, Nagle, and Aggleton, 1997). It receives input from the subiculum (Vogt, 1985; Witter, Ostendorf, and Groenwegen, 1990; Wyss and van Groen, 1992), representing the location of the animal (chapter 6), and from the anterior thalamic nuclei (Sripanidkulchai and Wyss, 1986; Bentivoglio, Kultas-Ilinsky, and Illinsky, 1993; van Groen, Vogt, and Wyss, 1993) and the postsubiculum (van Groen and Wyss, 1990; Wyss and van Groen, 1992; Finch, 1993), components of the head direction system (chapter 5). Cells in the posterior cingulate cortex (PCC) show head direction and behavioral correlates on the radial maze (Chen, 1991; Chen et al., 1994a, 1994b). The PCC also sends projections to motor cortices (Finch, 1993). Both Sutherland and Hoesing (1993) and Redish and Touretzky (1998a) have suggested that the posterior cingulate cortex is the long-term storage of routes. Lesions of the PCC strongly impair navigation in the water maze (Sutherland and Hoesing, 1993).[2] An important distinction needs to be noted between the anterior and posterior cingulate cortices. While posterior lesions affect spatial tasks, anterior lesions do not (Sutherland and Hoesing, 1993), and while anterior lesions affect classical conditioning (such as in a visual discrimination task), posterior lesions do not (Bussey, Everitt, and Robbins, 1997; Bussey et al., 1997). The exact role of the posterior cingulate cortex in navigation is still an open question, but its involvement in goal memory is not out of the realm of possibilities.

Nucleus Accumbens

Mogenson (1984) first suggested that the nucleus accumbens (NAcb) combines information from amygdala, the ventral tegmental area (VTA, containing dopamine cells), CA1, and subiculum to produce locomotor actions via the subpallidal regions. The nucleus accumbens is one of the major targets of the fornix (Witter, Ostendorf, and Groenwegen, 1990), which can carry place information from subiculum and CA1. Accumbens receives afferent fibers from amygdala (Aggleton, 1993;

Davis, Rainnie, and Cassell, 1994; Finch, 1996), which has been implicated in emotion and goal information by a number of studies (for reviews, see Aggleton, 1993; Davis, Rainnie, and Cassell, 1994), and the ventral tegmental area (Wolske et al., 1993), which contains mostly dopaminergic neurons and supplies dopaminergic input to the accumbens (Sesack and Pickel, 1990; Kiyatkin and Gratton, 1994; Wickens and Kotter, 1995). Dopamine has been implicated in signaling reward (Schultz et al., 1995b; Wickens and Kotter, 1995; Schultz, 1997). The NAcb also receives afferents from the medial prefrontal cortex (Sesack et al., 1989; Finch, 1996), which may supply contextual information (Kolb, 1990b). Finch (1996) has shown that many of these inputs (amygdala, hippocampal formation, medial prefrontal) converge on single neurons in the nucleus accumbens. Other studies have shown that dopaminergic and hippocampal afferents converge together at single spines (Sesack and Pickel, 1990). Additional studies have implicated NAcb as a locomotor structure (Jones and Mogenson, 1980; Mogenson, 1984; Mogenson and Nielsen, 1984), and particularly in locale navigation tasks such as the water maze (Annett, McGregor, and Robbins, 1989; Sutherland and Rodriguez, 1990) and the radial maze (Seamans and Phillips, 1994; Floresco, Seamans, and Phillips, 1997).

Injections of dopaminergic agonists into NAcb produce excessive locomotion (Isaacson, 1974; Whishaw and Mittleman, 1991), as does carbachol (a cholinergic agonist, acetylcholine is a major neurotransmitter in the basal ganglia; Graybiel, 1990). Glutamate antagonists reduce the locomotor activity produced by injections of carbachol into hippocampus (Mogenson and Nielsen, 1984).

The nucleus accumbens forms the ventral component of the basal ganglia, and is thus sometimes refered to as the *ventral striatum*. It therefore forms a ventral contrast to the dorsal striatum or caudate nucleus. The caudate nucleus has been implicated in stimulus-reward associations and taxon and praxic navigation (see chapter 4).

NAcb lesions produce deficits in naive rats on the hidden platform version of the water maze, but not in the visible platform or with pretrained rats (Annett, McGregor, and Robbins, 1989;

Sutherland and Rodriguez, 1990). The rats in the first study did eventually learn the task, although they were never as good as normals. We should note that the lesions were incomplete.

Floresco, Seamans, and Phillips (1997) did transient unilateral lesions of ventral hippocampus and subiculum combined with transient contralateral unilateral lesions of nucleus accumbens. These disconnection lesions produced errors in the nondelayed but not in the delayed versions of the radial maze, while similar lesions of ventral hippocampus and subiculum with prelimbic cortex produce errors on the delayed but not the nondelayed versions (Floresco, Seamans, and Phillips, 1997). Similarly, Seamans and Phillips (1994) found that lidocaine lesions of nucleus accumbens produced errors in spatial win-shift but not cued win-stay tasks.

Recording from NAcb cells in a standard working memory task on the radial-arm maze, Lavoie and Mizumori (1994) found three major correlations to firing rate: place, reward, and movement. Some of the reward-correlated cells were actually correlated to reward expectation, that is, they reduced their firing on finding reward, and some of them were also correlated with the magnitude of the reward.

A number of early experiments (see Isaacson, 1974) found that hippocampal lesions produced hyperactivity in open arenas. Whishaw and Mittleman tested hippocampal lesions combined with damage to the dopaminergic inputs to the caudate or nucleus accumbens. They found that combined hippocampal and caudate lesions decreased the number of stereotypical movements observed but increased locomotion while combined hippocampal and accumbens lesions decreased locomotion but increased stereotypic movements. This led Whishaw and Mittleman to suggest that caudate and accumbens are balanced to produce stereotypy and locomotion, respectively, and that hippocampus affects locomotion through accumbens. Given that the caudate is involved in route navigation strategies and other stimulus-reward associations, the basal ganglia may subserve the general purpose of associating movements with input representations to achieve a goal — the dorsal striatum (caudate) associating movements, motivational inputs, and processed sensory inputs, and the ventral striatum (accumbens) associating movements, motivational inputs, and location representations. The theory that the basal ganglia perform this sort of general *reinforcement learning* function is supported by a large literature (see Barto, 1995; Houk, Davis, and Beiser, 1995; Schultz et al., 1995a, 1995b; Wickens and Kotter, 1995).

Animals with fimbria-fornix lesions and septal grafts can still learn the hidden platform water maze (Nilsson et al., 1987), which suggests there must be alternate pathways from hippocampus to the motor structures. One candidate may be the posterior cingulate cortex (Sutherland and Hoesing, 1993). Although it is not clear what the role of the nucleus accumbens is relative to this alternative pathway, even grafted animals are impaired relative to normals (although they are much better than lesioned, nongrafted animals). Further work needs to be done to fully determine the role played by the nucleus accumbens in the navigation system.

8   Place Code

To navigate within a familiar environment, an animal must use a consistent representation of position from session to session. Because the visual cues that serve to inform the animal of its initial position may be ambiguous or incomplete, there must be a mechanism to settle on a consistent representation of location. The evidence suggests that the *place cells* of the hippocampus are well suited for this role.

Spikes fired by dentate granule cells, as well as CA3 and CA1 pyramidal cells are strongly correlated with the location of the rat: each cell fires when the animal is in a specific place (called the *place field* of the cell; see figure 8.1). These place cells are some of the most studied neurons in the rodent brain; they have been examined in a wide variety of environmental manipulations. The hippocampus is also probably the most extensively modeled system in the rodent brain.

PLACE CELL PROPERTIES

Because place cells show such clear correlations between firing rates and spatial variables, many experiments have been done to explore how they react to environmental manipulations (see appendix B for a review). Here I list only the key properties:

- When distal landmarks are moved, place fields also move proportionately (Muller and Kubie, 1987; O'Keefe and Speakman, 1987; McNaughton, Knierim, and Wilson, 1994; Knierim, Kudrimoti, and McNaughton, 1995; Cressant, Muller, and Poucet, 1997).

- Place cells continue to show clean place fields when landmarks are removed (O'Keefe and Conway, 1978; Muller and Kubie, 1987; O'Keefe and Speakman, 1987; Pico et al., 1985).

Figure 8.1
Place field. Animal randomly forages for food in the environment.
The cell predominantly shows spikes in a restricted portion of the environment, the *place field* of the cell. Darker shading indicates areas in
which more spikes were seen. (Data courtesy D. Nitz, C. Barnes, and
B. McNaughton.)

- Place cells continue to show compact fields in the dark
  (O'Keefe, 1976; McNaughton, Leonard, and Chen, 1989;
  Quirk, Muller, and Kubie, 1990; Markus et al., 1994).

- Firing rates of hippocampal granule and pyramidal cells are
  correlated to more than the location of the animal, including odor set (Eichenbaum et al., 1987; Eichenbaum and Cohen, 1988; Cohen and Eichenbaum, 1993), match/non-match
  of samples (Otto and Eichenbaum, 1992b), task (Markus
  et al., 1995), and stage of task (Eichenbaum et al., 1987;
  Otto and Eichenbaum, 1992b; Hampson, Heyser, and Deadwyler, 1993).

- Place cells show different place fields in different environments (O'Keefe and Conway, 1978; Kubie and Ranck, 1983;
  Muller and Kubie, 1987; Sharp, Kubie, and Muller, 1990;
  Bostock, Muller, and Kubie, 1991; Sharp et al., 1995;
  Sharp, 1997).

- Place cells are directional when an animal takes limited
  paths, but non-directional when wandering randomly on
  open fields. (McNaughton, Barnes, and O'Keefe, 1983;

Markus et al., 1994; Muller et al., 1994; Gothard, Skaggs, and McNaughton, 1996).

Although place cells have other properties (see appendix B), these are the key properties that will drive our understanding of place cell models.

MODELS OF PLACE CELLS

From the first discovery of place cells in the 1970s, people have questioned what drives hippocampal pyramidal cells to show place fields. There is no direct cue that tells the animal when it is at a certain location; it must use a combination of cues to determine its location. This was the original hypothesis proposed by O'Keefe and Nadel (1978): locale navigation depends on a combination of cues, in contrast to taxon or praxic navigation, which depends on a single cue.

Many theories of hippocampal function have been proposed. There are also a number of specific models of place cells, many including simulations and comparisons to data (Zipser, 1985, 1986; McNaughton and Morris, 1987; O'Keefe, 1989; McNaughton, 1989; McNaughton, Leonard, and Chen, 1989; Leonard and McNaughton, 1990; O'Keefe, 1991; Sharp, 1991; Treves, Miglino, and Parisi, 1992; Hetherington and Shapiro, 1993; Schmajuk and Blair, 1993; Shapiro and Hetherington, 1993; Burgess, Recce, and O'Keefe, 1994; Wan, Touretzky, and Redish, 1994b, 1994c; McNaughton, Knierim, and Wilson, 1994; Burgess and O'Keefe, 1996; O'Keefe and Burgess, 1996a; Recce and Harris, 1996; Touretzky and Redish, 1996; Redish and Touretzky, 1997a; Redish, 1997; Samsonovich and McNaughton, 1997; Samsonovich, 1997; Redish and Touretzky, 1998a; Fuhs, Redish, and Touretzky, 1998). These models fall into three major classes: (1) *local view models*, which depend solely on the local view to explain place cell firing; (2) *path integration models*, which depend on a combination of local view and path integration to form the place field; and (3) *associative memory models*, which depend on internal dynamics of the hippocampal network to produce the key place field properties.

Before discussing the models in depth, let us take note of some mathematical properties of space. Local view is a high-dimensional continuous space, representing spatial aspects of local and distal landmarks, such as distance and egocentric or allocentric bearing. Although local view is a high-dimensional space, in any single environment, the position of the animal at any point in time can be described by two variables (its coordinates on the plane). This means that the animal only experiences a two-dimensional manifold of the high-dimensional space. Both the local view representations and this manifold share an important property: they are continuous.[1] This means that a cell tuned to a compact section of the high-dimensional space will also be tuned to a compact section of the two-dimensional manifold, that is, it will be a *place cell* and will show a *place field*. Any learning mechanism that allows cells to distribute themselves around this two-dimensional manifold will produce place cells.

This also means that any sufficient subset of spatial cues will force cells to show small, compact fields, where "sufficient" means "enough to specify a point in space." For example, distance to three landmarks, distance and allocentric orientation to a single landmark, or allocentric orientation to two landmarks are all sufficient. It should also be noted that these properties do not have to be measured directly. Because distance is correlated with other aspects, such as retinal size and height relative to the horizon, other aspects could also be used instead of distance. Differentiating between these input sets would require highly accurate measurements of place cell activity as one manipulated single cues. Because of the recurrent interactions in hippocampus and the consequent auto-associative properties (see below), this would be extremely difficult and indeed might even be impossible.

Local View Models

The first neural model of place cells that included simulations was presented by Zipser (1985, 1986). In this radial basis function model, each cell is assumed to be tuned to a set of cues; the cell fires with a rate proportional to a sum of Gaussians dependent on retinal area subtended by the distal landmarks.

O'Keefe (1989, 1991) suggested a local view model based on egocentric bearing to landmarks. In this model, the hippocampus determines the location of the animal by taking the centroid of the bearing to three or more distal landmarks. However, O'Keefe reported no simulations, nor any direct comparisons to actual place fields.

McNaughton, Knierim, and Wilson (1994) proposed that each place cell could be understood as representing the vector from an animal to a specific landmark. Their hypothesis predicted that when two landmarks were separated by more during testing than during training, the place fields would dissociate, so that some fields follow one landmark, while other fields follow the other (McNaughton, Knierim, and Wilson, 1994). Data from Gothard, Skaggs, and McNaughton (1996) showing that the population of place fields always represents a coherent location when the length of a track has been shortened disproved this hypothesis.

Other local view models include those of Sharp (1991) which used inputs sensitive to distances to landmarks at the edge of the environment, Fuhs, Redish, and Touretzky (1998) which used retinal size as a distance correlate; and Burgess and colleagues (Burgess, Recce, and O'Keefe, 1994; Burgess and O'Keefe, 1996; O'Keefe and Burgess, 1996a) which incorporated a distance modifier: the closer the landmark, the more accurately distance was encoded.

Neither the Zipser, the O'Keefe, nor the Burgess and colleagues models incorporated learning. Other local view models did examine the effects of learning rules, including competitive learning (Sharp, 1991; Fuhs, Redish, and Touretzky, 1998), and genetic algorithms (Treves, Miglino, and Parisi, 1992). Learning mechanisms have minor effects on the place fields.

For example, Sharp (1991) used a limited field of 300° in her local view input. Combined with competitive learning, this makes place cells along repeated paths directional. If the rodent samples the local view at a place from a discrete number of directions, competitive learning separates views to represent the place differently at each discrete direction. Theoretically, at some level of sampling, the discrete directions will merge and become an omnidirectional place field. Sharp shows that her model place fields are directional in radial mazes, but remain omnidirectional in open fields. This theory predicts that cells in the center of the radial maze will not be directional, because all directions are sampled there. Markus et al. (1995) report that cells in the center of the radial maze are directional, which is inconsistent with the prediction.

Fuhs, Redish, and Touretzky (1998) showed that a product-of-Gaussians model based on noisy distance metrics such as retinal angle can produce excellent place cell models using real images, demonstrating place fields without explicit object recognition mechanisms. Using competitive learning, they trained cells on constant-colored blobs and showed place-like activity even from extremely noisy data taken from a robot camera.

All of these models share the property that they are driven solely by local view, which means they cannot explain place cell activity in the dark. One could hypothesize that place cell activity in the dark is driven by nonvisual sensory cues, but that hypothesis is disproved by observations from Quirk, Muller, and Kubie (1990) and Knierim, Kudrimoti, and McNaughton (1995) that place fields can drift.

Recce and Harris (1996) suggested what is essentially a local view model of hippocampal place cells based on storing *snapshots of cortical input*, but they assumed that the local view representations could be updated by path integration in the dark. They assume that there is an egocentric representation of landmarks in cortex and that the hippocampus is an autoassociator storing egocentric maps. To explain the continued activity of place cells in the dark, Recce and Harris hypothesize an extrahippocampal path integrator that updates the egocentric map. Updating representations of landmarks by path integration is equivalent to the *virtual landmark* hypothesis of Muller et al. (1991) and tends to be computationally unstable. *Virtual landmarks* are locations in space from which distance and bearing can be measured (just as from real landmarks), but instead of being identified with a perceptual feature, they must be tracked by path integration. Because each of the landmarks is being tracked separately in the Recce and Harris (1996) model, errors that do not build up identically in each representation will distort the overall map.

Path Integration Models

In contrast to the local view models, a number of authors have suggested that place cell firing in the absence of cues is the direct result of path integration (O'Keefe, 1976; Muller et al., 1991; Wan, Touretzky, and Redish, 1994c; McNaughton et al., 1996; Touretzky and Redish, 1996; Redish and Touretzky, 1997a; Redish, 1997; Samsonovich and McNaughton, 1997; Samsonovich, 1997).[2]

The first model to simulate place cells driven by both local view and path integrator information was that of Wan, Touretzky, and Redish (1994c, see also Touretzky and Redish, 1996).[3] Touretzky and Redish (1996) modeled place cell activity by a product of six Gaussians including two Gaussians tuned to distance, two to allocentric bearing, one to retinal angle between a pair of landmarks, and one to path integrator coordinates. Because local surface orientation was also included in the local view, some of the landmarks were surface landmarks (such as the arena wall). Distance and bearing to a surface landmark were calculated as the normal to the surface (i.e. the vector of the shortest distance between the animal and the landmark). This allowed the modeling of crescent-shaped fields.

Touretzky and Redish (1996) showed that their model is consistent with the existence and shape of both normal convex place fields and crescent-shaped fields, that place fields are tied to local landmarks, that they are unchanged when landmarks are removed, that place cells continue to show activation in the dark, and that place fields can be controlled by entry point. They simulated cue manipulations in radial maze tasks, disorientation in a rectangular arena, and navigation using arrays of local landmarks. They also hypothesized the existence of (but did not show simulations for) reference frames, which allowed them to explain directional place cells, place cells showing different place fields dependent on environment, task-dependent place fields, and goal-sensitive place fields using a single mechanism.

In an alternate model (McNaughton et al., 1996; Samsonovich and McNaughton, 1997), the hippocampus is, in fact, the path integrator proper. Taking the proposition that the synaptic weight between place cells is inversely proportional to the overlap of their place fields (Wilson and McNaughton, 1994, also known as the *cognitive graph*, Muller, Kubie, and Saypoff, 1991, 1996) as a basic starting point and proposed the existence of a loop between hippocampus and subiculum which performs path integration. However, this hypothesis has been weakened by recent data from Alyan et al. (1997) that animals can path integrate with hippocampal lesions, suggesting that the path integrator does not include hippocampus (see chapter 6 for review and discussion).

Associative Memory Models

In the third major class of place cell models, *associative memory models*, the place fields are assumed to be driven by local view input, but auto-associative properties in the hippocampus change the properties of place fields significantly.

The idea that the hippocampus has autoassociative properties can be traced back to early writings by Marr (1971) and McNaughton and Morris (1987; see also McNaughton, 1989; Leonard and McNaughton, 1990). Other autoassociative models include those of Rolls (1989, 1996), Hetherington and Shapiro (Hetherington and Shapiro, 1993; Shapiro and Hetherington, 1993), Levy and colleagues (Levy, 1989; Levy, 1996; Levy and Wu, 1996; Wu, Baxter, and Levy, 1996), McClelland and colleagues (O'Reilly and McClelland, 1994; McClelland and Goddard, 1996), and Hasselmo and colleagues (Hasselmo and Schnell, 1994; Hasselmo, Wyble, and Wallenstein, 1996; Sohal and Hasselmo,

1998). In these models, recurrent connections within the CA3 field are assumed to produce attractor states so that, given sufficient inputs, representations are *completed*.

Early models by McNaughton and colleagues (McNaughton and Morris, 1987; McNaughton, 1989; Leonard and McNaughton, 1990; McNaughton, Chen, and Markus, 1991; McNaughton, Knierim, and Wilson, 1994) hypothesized that the hippocampus functions as an associative memory, associating local views with movements to predict future local views. This forms a sort of transition table. This theory can be seen as a sort of path integrator in that it updates the representation of place with each movement, but it requires exploration before a rodent can show path integration abilities in an environment.

The Recce and Harris (1996) and Samsonovich and McNaughton (1997) models can be seen as associative memory models in that they require attractor states which complete incomplete inputs. Recce and Harris assume that local view inputs (corrected in the dark by path integration, external to the hippocampus) are input into the hippocampus and stored as stable states in a content-addressable memory. The prewired charts hypothesized by Samsonovich and McNaughton can be viewed as a continuous version of an auto-associative memory.

Another associative memory model is that of Hetherington and Shapiro (Hetherington and Shapiro, 1993; Shapiro and Hetherington, 1993). Here, place cells are identified with hidden units in a three-layer neural network with recurrent connections in the middle layer trained by the standard backpropagation algorithm (Rumelhart, Hinton, and Williams, 1986; Hertz, Krogh, and Palmer, 1991). Because of the recurrent connections, cells remain active in the dark. This model requires that the animal see the environment in the light before the lights are turned out; if the animal is placed into the environment in the dark, the cells will not be active. Quirk, Muller, and Kubie (1990) and Markus et al. (1994) report, however, that place cells sometimes continue to show normal place fields, even when an animal first enters an environment in the dark, which is inconsistent with this prediction.

The Three-Mode Place Code Model

The local view models share the idea that place fields are built from the combination of multiple spatial parameters. The path integration models share the idea that local view information is associated with path integrator information in the place code. The associative memory models suggest that the hippocampus can be understood to function as a content-addressable memory that stores associations among its input representations. These three aspects are not incompatible. Path integration can drive place cells originally; during exploration, local views can be associated with place cells; and then on reentry into an environment, local view can drive place cells when there is insufficient path integrator information to drive them directly. Local view information can also be used to correct for path integrator drift as the animal navigates around the environment. Associative memory properties allow the system to be insensitive to noise and to recall incomplete inputs.

Figure 8.2 shows a model of hippocampal function under three modes or conditions. An amalgam of ideas from previous place cell models, this model has the following key properties:

1. The path integrator (PI, *outside* the hippocampus; see chapter 6) sends strong pre-wired but random connections into the dentate gyrus (DG).[4]

2. Areas representing processed sensory input (LV, local view, also *outside* the hippocampus; see chapter 3) send strong pre-wired but random connections into the dentate gyrus (DG).[4]

3. During normal navigation, the dentate gyrus performs an *and* function on the PI and LV inputs so that a cell fires only if it gets sufficient activity from both inputs.

4. The dentate gyrus sends strong projections to CA3. Each DG cell projects to only a few CA3 cells and each CA3 cell receives only a few DG projections. The effect of these strong connections is that a single DG input can drive a CA3 cell to fire.[4]

5. Areas representing LV send direct connections into the hippocampus. These connections are modifiable via a Hebbian mechanism such as long-term potentiation (LTP).

6. Recurrent connections within the hippocampus are also modifiable via a Hebbian mechanism such as LTP.

7. The hippocampus (CA1, which receives input from CA3) sends projections back to the path integrator. These connections are modifiable via a Hebbian mechanism such as LTP.

8. The hippocampus has three different activation modes: *storage*, *recall*, and *replay*.

   Storage. During storage, LTP occurs in the hippocampal formation (between local view and hippocampus, within the recurrent connections in CA3, between hippocampus and the path integrator), but these same connections show little or no synaptic transmission.

   Recall. During recall, LTP does not occur anywhere in the hippocampal formation, but the connections that once showed LTP now show synaptic transmission. Moreover, dentate gyrus is assumed to be inactive, that is, it does not transmit information during recall.

   Replay. Replay is like recall, except that the local view and path integrator representations are assumed to be silent. They provide no information to the hippocampus, which acts from internal dynamics only.

The model described above has properties in common with all three of the preceding classes. It is similar to the path integrator models discussed above (Wan, Touretzky, and Redish, 1994c; McNaughton et al., 1996; Touretzky and Redish, 1996; Redish and Touretzky, 1997a; Samsonovich and McNaughton, 1997; Samsonovich, 1997) in that place cell activity is driven by both path integration and local view. It differs from models of McNaughton and colleagues (McNaughton et al., 1996;

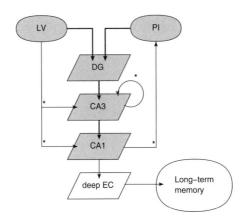

Storage

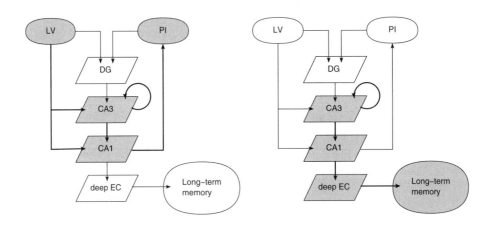

Recall   Replay

Samsonovich and McNaughton, 1997; Samsonovich, 1997) in that it assumes an extrinsic path integrator which works on a canonical map.

This model is also similar to the local view models in that it assumes that extrinsic local view input into the hippocampus helps drive place cell activity. It differs from them in that during *storage*, the local view alone is insufficient to drive place cell activity; path integrator input is also required. (In the dark, normalization processes driven by recurrent inhibition would allow place cells to be driven solely by path integration input. During *recall*, local view must be sufficient to drive place cells via the direct local view to hippocampal connections.)

This model is also similar to the associative memory models in that the role of the hippocampus is to associate local views with path integrator representations. As reviewed above, the idea that the hippocampus is completing inputs orthogonalized by the dentate gyrus was first proposed by McNaughton and Morris (1987), using a mechanism originally proposed by Marr (1969) for cerebellum. (See also Rolls, 1989; O'Reilly and McClelland, 1994; McClelland and Goddard, 1996; Rolls, 1996, for extensive discussions of this idea.)

The role of the dentate gyrus in this model is to force the system to use a new place code when the LV × PI association changes. This allows the system to handle multiple environments that differ in their local view inputs, and forces the system to use different hippocampal representations when the path integrator

---

Figure 8.2
Major components of the three-mode place code model. In each mode, pathways indicated by thick lines are hypothesized to transmit information, while those indicated by thin lines are not. Pathways marked with asterisks are hypothesized to show long-term potentiation. Structures involved in each mode are shaded. LV: local view; PI: path integrator; DG: dentate gyrus; EC: entorhinal cortex; CA3, CA1: hippocampus proper.

changes reference points (Redish, 1997; Redish and Touretzky, 1998b).

This model shares much with the Recce and Harris (1996) model in that the hippocampus is an associative memory that stores and recalls representations of location, but differs in that Recce and Harris assume the path integrator changes the local view external to the hippocampus, while in this model the path integrator representation is input directly into the place code.

The observation that the hippocampus shows multiple modes of activity was first made by Vanderwolf (1971). The hippocampus does show at least two modes of activity (Vanderwolf, 1971; O'Keefe and Nadel, 1978; Vanderwolf and Leung, 1983; Buzsáki, 1989; Stewart and Fox, 1990; Vanderwolf, 1990) differentiated by distinctive EEG traces: (1) during motion and REM sleep, the hippocampal EEG shows a 7–12 Hz rhythm called *theta*; and (2) during rest and slow-wave sleep, the hippocampal EEG shows irregular activity, called *large-amplitude irregular activity* (LIA), characterized by short-duration *sharp waves*.

During LIA, hippocampal pyramidal cells tend to fire in synchrony with sharp waves, but are then mostly all silent (Buzsáki, 1989; Ylinen et al., 1995). During theta, each cell fires only when the animal is in the corresponding place field. Because each cell has a different place field, cells fire a few at a time.

Chrobak and Buzsáki (1994) have shown that during theta, cells in superficial layers of entorhinal cortex (EC) fire in a pattern correlated to the theta rhythm, while cells in deep layers of EC do not. In contrast, during LIA, cells in deep layers of EC fire in a pattern correlated to the sharp waves, while cells in superficial EC do not.

A number of models have included suggestions that the hippocampus shows two modes: *storage* and *replay* (see, for example, Marr, 1970, 1971; Buzsáki, 1989; Hasselmo and Schnell, 1994; Wilson and McNaughton, 1994; McClelland, McNaughton, and O'Reilly, 1995; McClelland and Goddard, 1996; Skaggs and McNaughton, 1996; Shen and McNaughton, 1996), and, in many of these, that storage occurs during theta, while replay occurs during LIA.

Some models have included storage and recall-like properties, but have not separated the two modes (Burgess, O'Keefe, and Recce, 1993; Burgess, Recce, and O'Keefe, 1994; Brown and Sharp, 1995; Blum and Abbott, 1996; Sharp, Blair, and Brown, 1996; McNaughton et al., 1996; Gerstner and Abbott, 1997; Samsonovich and McNaughton, 1997; Samsonovich, 1997). I refer to these models as *online* models because they include the idea that recall occurs "online" during navigation.

Other researchers have previously hypothesized that the hippocampus does show explicit modes: *storage* and *recall* (Hasselmo and Bower, 1993; Hasselmo and Schnell, 1994; Nadel, 1995; Hasselmo, Wyble, and Wallenstein, 1996; Recce and Harris, 1996; Rotenberg et al., 1996; Touretzky and Redish, 1996; Redish and Touretzky, 1997a). This issue is also related to the concept of *recognition memory* and the detection of novelty, particular novel environments (Gaffan, 1972, 1974; O'Keefe and Nadel, 1978; Nadel and Willner, 1980; Mishkin and Murray, 1994; Murray and Mishkin, 1996).

This theory requires the hippocampus to show three modes of activation: *storage*, *recall*, and *replay* — the storage mode during theta as an animal explores around the environment; the recall mode on a significant context switch, such as when an animal is returned to an environment; and the replay mode during sleep.

PLACE CELL PROPERTIES REVISITED

This synthesized theory brings together aspects of all three kinds of hippocampal models (local view models, path integrator models, associative memory models). While there is not room to show the hundreds of place cell experiments (or even to list them), the theory is compatible with the major results.

- *When distal landmarks are moved, place fields also move proportionately.* On returning to an environment, the place code is used to reset the path integrator representation so that it is compatible with the local view. This reset will have the effect of shifting the entire population of place fields to be compatible with displaced landmarks. This, of course, assumes that all of the landmarks have been displaced in tandem. If only some landmarks have been displaced, then the place code will either shift with the most salient landmarks, ignoring the moved landmarks, or the entire map might change (see chapter 10).

- *Place cells continue to show clean place fields when landmarks are removed or in the dark.* Once the animal has reset its path integrator representation, the place fields can be driven by path integrator input. This will allow the animal to remember its location even when some or all the landmarks are removed. According to this theory, navigation in the dark is equivalent to navigation with no landmark cues.

- *Firing rates of hippocampal granule and pyramidal cells are correlated to more than the location of the animal, including environment, odor set, match/nonmatch of samples, task, and stage of task.* Whenever the LV × PI changes, the place code will have to change completely. Essentially, these aspects can all be explained because the animal is changing the reference point on which the path integrator is based, thus changing the path integrator representation. This is the *multiple-map theory of hippocampus* (O'Keefe and Nadel, 1978; Muller and Kubie, 1987; McNaughton et al., 1996; Touretzky and Redish, 1996; Redish, 1997) and is described in detail in chapter 10.

Although these key properties drove the synthesized model, there are a number of other place cell properties which should be discussed here (see appendix B for a review of other major place cell results).

- *Place cells are directional when animals traverse limited paths, but not when animals search open fields randomly* (McNaughton, Barnes, and O'Keefe, 1983; Markus et al., 1994; Muller et al., 1994; Gothard, Skaggs, and McNaughton, 1996). There are two important issues here: (1) why do cells show directional place fields when traversing repeated paths, and (2) why do cells not show directional place fields when wandering randomly over open fields?

An early suggestion and model was presented by Sharp (1991) who suggested that competitive learning combined with a limited local view (covering only 300°) would produce directional place fields on linear tracks and radial mazes but not when animals wandered randomly on open fields. However, this theory predicted that place fields would not be directional on the central dais of a radial maze, while Markus et al. (1994) report that they are. The theory also predicts that place cells should be initially nondirectional and directionality should develop over time. This prediction has not yet been tested.

McNaughton and colleagues (McNaughton, Knierim, and Wilson, 1994; Markus et al., 1995) oriosed that on linear tracks, animals attended to specific landmarks that were different for each direction, but when wandering randomly on open, animals shifted attention between many landmarks continuously. Thus the place fields appeared nondirectional.

Finally, Wan, Touretzky, and Redish (1994c; see also Touretzky and Redish, 1996; Redish and Touretzky, 1997a) proposed that different *reference frames* were being used for each direction on the linear track, but on the open field, a single reference frame was being used. A similar proposal has now been put forward by McNaughton and colleagues (McNaughton et al., 1996; Samsonovich and McNaughton, 1997; Samsonovich, 1997).

Although this last proposal is the most parsimonious with the data, its predictions have not been fully tested. For example, it predicts that there will be a *map transition* at the ends of the linear track. It also predicts that place cells will be equally reliable in both directions, and in both environments (the linear track and the open field).

- *Some place fields are crescent-shaped and hug the arena walls* (Muller, Kubie, and Ranck, 1987). There are three possible explanations for this result: (1) cells with crescent-shaped place fields might be sensitive to distal landmarks, with the center of the place field be external to the maze and only a small edge of the place field accessible to the animal (Sharp, 1991); (2) crescent-shaped place fields might be small, compact (Gaussian-shaped) fields that drift in orientation due to drift in the head direction system (B. McNaughton, personal communication); (3) place cells could be sensitive to the surface orientation of the wall (Touretzky and Redish, 1996).

The first explanation is unlikely to be correct because it would give rise only to place fields with convex sides — not concave — and the interior edges of these fields are concave. The second explanation implies that the place fields should appear as small, compact, convex fields when integrated over small time courses; and that simultaneously recorded place fields with locations near the wall should all stretch in synchrony. Both of these propositions are as yet untested. Nevertheless, the second explanation is unlikely to be correct because it also implies that cells away from the wall would occasionally form arcs at a constant distance from the wall. No such cells have ever been reported in normal animals.

The most parsimonious explanation is the third which fits the available data. An alternative version of this explanation has been proposed by McNaughton (B. McNaughton, personal communication): the sensory cue provided by the wall might become associated with place cells representing a specific location, at which point, the wall cue would drags the activity packet. However, this is just another way of saying that the cells at that location are *sensitive* to the wall.

- *Some place cells show multiple subfields in a single environment* (see appendix B for an example). The explanation of these fields is simple in this model: some CA3 cells receive multiple inputs from active DG cells. In this theory, there is no difference between multiple place fields in a single environment and place fields in different environments (McNaughton et al., 1996; Redish, 1997;

Samsonovich and McNaughton, 1997; Samsonovich, 1997; see chapter 10).

WHAT SEPARATES THESE MODES?

The three computational modes that the hippocampus has been hypothesized to show occur during awake theta (*storage*), during awake sharp waves (*recall*), and during slow-wave sleep (*replay*). There is also a fourth mode ocurring during REM sleep (*sleep theta*), but the role of REM sleep is still an open question. (The issue of REM sleep will be discussed in depth in chapter 12.)

It is unclear what exactly separates these modes, but there is extensive evidence that theta and LIA are separated by the presence (and absence) of acetylcholine in the hippocampus (Vanderwolf, 1971; O'Keefe and Nadel, 1978; Vanderwolf and Leung, 1983; Stewart and Fox, 1990; Vanderwolf, 1990; Hodges et al., 1991a, 1991b; Huerta and Lisman, 1993; Fox et al., 1997). This can separate out storage and recall modes (Buzsáki, 1989; Hasselmo and Bower, 1993; Hasselmo and Schnell, 1994). Norepinephrine and serotonin may also play some role (Flicker and Geyer, 1982; Plaznik, Danysz, and Kostowski, 1983; Bjorklund, Nilsson, and Kalen, 1990; Vanderwolf, 1990; Decker and McGaugh, 1991; Buhot and Naili, 1995).

The only difference necessary to separate out the recall from the replay modes is the presence and absence of local view inputs. When the local view provides candidate locations, the system will show a recall of previous representations of position compatible with that local view (*self-localization*; McNaughton et al., 1996; Touretzky and Redish, 1996; Redish and Touretzky, 1997a; Samsonovich and McNaughton, 1997, see chapter 9). On the other hand, in the absence of local view inputs, the system will still settle to a stable state but will then retrace recently traveled routes (*route replay*; Levy, 1996; Shen and McNaughton, 1996; Redish and Touretzky, 1998a; see chapter 11). Again, neuromodulators may play some role, but what that role might be is not yet understood.

An important question that remains unresolved (both theoretically and experimentally) is whether route replay can occur
during awake LIA states. Although Redish and Touretzky (1997a;
1998a) suggested that self-localization occurs during awake LIA,
the time course of self-localization only requires a single sharp
wave. One possibility is that during sustained awake LIA, the
system shows replay but that there are occasional states with the
time course of a single sharp wave (100–200 ms) during which
the system self-localizes.

9   Self-Localization

When an animal returns to a familiar environment, the role of the place code is to reset the path integrator representation so that the animal can use the same coordinate system from one experience to the next. In a sense, given the local view inputs, the place code *recalls* the previous representation.

As reviewed in the previous chapter, many models include the idea that the local view influences the place code. Other models include the idea that the hippocampus serves as an associative memory, recalling representations based on sensory cues, but these other models are all *online* models in that they assume the hippocampus is constantly using the local view to check and reset the hippocampal representation.

Because recent data suggests that place fields are only unstable across removal and reentry into an environment, some researchers are now considering that the recall process may only occur on reentry into an environment (Bostock, Muller, and Kubie, 1991; Rotenberg et al., 1996; Barnes et al., 1997; for similar effects in the primate literature see also Scoville, 1968; Milner, Corkin, and Teuber, 1968; Sacks, 1985; Cohen and Eichenbaum, 1993; Murray and Mishkin, 1996). The idea that the hippocampus is only necessary to reinstantiate context (i.e., that the recall process occurs on a *context switch*) has much in common with ideas of *contextual retrieval* (Hirsh, 1974; Nadel and Willner, 1980; Nadel, 1994, 1995; see also Rotenberg et al., 1996) *temporal discontiguity* (Rawlins, 1985), and *recognition memory* (Gaffan, 1972, 1974).

Self-localization can also be seen as an instance of *recalling a memory*. Other hippocampal models have included the concept of a general recall process without being models of navigation. Instead, they purport to be models of episodic memory and only deal with retrieval of binary vectors (e.g. Marr, 1971;

McNaughton and Morris, 1987; Rolls, 1989; Hasselmo and Bower, 1993; Hasselmo and Schnell, 1994; Rolls, 1996). (The similarities and differences between all of these theories will be discussed in chapter 13.)

THE SELF-LOCALIZATION PROCESS

In their early models, Touretzky and colleagues (Wan, Touretzky, and Redish, 1994a, 1994b, 1994c; Touretzky and Redish, 1996; Redish and Touretzky, 1997c), proposed an abstract implementation in which place cells provided candidate locations into the path integrator, which (because the path integrator could only represent a single location) limited the number of candidates. By slowly tuning the place cell's sensitivity to the path integrator, one candidate location eventually won out.

A more neural implementation of the self-localization process can occur as a consequence of local excitation and global inhibition in the hippocampus (McNaughton et al., 1996; Shen and McNaughton, 1996; Zhang, 1996; Redish and Touretzky, 1997a; Samsonovich, 1997; Samsonovich and McNaughton, 1997; Redish, 1997; see also Kohonen, 1982, 1984; Droulez and Berthoz, 1991; Munoz, Pélisson, and Guitton, 1991). Place cells that encode nearby locations support each other. When combined with global inhibition, this produces competitive dynamics similar to winner-take-all dynamics.

The final state of this system is an *activity bubble* (Kohonen's term) or *hill* of activation on the neural sheet represented by the cells. Cells with preferred locations near the represented location are very strongly active and cells with preferred locations farther from the represented location are progressively less and less active. (Code for and examples of a one-dimensional version of this process are given in appendix A; an example of this stable state in two dimensions is shown in the final panel of figure 9.2.) Because the place cells are not laid out topologically[1] (McNaughton, 1989), the neural sheet has to be understood as occurring in the space of the represented position of the cells and not anatomically (McNaughton et al., 1996; Redish, 1997; Samsonovich and McNaughton, 1997).

Because the final stable state of this system is not a single active cell, but a population of cells that encode a single location, I refer to this as *pseudo winner-take-all* (pWTA) dynamics. It can be understood as winner-take-all (WTA) dynamics in the context of location represented by the place code, but the final stable state is not one cell completely active (as would be true WTA dynamics), nor is it k cells completely active (as would be true k-WTA dynamics).

That local excitation and global inhibition produces a single pocket of activation in one-dimension was first shown mathematically by Wilson and Cowan (1973; see also Amari, 1977; Ermentrout and Cowan, 1979; Kishimoto and Amari, 1979). The first simulations of this pWTA process were reported by Kohonen (1982, 1984), who showed simulations in both one and two dimensions.

There have been three models that explicitly use the pWTA process as a means of recalling a location: (1) Samsonovich and McNaughton (McNaughton et al., 1996; Samsonovich and McNaughton, 1997; Samsonovich, 1997), (2) Shen and McNaughton (1996), and (3) Redish and Touretzky (Redish, 1997; Redish and Touretzky, 1998a). In the Samsonovich and McNaughton model, the hippocampus is the path integrator, and local view input influences it (see chapter 6 for a discussion of this hypothesis and some of its implications). In the Shen and McNaughton (1996) model, learned biases in intrahippocampal connections (or on the cells themselves) replay recent memories (details of this will be discussed in chapter 11). Although the local view influence on the hippocampus is ongoing in the first two models, the mechanism of the local view providing biases to a pWTA process is identical to that used in the third model (Redish and Touretzky), which is the one described here.

DATA SUPPORT

The self-localization process requires a connection function combining (1) support between place cells representing nearby locations with (2) global nonspecific inhibition. Recording from more than a hundred hippocampal place cells simultaneously as the animal explored an environment, Wilson and McNaughton (1994) found that the correlation between the specific timing of place cell spikes was stronger between cells with overlapping fields than between cells with widely separated fields. This suggests that the synaptic efficacies between them are also stronger, and that (after exploration) the necessary local excitation exists within the place cells.

There are inhibitory neurons in the hippocampus with very broad arborizations (Freund and Buzsáki, 1996). Inhibitory interneurons in the hippocampus also tend to fire over large portions of the environment (McNaughton, Barnes, and O'Keefe, 1983; Christian and Deadwyler, 1986; Kubie, Muller, and Bostock, 1990; Leonard and McNaughton, 1990; Mizumori, Barnes, and McNaughton, 1990; Muller et al., 1991; Wilson and McNaughton, 1993), implying that they are very nonspecific. This can provide the global nonspecific inhibition.

The local excitation component can be learned by correlational long-term potentiation (LTP) and can be seen on a neural level as increased synaptic efficacy between place cells with overlapping place fields. It can be realized in the intra-CA3 connections if the synaptic efficacies between place cells are inversely related to the distance between the centers of their place fields (Muller, Kubie, and Saypoff, 1991; Wilson and McNaughton, 1994). Muller and colleagues (Muller, Kubie, and Saypoff, 1991; Muller, Stead, and Pach, 1996) call this the *cognitive graph*. It can be learned by correlational LTP combined with random exploration of an environment. As an animal wanders around its environment, cells with overlapping place fields are more likely to be coactive than cells with well-separated fields. Combined with correlational LTP, in which the synaptic efficacy is increased when both cells are simultaneously active, the CA3 recurrent connections will be inversely related to the distance between the place field centers after a session of wandering an environment.[2]

Hebb (1949) first suggested a correlational learning rule between neurons. Data suggesting that LTP is correlational (i.e. that the synaptic weight between two cells is increased only with presynaptic firing and postsynaptic depolarization) have been well established (for reviews, see Landfield and Deadwyler, 1988; Brown et al., 1991; McNaughton, 1993; Malenka, 1995). LTP specifically has been shown in the recurrent connections in CA3, and in the Schaffer collaterals connecting CA3 to CA1 (for reviews, see Landfield and Deadwyler, 1988; Brown et al., 1991; McNaughton, 1993; Malenka, 1995).

An important aspect of this learning rule is that it will also produce local excitation within a single map. In chapter 10, I will argue that the hippocampus represents space on different maps.[3] In order to navigate within an environment, an animal must self-localize to the correct map as well as to the correct location on that map. Two cells will be strongly connected if they have place fields near each other in one experienced map whether or not they have place fields near each other in another. This means that the correlational learning rule will produce pWTA dynamics within each map as well as competition between maps.

The key point is that local excitation in location space forms from random navigation (i.e. cells that represent nearby locations in the same map are more strongly connected than cells that represent positions distant from each other). A local excitation/global inhibition structure has stable states that represent coherent locations in space (Wilson and Cowan, 1973; Amari, 1977; Kohonen, 1982, 1984; see appendix A).

ALIGNING LOCAL VIEW AND PATH INTEGRATOR REPRESENTATIONS IN THE PLACE CODE

During normal navigation, both the path integrator and local view subsystems will provide excitatory input onto the same place cells. When this happens, we say that the representations are *consistent* with each other. When these representations become misaligned, it is the role of the place code to make them consistent again. This can be done either by resetting the path integrator, which corresponds to the *self-localization* process (*recall*), or by changing the LV × PI association stored in the place code, which corresponds to deciding that the environment is novel which requires exploration (*storage*).

When an animal is placed into a familiar environment by an experimenter, the path integrator will presumably be tracking the animal's position relative to the previous environment. This means that the LV × PI association will be inconsistent. If we assume that the environment is familiar and the animal is unfamiliar with the spatial relationship between the two environments, then the animal must self-localize. In many experimental paradigms, animals are disoriented before being placed into an environment; in other paradigms, they are placed into a random location in the environment. In both these cases, the animal has no information except local view with which to reset the path integrator representation. On the other hand, if the animal is always put into the environment at the same location, it could use additional information by priming the path integrator before the self-localization process. All this does is provide additional candidate biases to the self-localization process.

What happens when the animal does not change environments, but still finds an inconsistency between local view and path integrator? Gothard, Skaggs, and McNaughton (1996) trained rats to run back and forth on a linear track, and then shortened the track. By recording multiple place cells simultaneously, they could observe how the place code handles inconsistencies in the local view and path integrator. They found two effects: either the place code precessed faster along the track than the animal ran, so that the represented position eventually caught up with the animal; or the place code jumped to match the actual position. As pointed out by Gothard, Skaggs, and McNaughton (1996; see also Samsonovich and McNaughton, 1997; Samsonovich, 1997), these two effects correspond to the two possible modes shown by the attractor networks in appendix A: either the system precesses when the two inputs represent similar (but not identical)

positions (figure A.2) or it jumps when the two representations
are very different (figure A.4).

Novel versus Familiar Environments

In Gothard, Skaggs, and McNaughton (1996), the animal has not
re-encoded the LV × PI association, that is, it has not decided the
environment is novel. (We know this because many of the same
place fields appear in the same topological relation to each other;
if the environment had been treated as novel, the topology of
the place fields would have changed dramatically.) But there are
experiments in which inconsistency is resolved by treating the
new environment as novel (e.g. Kubie and Ranck, 1983; Muller
and Kubie, 1987; Thompson and Best, 1989; Bostock, Muller, and
Kubie, 1991). When does an animal resolve the inconsistency
by changing the path integrator representation and when does
it resolve the inconsistency by treating the change as a novel
environment?

An animal that treated an environment as novel whenever
a single cue appeared out of place would never see a familiar
environment. On the other hand, if enough has changed that
the environment really is novel, the animal will be best served
by treating all of the cues it sees as novel as well. This issue
can be phrased in terms of *completion* and *separation* and is detailed in figure 9.1. Sensory information from each environment
is assumed to be represented as a distributed pattern of activity
over a population of cells. Above some threshold of overlap of
the current representation with a remembered representation, the
system should complete the new representation based on the old,
while below that threshold, the system should separate the two
representations as much as possible to prevent memory interference.

This is discussed by McClelland and Colleagues (O'Reilly and
McClelland, 1994; McClelland, McNaughton, and O'Reilly, 1995;
McClelland and Goddard, 1996), who suggest the dentate
gyrus (DG) is well suited for separation and CA3 for completion. McNaughton and Morris (1987, see also Marr, 1969;

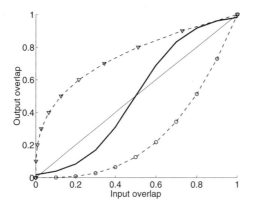

Figure 9.1
Correlation between two output patterns as a function of correlation between two input patterns. Thin solid line indicates 1:1 mapping. Dashed
line marked with small triangles indicates completion: output patterns
are more similar than input; dashed line with small circles indicates separation: output patterns are less similar than input. An optimal balance
between separation and completion requires that dissimilar patterns
be made more dissimilar while similar patterns be made more similar
(thick solid line). This figure does not show simulation or experiment, it
is meant to be explanatory only. (After O'Reilly and McClelland, 1994.)

McNaughton, 1989; Rolls, 1989, 1996) made similar suggestions that DG separates inputs from entorhinal cortex (EC) into
orthogonal representations, while the recurrent collaterals in
CA3 form an associative memory to complete input representations. It has been shown that the activity of DG cells is
much lower than the CA3 and CA1 representations (Jung and
McNaughton, 1993), and that DG is required for learning spatial
tasks, but not for their performance (McNaughton et al., 1989;
Sutherland and Hoesing, 1993).

Neuropharmacology: Acetylcholine

When learning a new environment, the recurrent connections
within CA3 will still drive the new representation toward an
already stored one, causing interference between the two rep-

resentations (Hasselmo and Bower, 1993; Hasselmo, 1993). As discussed above, place cells in CA3 are most strongly connected to other cells that represent similar locations. This means that CA3 can be understood as an associative memory and the self-localization process can be understood as a recall of place and reference frame from an associative memory.

An important problem with autoassociative memories is that if synaptic transmission continues to occur across recurrent connections when a memory is being stored in the system then incorrect correlations will occur between two memories that share neurons. This is called *interference* (Hasselmo and Bower, 1993). To fix the problem of interference, when LTP occurs in the system (i.e., when the system is storing a memory), the recurrent connections should be ineffective.

Hasselmo and Schnell (1994) report that carbachol (a cholinergic agonist) infused into hippocampal slices reduces the size of the excitatory postsynaptic potential (EPSP)[4] in CA1 produced by stimulating Schaffer collaterals by 90 percent, while only reducing that produced by stimulating the perforant path by 40 percent. That the Schaffer collateral axons also form the CA3 excitatory feedback pathway suggests that acetylcholine (ACh) may shut off these recurrent connections. Returning to the conceptual framework above, we can say that ACh turns off pattern completion while not affecting pattern separation. ACh also has an effect on learning: although it suppresses synaptic transmission, ACh enhances LTP in DG, CA1, and other structures (see Hasselmo, 1995, for a review). This means that ACh should enhance the learning and separation of place codes.

HIPPOCAMPAL MODES

As we have noted, the hippocampus shows multiple modes of activity. In the current model, the storage mode corresponds to hippocampal theta (in agreement with a number of models; see previous chapter), and recall occurs during sharp waves occurring during awake states.

There are two hypotheses being put forward here: (1) that there is an explicit recall process occurring on reentry into an environment and (2) that the recall process occurs during sharp waves. While one can make predictions from each of these hypotheses, disproof of the second hypothesis does not constitute disproof of the first.

During exploration (according to this theory), the rodent navigation system must learn three things:

1. a mapping from local views to place codes (realized by long-term potentiation (LTP) in the local view $\rightarrow$ hippocampus connections in the model presented in the previous chapter);

2. a connection function that enforces the place code to always consist of a coherent representation of location (realized by LTP within the recurrent connections of CA3 and between CA3 and CA1); and

3. a mapping from place codes to path integrator coordinates (realized by LTP between CA1 and the path integrator).

In this model, on entering an environment, the following sequence occurs:

1. The hippocampal and path integrator systems are initially noisy.

2. Sensory cues in local view areas such as parietal cortex are passed through superficial EC into the hippocampus proper, biasing the random firing rates with candidate locations.

3. The recurrent connections in CA3 allow one of these candidate locations to win out, forming a coherent code in hippocampus.

4. The connections between CA1 and subiculum reset the path integrator to the correct representation of the animal's location in path integrator coordinates.

Redish and Touretzky (1998a; see also Redish and Touretzky, 1997a; Redish, 1997), who refer to this sequence as the *self-localization* or *recall* process[5] suggest that it occurs within the course of a single sharp wave. In their simulations, the place code in CA3 is coherent within 50–100 ms. (Figure 9.2 shows the first 70 ms of a simulated self-localization sequence.) During a sharp wave, place cells do not show normal place fields; many cells are simultaneously active (many more than during theta; Buzsáki, 1989).

This model also requires that the superficial and deep layers of entorhinal cortex be active at different times. As the intrahippocampal connections are learning (during theta), activity should not be transmitted out from hippocampus (through deep EC). During the self-localization procedure, the hippocampus should show LIA, but superficial EC cells should fire at a constant rate and still be uncorrelated to LIA. Consistent with this hypothesis is data showing that while superficial EC cells are phase-locked to the theta rhythm, they are uncorrelated to LIA, and conversely, while deep EC cells are uncorrelated to theta, they are correlated to the LIA EEG signal (Chrobak and Buzsáki, 1994).

PREDICTIONS

The key prediction we can take from this theory about the role of the place code is that when the animal returns to a familiar environment, it should show the self-localization process.

Sharp Waves on Entry

If the recall process is realized by sharp waves, then we can predict that animals will show at least one sharp wave on entry into a familiar environment. (Note that this says nothing about what happens when the animal enters a *novel* environment.)

Coherency Changes on Entry

We can also predict that during the last sharp wave before the animal begins moving, the representation in CA3 will begin in an incoherent state and become coherent over the course of the sharp wave. At the end of the sharp wave, the place cells will

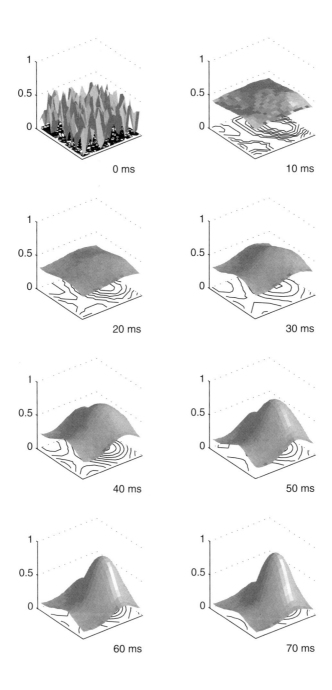

encode the animal's current location accurately, and these cells will be the initial ones active during the first theta cycles.

We can define the coherency of a representation mathematically as the inverse of the width of the confidence interval of the position represented by the population. Given enough cells, it can be measured by the bootstrap algorithm (Efron, 1982). The simultaneous recording of a hundred cells described by Wilson and McNaughton (1993) should be sufficient.

Another way to view the coherency of a population is to plot the sum of the place fields of each cell, weighted by their current firing rates. A coherent representation of position will show up clearly as a single pocket of activity.

The Resolution Issue

A third prediction we can make is that when the candidate locations are near each other (within the radius of a single place field), they will be averaged together, but when the candidate locations are far apart only one of them will be chosen and no interaction effect will be seen. This is because the hill of activity will precess toward nearby representations, but will suppress distal represen-

Figure 9.2
Simulation of self-localization. Each panel shows the firing rates of all of the simulated CA3 place cells at a single moment in time. The cells are laid out in a two-dimensional sheet with their locations in the sheet corresponding to the centers of their place fields in the environment. Intensity values have been interpolated for clarity. At time 0, the simulation is primed with noise and small biases toward candidate locations at three points in the environment. The recurrent connections force it to settle to a single one of those candidate locations. Adapted from Redish and Touretzky (1998a, which see for simulation details). Similar results occur in the models of Zhang (1996), Samsonovich and McNaughton (1997), and Shen and McNaughton (1996). Used with permission of publisher.

tations that are too weak to overrule it. (See appendix A for a discussion of this issue.)

WHEN DOES SELF-LOCALIZATION OCCUR?

Both behavioral and neurophysiological evidence supports the hypothesis that self-localization occurs uniquely on reentry into an environment.[6] As noted above, place cells continue to track an animal's position after the room lights are extinguished (Quirk, Muller, and Kubie, 1990; Markus et al., 1995), or after cues are removed (O'Keefe and Conway, 1978; O'Keefe and Speakman, 1987). That place fields drift in the dark implies that error correction does occur in the light (Quirk, Muller, and Kubie, 1990).

Behaviorally, in an already well-explored environment, a short flash at the beginning of a trial is sufficient to allow an animal to find a goal (Collett, Cartwright, and Smith, 1986). In the water maze, 100 ms flashes occurring at 1 Hz (i.e., 10 percent of the swim time) are sufficient to guide navigation to the platform (Bures, 1996). Arolfo et al. (1994) found that although animals could learn to find a location in darkness if they had been pre-trained in the light and began in the light, animals were impaired relative to those given complete light. Animals deprived of light whenever they were more than 20 cm from the wall were even more impaired. Again, this implies that some error correction is occurring in the normal condition.

IMPLICATIONS FOR EXPLORATION

While there is not room to go into depth about the relationship between exploration and navigation or between hippocampal lesions and exploration (for reviews, see Archer and Birke, 1983; especially Birke, 1983; O'Keefe and Nadel, 1978; and Renner, 1990), the hypothesized self-localization role has some intriguing implications for exploration. It suggests a reason why animals might establish *home bases*.

Animals spend large portions of their time in specific locations, called *home bases*, as they explore an environment (Chance and Mead, 1955; Birke, 1983). A similar behavior has been observed by Leonard and McNaughton (1990), who report that animals begin exploration by making small excursions from the initial entry point, and by Whishaw (1992), who notes that rats begin with small lateral head movements before venturing out into the world. More recently, Golani and colleagues (Eilam and Golani, 1989; Golani, Benjamini, and Eilam, 1993) have shown that not only do animals (female hooded rats) spend more time at these home bases, but they also visit the home base more than any other site in the environment. Touretzky and colleagues found similar effects in gerbils exploring a large (cue-rich) open arena (Touretzky, Gaulin, and Redish, 1996; Redish, 1997). Animals rear more frequently and spend more time grooming themselves at these home bases then elsewhere in the environment (Eilam and Golani, 1989; Golani, Benjamini, and Eilam, 1993).

One possible explanation is that animals are making an association between local view and path integrator representations in the place code (Touretzky and Redish, 1996). If the path integrator drifts significantly as an animal explores the environment, then the wrong association will be made. Indeed, Samsonovich (1997) has suggested that unless the path integrator is very accurate, the association between local view representations and path integrator coordinates must be made directly and cannot be made using an intermediate representation, and that the hippocampus must therefore update its information by path integration. The home base behavior of exploring animals can, however, counteract path integrator drift even if there is an intermediate representation associating the local view and an extrahippocampal path integrator.

At the home base, the animal has presumably learned an appropriate association between the local view and the path integrator. Then, as it makes a foray into the environment, the path integrator drifts. Near the home base, the drift will not be serious, but as the animal moves farther into the environment, the drift will worsen, the assocaition will no longer be accurate, and the animal will have to return to the base. By constantly returning to an area in which the association has been made, the animal is able to correct for any inaccuracies in its path integration ability. In a sense, we can say that the animal is inductively exploring the environment, constantly adding novel portions to its known area.

Chapter 9

10 Multiple Maps

Place cells allow an animal to self-localize and thus resolve ambiguous local views, that is to plan a path to a goal when some cues have been moved or even removed entirely from the environment. This suggests that place cells have to be sensitive to environment: anytime the association between local view and path integrator changes significantly, the place code will have to change entirely. It does. In different environments, cells show different place fields that are not topologically related to each other (O'Keefe and Conway, 1978; Kubie and Ranck, 1983; Muller and Kubie, 1987; Thompson and Best, 1989)

But place cells are also sensitive to a host of other factors, including direction along repeated paths (McNaughton, Barnes, and O'Keefe, 1983; Markus et al., 1995), task (Markus et al., 1995), and subtask (Eichenbaum et al., 1987; Otto and Eichenbaum, 1992b; Cohen and Eichenbaum, 1993; Hampson, Heyser, and Deadwyler, 1993; Gothard, Skaggs, and McNaughton, 1996; Gothard et al., 1996). In this chapter, I will argue that place cell sensitivity to all of these nonspatial factors (environment, task, etc.) can be understood as realizations of a single effect: that of *changing maps* within the hippocampus.

To say that a cell is *sensitive to a nonspatial aspect* (such as task), means that if it has a place field under one condition, it may or may not show a place field under the other, and that if two cells both show place fields under both conditions, then the spatial relationships between the fields may change drastically from one condition to the other. Essentially, a cell's place field (or even whether it has a place field at all) on one map is independent of its field in other maps.

Note how this differs from the head direction (chapter 5) and path integration (chapter 6) representations. Although the *reference orientation* (for the head direction system) or the *reference point* (for the path integration system) may change from one environment to the next, the topology of the representation does not change. Whenever two postsubicular or anterior thalamic head direction cells have been recorded simultaneously, the difference between their preferred directions never changes, even though the actual preferred directions may rotate when distal cues are moved (Taube, Muller, and Ranck, 1990b; Taube, 1995a; Taube et al., 1996). Similarly, the place fields of entorhinal cells do not change between two similar environments (Quirk et al., 1992), nor do the place fields of subiculum cells (Sharp, 1997), unlike those of hippocampal CA3 or CA1 cells (O'Keefe and Conway, 1978; Kubie and Ranck, 1983; Muller and Kubie, 1987; Kubie and Muller, 1991; Thompson and Best, 1989).

REFERENCE FRAMES

Together, a *reference point*, a *reference orientation*, and a *distance metric* define a coordinate system. These components form a *reference frame*. Each location in each reference frame is represented in the hippocampus by a different set of place cells, the place code in hippocampus represents, not just location, but location *within a reference frame*.[1]

The earliest theoretical descriptions of the cognitive map hypothesis included the idea that different environments would be encoded by different maps. O'Keefe and Nadel (1978) pointed out that the cognitive map had to be internally consistent: if some of the cues moved while others did not, the map should rigidly translate, rotate to follow some consistent subset of cues, or both. If too many of the cues changed, a new map would be needed.

One way to understand this is that in each map there are a different set of potential place fields in the hippocampus. For example, Muller and Kubie (1987) have suggested that different environments have different *active subsets* of place cells, each subset forming a set of potential place fields from which the specific cells active at each location in the environment are drawn.

McNaughton and colleagues (McNaughton et al., 1996; Samsonovich and McNaughton, 1997; Samsonovich, 1997) have suggested that there are a set of *charts* in the hippocampus, which are used for different environments, that the charts are prewired in the hippocampus and that external cues are associated with representations of location on a chart. Thus, in their model, the hippocampus represents, not location per se, but *coordinates within a chart.*

I prefer to think of the issue of reference frame as a property of the whole system and not just the hippocampus. For example, if the path integrator reference point changes, then the LV $\times$ PI association will change and the place code will have to change to accommodate it.[2] One explanation of the results of Barnes et al. (1997), that old rats do not always use the same map to encode an environment, while young rats do, is that the reference point is reset to the incorrect value in old animals, which changes the LV $\times$ PI association (Redish, 1997; Redish and Touretzky, 1998b).

A number of authors (McNaughton, Chen, and Markus, 1991; Muller et al., 1991; McNaughton, Knierim, and Wilson, 1994; Markus et al., 1995; Recce and Harris, 1996) have suggested that some of the sensitivity of place cells to cues other than visible landmarks can be attributed to changes in attention to *virtual landmarks*, locations in space from which distance and bearing information can be derived, just as for real landmarks. Because, however, virtual landmarks are not tied to perceivable objects, they must be tracked by path integration. Although a reference frame could be said to employ a virtual landmark as the reference point, reference frames also include a canonical orientation; thus the two proposals are not equivalent. Questions of how many virtual landmarks can be tracked by the system depend solely on processing power issues, much like questions of how many normal landmarks can comprise a local view. In contrast, because the animal has only one path integrator and one head direction code, it should only be able to represent a single reference frame.

Reference frames can be selected based on changes in the local view, the path integrator, and *mental set*, which must represent aspects of the goal or other key task parameters. The *multiple map* hypothesis (*multiple maps in the hippocampus*, O'Keefe and Nadel, 1978; *active subsets*, Muller and Kubie, 1987; *refer-*

ence frames, Wan, Touretzky, and Redish, 1994b, 1994c; Touretzky and Redish, 1996; Redish and Touretzky, 1997a; Redish, 1997; Redish and Touretzky, 1998b; *charts*, McNaughton et al., 1996; Samsonovich and McNaughton, 1997; Samsonovich, 1997) can explain most of the nonspatial aspects seen in place cell recordings. In the next section, we review the experimental data showing place cell correlations to aspects beyond the location of the animal, and note how the multiple-map hypothesis explains each one.

NONSPATIAL ASPECTS OF PLACE CELLS

Environmental Manipulations

Because different environments will require different LV × PI associations, they will require different place codes. The topology of place fields changes between two environments (O'Keefe and Conway, 1978; Kubie and Ranck, 1983; Muller and Kubie, 1987; Thompson and Best, 1989; see figure 10.1 for an example).

All of these experiments show that when the animal is returned to an environment, the place fields return to the representation encoding that environment. In other words, place fields are usually stable from session to session (Muller, Kubie, and Ranck, 1987), particularly for normal animals that are very familiar with the environment. For example, Thompson and Best (1990) report recording a stable place field for months.

Barnes et al. (1997) report differences between animals of different ages. For young animals, the ensemble correlation between the place fields seen during two subsequent 25-minute experiences shows a unimodal distribution (around 0.7, indicating a similar representation between experiences). For senescent animals, however, the ensemble correlation was bimodal (around 0, indicating a complete remapping, and around 0.7, indicating a similar representation between experiences). Within a single 25-minute run, the ensemble correlation (taken between two halves of the run) was always high (around 0.8; see figure 10.2). This is consistent with the hypothesis that animals must self-localize

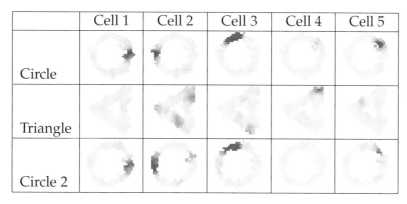

	Cell 1	Cell 2	Cell 3	Cell 4	Cell 5
Circle					
Triangle					
Circle 2					

Figure 10.1
Place fields of five simultaneously recorded cells in two environments. The animal was first allowed to run around a circular track, then was transferred to a triangular track, after which it was returned to the circular track. Shading indicates firing rate within that region (black is high; gray low). Scale is normalized for column (i.e., each cell). (Data courtesy G. Poe, C. Barnes, and B. McNaughton.)

on returning to the environment, but not while traveling through the environment and suggests that old rats were occasionally self-localizing to a different map when they were returned to the track.

This same stability within a given session but instability across sessions has been seen in animals with genetic deficits to NMDA receptors (Rotenberg et al., 1996).

Bostock, Muller, and Kubie (1991) recorded from place cells in a cylindrical arena, first with a white cue card, then with a black cue card, removing the animal from the environment after each session. Sometimes the place fields were similar, and sometimes they were unrelated (as if the two situations were encoded as different environments). Nevertheless, once a place field changed when the cue card was changed, all other place fields recorded subsequently from the same animal changed with the cue cards. When the white cue card was returned, the place field returned to its original configuration. This implies that after the two cards are represented differently, they are always represented by two different reference frames.

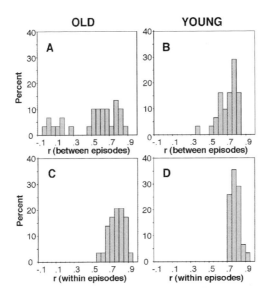

Figure 10.2
Histogram of correlation between two subsequent experiences in a single environment (panels A and B) or between the two halves of a single experience in an environment (panels C and D) for old (panels A and C) and young (panels B and D) rats. Reprinted by permission from *Nature*. (From Barnes et al., 1997, with permission of author and publisher. Copyright ©1997 Macmillan Magazines Ltd.)

On the other hand, reference frame transitions have been shown even within a single session. For example, Sharp et al. (1995) measured place cells in a circular arena with a four-way symmetrical local view. Halfway through the session, they rotated the arena by 90° (which left the local view unchanged). Like Bostock, Muller, and Kubie (1991), they found that the place fields first followed the rotation, then, after a number of sessions, changed suddenly and dramatically after the rotation. As in Bostock, Muller, and Kubie (1991), once the fields began remapping, they always remapped after the experience.

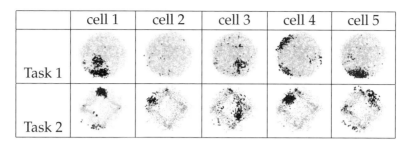

Figure 10.3
Place fields of five simultaneously recorded cells in each of two tasks in a single environment. Task 1: Animals searched randomly for food. Task 2: Animals found food at the four corners of a square. (From figure 9 of Markus et al., 1995. Used with permission of author and publisher.)

Task Manipulations

Wible et al. (1986) were among the first to report that hippocampal cells were task-dependent. Testing animals in two tasks within a Y-maze, they found that some cells fired in different portions of the environment in the two tasks.

Markus et al. (1995) also found that within-session task manipulations could produce map transitions (see figure 10.3). When rats were trained to search for food on a large elevated platform either randomly or at the corners of a diamond, different subsets of place cells were active for each task, and some cells that were active for both tasks had different place fields, as if the animals were encoding the tasks as different environments. When animals switched between these two tasks, the change between representations was rapid, suggesting a shift in a property encompassing the entire system.

Markus et al. also found some cells with similar fields in both tasks, suggesting that there may be two levels of representation here: the physical environment and the task within the environment. This does not imply, however, that there are two simultaneously active reference frames. Because the two tasks are occurring in the same environment, some cells may be tuned to the same cues in both tasks. The place fields of these cells would not change from task to task. On the other hand, the topology of the overall place code still changed dramatically from one task to the other. An alternative possibility is that some of the animals may have been using a new map, while others used the same map. This would predict that either all cells would show similar fields or none of them would (as observed by Barnes et al., 1997); Markus et al. (1995) did not specifically examine this question.

In more complex tasks than simply finding food scattered on the floor of the arena, place cells do not always fire when the animal is in the place field. Eichenbaum and colleagues (Eichenbaum et al., 1987; Eichenbaum and Cohen, 1988; Cohen and Eichenbaum, 1993) tested rats in an odor detection task and found that some place cells were dependent on whether the rat was going to the reward location. In a similar task, Eichenbaum and colleagues (Otto and Eichenbaum, 1992b; Cohen and Eichenbaum, 1993) found that cells responded when two odors matched in a delayed match-to-sample task, but not when they didn't. Animals in the Eichenbaum et al. (1987) task had been trained to go to a reward location given one set of odors (S^+) but not given another (S^-). This meant that the animals were learning to take two different paths to reward, depending on whether the odor was in the S^+ or S^- set. Eichenbaum et al. (1987) report that hippocampal pyramidal cells (i.e. place cells) are odor sensitive. However, they are not sensitive to different odors as such; rather they are sensitive to different reward conditions, indicated in this experiment by different *odor sets*.

This means that the Eichenbaum and colleagues tasks can be explained by map transitions (Touretzky and Redish, 1996; Redish and Touretzky, 1997a). Somehow, the animals associate the S^+ or S^- odor sets with different reference frames (presumably because different odor sets imply the animals should take different paths to reward). Equivalently, Otto and Eichenbaum (1992b) found place cells sensitive to S^+ and S^- odor pairs.

In addition to sensitivity to reward availability, Eichenbaum and colleagues report that some cells are correlated with location during stage of a task. For example, one cell might show a place field when the animal is approaching a sniff port to sample the odor (to determine whether it is an S^+ or an S^- odor), but not when the animal leaves the sniff port to go either to the reward location or back to the starting point. Again, this can be explained by reference frame transitions that occur between stages of the task (Touretzky and Redish, 1996; Redish and Touretzky, 1997a).

Consistent with this hypothesis, Otto and Eichenbaum (1992a) report that hippocampal cells were not sensitive to individual odors, but were sensitive to whether the odors matched (the key parameter in their task). This is what we would expect if the animal were switching maps between the two conditions. Cells would depend on condition, but because each condition is handled within a single map, cell firing would not correlate with odor differences within a given condition. Similarly, while Sakurai (1990a) found sensory correlates to auditory tones in an auditory nonmatch-to-sample task in entorhinal and auditory cortex cells, he found no significant sensory correlates in any CA1 cells. Instead, he found CA1 cells that differentiated the match or non-match at each sample.

When they trained rats to do a delayed match-to-sample task (between two available levers), Hampson, Heyser, and Deadwyler (1993) found place cells dependent on whether a lever had already been pressed and which lever had been pressed (thus which lever had to be pressed to receive reward). Again, because these stages of the task require different path integration reference points, they might require different reference frames, and might also be expected to be encoded by different hippocampal maps (Touretzky and Redish, 1996; Redish and Touretzky, 1997a).

All of these task manipulations share one important trait in common: the different reference frames all occur when the animal is learning to take different routes to reward. In the Markus et al. (1995) task, the food was distributed either randomly (and approximately uniformly) across the environment or at the four corners of a square. In the Eichenbaum et al. (1987) task, when the rat detected an S^+ odor, reward was unavailable. Similarly, in the Otto and Eichenbaum (1992a) and Sakurai (1990a) tasks, a nonmatching pair implied reward was available, while a matching one did not. In the Hampson, Heyser, and Deadwyler (1993) task, different levers had to be pressed to produce reward.

Directional Place Cells

An early debate in the place cell literature was over whether place cells were directional or not: they appeared to be directional on the radial maze (McNaughton, Barnes, and O'Keefe, 1983), but not in open arenas (Muller, Kubie, and Ranck, 1987; Muller et al., 1994). This debate was partially resolved by data showing that place cells were directional when the animal took repeated, restricted movement paths, but not when it had complete freedom and crisscrossed its path from every direction (Markus et al., 1995). In other words, when the animal only entered a place field from a few discrete directions, place fields were highly directional, but when it entered the field from a continuum of directions, the fields were not directional at all.

One possible explanation for the directionality of place cells on linear tracks is that animals use two reference frames to encode the track (Wan, Touretzky, and Redish, 1994c; Gothard, Skaggs, and McNaughton, 1996; McNaughton et al., 1996; Touretzky and Redish, 1996; Redish and Touretzky, 1997a; Samsonovich and McNaughton, 1997). When the animal runs back and forth along a linear track, it defines a reference point for each end of the path. When the animal travels in one direction, one reference frame is active, but when the animal travels in the other direction, the other frame is active. Because location within each reference frame is encoded by a different representation, place fields appear directional. In contrast, because they use a single map to encode the environment when animals wander around open arenas, place cells would be nondirectional (Wan, Touretzky, and Redish, 1994c; McNaughton et al., 1996; Touretzky and Redish, 1996; Redish and Touretzky, 1997a; Samsonovich and McNaughton, 1997).

A number of early explanations of place cell directionality included *shifting attention* between directions (e.g. McNaughton, Knierim, and Wilson, 1994; Markus et al., 1995) but these theories explained the nondirectionality of place cells in tasks like those used by Muller et al. (1994) by *quickly shifting attention* among landmarks (McNaughton, Knierim, and Wilson, 1994), which is not equivalent to the single reference frame hypothesis.

While the multiple map hypothesis explains how place cells can be directional in some tasks but not in others, it does not explain why. Chapter 11 will review data that the hippocampus stores recently traveled routes in asymmetries in the synaptic weights between place cells and replays them during slow-wave sleep. As pointed out by Mehta, Barnes, and McNaughton (1997), if the two directions on a linear track are both represented by a single map, then the asymmetries will cancel out, which may be why the system requires two different maps for certain tasks, but only one for others.

ANATOMY

Maps can be differentiated based on local view (such as which landmarks are present), on routes traveled, and on other sensory cues (such as olfactory information). These cues enter the hippocampus, are mixed with location information (spatial aspects of landmarks represented in the local view) and path integrator representations in the dentate gyrus (DG), and are then passed into CA3, which represents a specific position in a specific reference frame.

Let us begin by examining where each of these aspects is represented and follow the anatomical pathways from those representations into the hippocampal formation. As discussed in chapter 3, spatial aspects of landmarks are represented in the posterior parietal cortex and passed through the postrhinal cortex to the superficial layers of the entorhinal cortex (ECs), and from there into DG and CA3 via the perforant path.

Chapter 3 reviewed data suggesting that visual information was divided into a dorsal and a ventral stream in the primate and probably also in the rodent. Spatial aspects of the local view are likely to be represented in the dorsal stream, which includes parietal cortex, and ends in the postrhinal cortex, while nonspatial aspects are represented in the ventral stream, which includes the inferotemporal cortex in the monkey and area Te2 in the rodent, and ends in the perirhinal cortex.

Olfactory information enters the system from the piriform cortex via the lateral olfactory tract. It seems to be more strongly represented in the lateral entorhinal cortex (LEC) than in the medial (MEC). Stimulation of the lateral olfactory tract (LOT), which carries input from the olfactory cortex into the entorhinal cortex, evokes responses in the hippocampus, report Wilson and Steward (1978), although the LOT is polysynaptic through the lateral entorhinal cortex. LEC lesions eliminate the response, paired-pulse potentiation can be evoked between the LOT and LEC, and identical cells were stimulated by LOT and LEC stimulation. In an odor-to-place matching task, LEC lesions produced incorrect odor-to-place matches, but when the LEC lesions encroached on MEC, the rats also made spatial errors as well (Otto et al., 1996).

An interesting possibility is that while the location information may enter the system through MEC, the map selection information (such as object identity, olfactory information, etc.) may enter via LEC. Because they can be carried on the wind, odors are much more useful for determining issues such as general environment or task (i.e., map selection) than location. One explanation for the Otto et al. results is that LEC lesions preferentially disrupted map selection, while MEC lesions preferentially disrupted the location input. When Quirk et al. (1992) recorded from MEC cells, they found broad placelike behavior, but no sensitivity to environment. No one has (to my knowledge) recorded from LEC cells.

Another interesting possibility is that the location information may enter via the postrhinal cortex, while map selection may pass through perirhinal cortex. Postrhinal cortex receives input from parietal areas, while perirhinal receives input from ventral visual areas and other secondary sensory cortices (including auditory, olfactory, etc.; Burwell, Witter, and Amaral, 1995; Witter et al., 1989; Suzuki, 1996). While perirhinal cortex projects almost exclusively to lateral entorhinal cortex, postrhinal projects strongly to both LEC and MEC (Burwell and Amaral, 1998). Burwell and Eichenbaum (1997) recorded from perirhinal cortex on a plus maze and did not find spatial correlations, whereas Young et al. (1997) found odor sensitivity and selectivity. However, no one has recorded from rodent postrhinal cortex, where one would expect spatial correlations undifferentiated by map; or from rodent perirhinal cortex in multiple tasks, where one would expect stronger map selection correlations than spatial correlations.

REFERENCE FRAME TRANSITIONS

There are two important cases in which a reference frame transition can occur: (1) when an animal has just entered an environment (e.g., when it is placed into the water in the water maze task); and (2) when something has changed within a single environment that produces a map transition (e.g., when an animal reaches the end of a linear track and turns around).

These two cases differ in the amount of knowledge the animal has of the relationship between the reference frames. In case 1, the animal has no information about the spatial relationship between its position before and after the transition. Thus it must determine its location entirely from external cues (local view). In case 2, there is a constant relationship between the coordinates in the pre- and posttransition reference frames. Each of these cases can occur in novel or familiar environments.

Returning to a Familiar Environment

Chapter 9 has already discussed how an animal self-localizes on returning to a familiar environment. This process is dependent on a connection structure within CA3 such that each cell has the strongest synaptic ties to cells that represent similar locations. Because place cells are only coactive when they have overlapping place fields within a map, correlational LTP will produce a connection matrix such that each cell actually has the strongest synaptic ties to cells that represent similar locations *within a reference frame*. This means that the self-localization process described in chapter 9 will settle not only to a representation of location, but also to a reference frame (Shen and McNaughton, 1996; Redish, 1997; Samsonovich and McNaughton, 1997; Samsonovich, 1997).

Entering a Novel Environment

When an animal enters a novel environment, there will be no stored LV × PI association, so a new one will need to be learned. The system needs to use a new map (i.e., a new place code sufficiently independent of previously learned ones) and to store a new association to and from that place code. There are two possible mechanisms by which this association can be learned: either the reference frames can be separated by an attractor process in CA3 (McNaughton et al., 1996; Samsonovich and McNaughton, 1997; Samsonovich, 1997) or they can be separated by an orthogonalization process in dentate gyrus (DG; as originally suggested by McNaughton and Morris, 1987; see also Marr, 1969; McNaughton, 1989; Rolls, 1989; O'Reilly and McClelland, 1994; Rolls, 1996; Redish, 1997).

We can best understand each of these hypotheses by examining how they explain the Barnes et al. (1997) finding that old animals show unstable place field representations. Barnes et al. allowed an animal to explore an environment, removed it from the environment for an hour, and then returned the animal to the same environment. They found that old animals sometimes return to a different map. After enough experience, normal young animals always used the same map between experiences.

CA3 Hypothesis

The key idea of this hypothesis is that the connection structure described as a means of dealing with entering familiar environments above is prewired in the hippocampus. This means that when an animal enters a novel environment, the settling process will coalesce on a representation of one of the previously available maps (Samsonovich and McNaughton, 1997). Because old animals have deficient LTP, the local view does not force them into the same map as before. Instead, the system falls into a random basin of attraction – sometimes the same one, sometimes a different one.

On entering a novel environment, one location on one map will win the competition. As young animals explore the environment, a representation of the local view gets bound to the currently active chart. On returning to the environment, the local view representation biases the pseudo-winner-take-all (pWTA) dynamics in the hippocampus, and the same representation of location on the same map is reinstantiated. Because old animals have LTP deficiencies (for reviews, see Barnes, 1994; Barnes, Rao, and McNaughton, 1996; Barnes, 1998), the local view would not become as tightly bound to the currently active chart in the old animals. Thus, on returning to the environment, there would be a much weaker bias to select the same location on the same chart.

DG Hypothesis

The key idea here is that a DG cell fires given a specific PI representation and a specific LV representation (due to random pre-wired connections), in other words, it *orthogonalizes*[3] the two representations (McNaughton and Morris, 1987; Redish, 1997). Evidence supporting the dentate gyrus orthogonalization hypothesis was discussed in chapter 8. According to this theory, the Barnes et al. (1997) finding is not a consequence of prewired map selection within the CA3 population, but rather an interaction between the nonlinearity of the path integrator and the orthogonalization properties of dentate gyrus (Redish, 1997; Redish and Touretzky, 1998b).

When a young animal returns to the environment, long-term potentiation (LTP) has created associations between local view and hippocampus and between hippocampus and the path integrator. Thus during the self-localization process, the local view representation instantiates representations in hippocampus, which force the path integrator to reset to the same representation of location as in the young animal's previous experience. In an old animal, however, LTP is deficient (as reviewed by Barnes, 1994;

Barnes, Rao, and McNaughton, 1996; Barnes, 1998) and thus there is little or no bias to reset the path integrator to the same location. Because each dentate gyrus (DG) cell performs a logical *and* function of its path integrator (PI) and local view (LV) inputs, a change in PI representation will produce a dramatic change in DG representation, which will be seen in hippocampus as a low overlap between each experience.

This second hypothesis demonstrates the necessity of understanding reference frame in terms of the entire system. According to it, old animals use different maps in their hippocampi because they are (sometimes) using an incorrect path integrator reference point.

These two hypotheses have some similarities and some crucial differences. Because place cells are active on initial entry into the environment (Hill, 1978; Austin, Fortin, and Shapiro, 1990; Wilson and McNaughton, 1994; Tanila et al., 1997b), there must be some prewired connections producing place field activity. In the CA3 hypothesis, the prewired connections are within the CA3 structure of the hippocampus and must have a predefined structure between them. In the DG hypothesis, prewired connections between PI→DG, LV→DG, and DG→CA3 produce place cells with stable place fields on initial entry into the environment. The prewired connections in the DG hypothesis are totally random; there does not have to be any predefined correlation between them (Redish, 1997; Redish and Touretzky, 1998b).

Because the place cell instability observed by Barnes et al. is bimodal in older animals, there must be some sort of nonlinear process. According to the CA3-hypothesis, this nonlinearity occurs by winner-take-all competitive dynamics between charts in CA3; according to the DG-model, it occurs because of nonlinearities in the settling of the path integrator combined with orthogonalization properties of DG.

Because the place cell instability observed by Barnes et al. only occurs on entry into the environment, there must be something special about entry into the environment. The self-localization process hypothesized to occur on entry into the environment would explain this. During normal navigation, the path integrator does not reset, it continues to be driven by internal dynamics more than external. But during self-localization, the path integrator is reset and external dynamics can have a strong influence.

Within a Familiar Environment

Let us assume that an animal has been representing an environment by multiple maps (such as the two directions on a linear track). How does it change from one to another when it switches directions? There are two possible mechanisms that cannot be distinguished with the current data, but that make predictions by which we can distinguish them.

The first is an explicit transition mechanism: some system recognizes an inconsistency between local view and path integrator coordinates (presumably by an incoherency in the place code; Touretzky and Redish, 1996) and forces a new self-localization process. Because the animal has not been disoriented or dislocated between this transition (it presumably happens without experimenter interference), the current path integrator representation can be used to prime the system. The combination of the new local view and path integrator representation will force the system to settle to the new reference frame.

The alternative is an implicit transition mechanism, based on the internal dynamics of the attractor described in appendix A (see also Samsonovich and McNaughton, 1997; Samsonovich, 1997). The change in local view produces a new *candidate location* represented on a new *candidate map*. If this new representation is strong enough it will produce a jump in the representation (as shown in figure A.4).

An intriguing question is whether the dentate gyrus is necessary for this kind of reference frame transition or whether the jump can be driven from learned connections. Findings from McNaughton et al. (1989) that even after DG lesions (by colchicine) place cells are directional imply that DG may not be necessary for this kind of reference frame transition. Knierim and McNaughton (1995) found that after colchicine lesions, CA3 and CA1 fields remain directional in thin tracks, whereas they become annular in open fields (as if the cells were not receiving head direction input). This suggests that whatever keeps place cells directional on the linear track is different from whatever keeps place fields small on the open arena.

If the explicit transition mechanism hypothesis is true, then there should be a self-localization process that occurs at reference frame transitions. For example, a single sharp wave may occur within what otherwise appears to be a normal theta state. While the explicit hypothesis cannot say whether a sharp wave will be necessary or whether some more subtle change can occur, it does require that some specific change occur. The implicit hypothesis does not. Gothard, Skaggs, and McNaughton (1996) may have seen a reference frame transition (see figure 10.4) but they do not report any abnormal processes occurring at the transition. This supports the implicit transition mechanism hypothesis, although Gothard, Skaggs, and McNaughton were not explicitly looking for such a process and may not have seen it if it is relatively subtle.

Within a Novel Environment

How quickly and in what manner do different intraenvironmental reference frames get separated? Findings by Sharp et al. (1995) imply that the difference is sometimes learned over time. Sharp et al. measured place cells in a small cylinder and rotated the environment (or part of the environment) 20 minutes into a 40-minute recording session. They found that in some sessions the fields followed the manipulation, but in other sessions (independent of the manipulation), the field changed location dramatically (or disappeared completely) when the manipulation occurred. The probability of a radical change or disappearance occurring increased over the sessions. As was discussed earlier, a change in or disappearance of a place field is one indication of a possible map change.

This issue is reminiscent of the question of how quickly place cells show their place fields in a novel environment. Some authors report that they appear very quickly (Hill, 1978;

Wilson and McNaughton, 1994), while others report that they can take hours to fill out (Austin, White, and Shapiro, 1993; Tanila et al., 1997b). Although the mechanism by which intraenvironmental references frames are separated is not known at this time, one mechanism could be a combination of the hypotheses on transitions within a familiar environment with those on exploration of a novel environment. Either of the two novel environment hypotheses can be combined with either of the two within-environment hypotheses. This is an open question and experiments examining the onset of directionality (particularly at the transition points such as the ends of a linear track) would be well worth undertaking.

DETECTING MAP TRANSITIONS

The central idea of the multiple map hypothesis is that maps are independent, that the place fields on each map are uncorrelated, which means that one should be able to detect map transitions explicitly. One way to do so is to look for that decorrelation.

An important aspect of the multiple map hypothesis is that when one looks at two locations a and b in an environment that are farther apart than the width of any place field, it is impossible to tell from the two representations whether the two locations are on the same or on different maps. In both cases (same or different maps), the representations will be uncorrelated. If, however, one looks at any two nearby locations on the same map, the representation should be highly correlated. Therefore, as an animal journeys from location a to location b, if the animal is on a single map, there will never be a moment of decorrelation. In contrast, if the animal switches maps between locations a and b there will be a moment of decorrelation. Therefore a transition between maps can be observed by a decorrelation between the place fields at the transition. (The following analysis method is due to B. McNaughton, personal communication.)

Because place fields cover continuous areas with a finite spatial extent, the firing rates of the population of cells at position x and those at position $x + x$ will be highly correlated as long

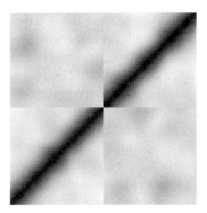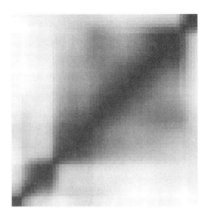

Figure 10.4
Pinch point phenomenon. Left panel: Simulation showing an idealized
pinch point. Each pixel shows the ensemble crosscorrelation between
the population of recorded place cells at each point in the environment
with each other point in the environment. Thus the diagonal consists
of correlations of 1.0. A map transition occurs at the halfway point
and this is indicated by a clear pinch point. Right panel: Pinch point,
possibly indicative of a reference frame transition, visible approximately
one-quarter of the way up the diagonal. Whether this pinch point is an
actual map transition or whether it is an artifact of a limited sample
size is not yet known. (From Gothard, Skaggs, and McNaughton, 1996.
Used by permission of author and publisher.)

as x is less than the average size of a place field. But the place
fields between two maps are independent. Therefore, after a map
transition, the population of place fields will be uncorrelated. I
have used this idea earlier (see *Environmental Manipulations*) to
argue that the Barnes et al. (1997) data showed that naive animals
sometimes returned to the wrong map.

The map transition can be seen by plotting the ensemble correlation of the population activity of cells at time t with the same
population at time s for all times t and s throughout a journey.
If the journey is represented by a single reference frame, the plot
will show high correlation along the diagonal. The decorrelation
can be seen as a *pinch point* (see figure 10.4).

REFERENCE FRAMES AND CONTEXT

Hippocampal place cells are sensitive to a host of nonspatial factors such as environment, direction, task, and subtask. We have seen how sensitivity to each of these factors can be explained by the concept of *reference frames*. These factors form the *context* in which the behavior occurs. An important question is whether place cells should still be considered primarily as *place* cells instead of more general *context* cells. According to the multiple map hypothesis, there is a fundamental difference between the representation of spatial coordinates and the representation of reference frame. When a small change occurs in spatial location, a correspondingly small change occurs in the activity of the place cell population; as the change increases, the place cell representation changes continuously. On the other hand, when a small change occurs in reference frame, no change occurs in the place cells; as the change increases, there is a sharp and sudden change in the representation. If the hippocampus were merely representing the context, then changes in nonspatial variables should be encoded identically with spatial. They are not. Therefore, I believe that it is still useful to consider place cells as representing location, albeit location within a reference frame.

WHY MULTIPLE MAPS WITHIN AN ENVIRONMENT?

As we noted at the beginning of this chapter, in order to minimize confusion during self-localization in similar environments, locations within different environments should be represented by uncorrelated codes. But why would it be useful for a system to separate different tasks within a single environment, or different directions on a linear track?

There are two important computational reasons why having multiple maps within a single environment would be useful. First, determining the path to the goal requires input of both task and location. It is true that these can be combined in the goal memory (chapter 7), but it might be useful to allow the place code to incorporate this information as well. For example, different tasks may require attending to different landmarks.

Second, as will be discussed in chapter 11, the hippocampus stores and replays recently traveled routes in asymmetric connection strengths in CA3. If both directions were represented by a single map, the asymmetries would cancel out (Mehta, Barnes, and McNaughton, 1997). By separating the two directions, the system can store routes in both directions.

Redish and Touretzky (1997a) hypothesized that multiple reference frames could be separated in a single environment because an animal had to represent different routes to goals — that all cases of multiple reference frames in a single environment occurred because the reward distribution had changed between the two cases. Directionality would then be explained by alternating goals. This is not entirely the case because place fields are still directional when food is scattered randomly (Markus et al., 1995). We have seen directional place cells even when food was only available at one end of a linear track (Redish, Weaver-Sommers, Barnes, and McNaughton, unpublished results). It may be that the thinness of the track is sufficient to produce subgoals at each end of the track independent of the actual reward distribution.

11   Route Replay

The place code in the hippocampus allows an animal to self-localize to a specific location in a specific reference frame when it returns to a familiar environment. Once there is a coherent representation in the place code, the goal memory can plan a trajectory to a goal. The hippocampus has also been implicated in the storage and replay of sequences and recent memories both theoretically (Marr, 1970, 1971; Cohen and Eichenbaum, 1993; McClelland, McNaughton, and O'Reilly, 1995; Squire and Alvarez, 1995; Levy, 1996; Shen and McNaughton, 1996; Redish and Touretzky, 1998a) and experimentally (Pavlides and Winson, 1989; Wilson and McNaughton, 1994; Skaggs and McNaughton, 1996). In the context of rodent navigation, sequence storage and replay appears as storage and replay of *routes* traveled (Levy, 1989; Abbott and Blum, 1996; Blum and Abbott, 1996; Levy, 1996; Skaggs and McNaughton, 1996; Shen and McNaughton, 1996; Gerstner and Abbott, 1997; Redish, 1997; Redish and Touretzky, 1998a).

The issue of storage and replay of recent routes is related to the issue of memory consolidation, discussed in depth in chapter 12. One explanation for the limited retrograde amnesia seen after hippocampal formation lesions is that memories are stored in the hippocampal formation and replayed into cortex over time[1] (Scoville and Milner, 1957; Marr, 1970, 1971; Squire, 1987; Squire and Zola-Morgan, 1988, 1991; Squire, 1992; Cohen and Eichenbaum, 1993; Zola-Morgan and Squire, 1993; McClelland, McNaughton, and O'Reilly, 1995; Squire and Alvarez, 1995; Redish and Touretzky, 1998a). Recent data suggest that the location of the hidden platform in the water maze is never consolidated from hippocampus (Koerner et al., 1996; Weisend, Astur, and Sutherland, 1996; Koerner et al., 1997). Chapter 12 will also address the question of whether the hippocampus proper or adjacent structures serve as the short-term memory store (Bohbot, 1997; Nadel and Moscovitch, 1997; Tulving and Markowitsch, 1997).

Whatever the hippocampal role is in memory consolidation, there is evidence that the hippocampus stores and replays recently traveled routes (Wilson and McNaughton, 1994; Skaggs and McNaughton, 1996; Qin et al., 1997). The key to this storage and replay mechanism is believed to be asymmetries in the connection structure within the recurrent connections of CA3 (Levy, 1996; Skaggs et al., 1996; Redish and Touretzky, 1998a). This might seem to some to suggest an incompatibility with the self-localization process discussed in chapter 9 (which requires symmetric connections), but simulations suggest that the two modes are not incompatible because local view information serves to counteract the asymmetries.

Evidence that the hippocampus replays routes does not imply that these routes are written out to a long-term cortex elsewhere. It is possible that the replay effect is a general property of the mammalian brain and may appear in numerous cortical structures. Qin et al. (1997) have shown evidence for replay in neocortex, hippocampus, and the interactions between them. Due to technological constraints, they recorded from the neocortical areas that lie just dorsal to hippocampus. Although they did not report exactly which areas, but posterior parietal and posterior cingulate cortices lie just dorsal to hippocampus (Zilles, 1990; McNaughton et al., 1994), and both of these areas are involved in spatial processing (Sutherland and Hoesing, 1993; Chen et al., 1994a, 1994b; McNaughton et al., 1994). Whether the hippocampus is actually a temporary memory store and whether replay of memories during sleep is hippocampally dependent or a general property of cortex remain open questions.

EVIDENCE FOR ROUTE REPLAY

Neurophysiological data supporting a replay of recent experience in hippocampus during sleep has been reported by Pavlides and Winson (1989), Wilson and McNaughton (1994), Skaggs and

McNaughton (1996), and Qin et al. (1997). Pavlides and Winson found that cells with recently visited place fields were more active during subsequent REM sleep than cells whose fields had not been recently visited. Wilson and McNaughton found that during slow-wave sleep (SWS) cells that showed correlated firing during a session in an environment (because their place fields overlapped) also showed a stronger correlation during sleep immediately after the session. Skaggs and McNaughton explicitly examined the temporal nature of replay during sharp waves in slow-wave sleep. They defined the *temporal bias* B_{ij} between two cells i and j to be the difference between the integrated cross-correlation for the 200 ms after each spike of cell j and the integrated cross-correlation for the 200 ms before each spike of cell j. Thus if cell i generally fires after cell j rather than before, B_{ij} will be greater than 0. Skaggs and McNaughton report that the temporal bias during sleep after running on a linear track is strongly correlated with the temporal bias seen while the animal was running on the track. Qin et al. used similar cross-correlation measures on interactions between hippocampal and neocortical cells.

STORING ROUTES

There are four neurophysiological effects that allow the hippocampus to store routes as the animal travels:

1. *Long-term potentiation is preferentially asymmetric* (for reviews see Abbott and Blum, 1996, and Levy, 1996). If neuron a fires shortly before neuron b then it is the $a \rightarrow b$ connection that is potentiated, not the $b \rightarrow a$ connection.

2. *The actual timing of spikes fired by hippocampal place cells precesses along the theta cycle* (O'Keefe and Recce, 1993; Skaggs et al., 1996). Effectively, the position represented in the place code sweeps across the actual position from back to front with each theta cycle (Tsodyks et al., 1996).

3. *Long-term potentiation is correlational* (for reviews, see McNaughton and Morris, 1987; Bliss and Lynch, 1988;

Brown et al., 1991; McNaughton, 1993; Malenka, 1995). The connection between two neurons is potentiated only when spikes in the presynaptic neuron are combined with a depolarization of the postsynaptic neuron. Thus the increase in connection strength between two neurons a and b is proportional to the product of their firing rates F_a and F_b.

4. *Cells near the route will have higher-firing neighbors closer to the route.* A cell with a place field not centered at the location of the animal will covary more strongly with cells that have place fields centered at the location of the animal than with cells that have distant place fields.

Effects 1 and 2 combine to produce asymmetries along the routes traveled; effects 3 and 4 combine to produce asymmetries leading toward those routes.

Asymmetries along the Route Traveled

O'Keefe and Recce (1993) and Skaggs et al. (1996) have shown that the timing of action potentials fired by place cells has an interesting interaction with the theta rhythm. As an animal moves through the place field, the cell generally fires its spikes earlier and earlier in the theta cycle. Figure 11.1 shows an example of a place cell on a linear track in which the spikes precess along the theta rhythm.

Because cells with place fields centered in front of the animal fire later in the theta cycle than cells with place fields centered behind the animal, the position represented by the population of active cells sweeps across the animal from back to front with each cycle. When combined with the biophysical time course of LTP (effect 1), this will favor connections pointing along recently traveled routes (Skaggs, 1995; Skaggs et al., 1996; Redish and Touretzky, 1998a).

A number of mechanisms have been put forward to explain the phase precession effect, including that it is an intrinsic process formed by an interaction of two rhythms with similar frequencies just different enough to produce beats (O'Keefe and Recce,

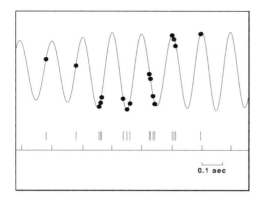

Figure 11.1
Phase precession of a CA1 place cell. EEG filtered between 6 and 10 Hz
(top), with times at which the cell fired a spike marked (bottom). (From
Shen et al., 1997, used with permission of the author and publisher.)
Similar results have been shown by O'Keefe and Recce (1993), and
Skaggs et al. (Skaggs, 1995; Skaggs et al., 1996).

1993), that it can be generated by asymmetric connections in CA3
(Tsodyks et al., 1996), that it is a consequence of attention sweeping from back to front (Burgess, Recce, and O'Keefe, 1994), and
that it is a consequence of an interaction between path integration
mechanisms and internal neural dynamics (Samsonovich, 1997).

Although any of these proposed mechanisms could play a
role in generating phase precession, none can fully explain the
data. The O'Keefe and Recce mechanism cannot explain why
place cells always start firing at a phase of 90°–120° after the theta
peak.

The Tsodyks et al. (1996) mechanism requires the asymmetric connections to precede the phase precession, but phase precession occurs from the first traversal through an environment,
before the asymmetric connections have had time to be trained
(B. McNaughton, personal communication). In addition, Skaggs
et al. (1996) report that DG cells also show phase precession, and
Bragin et al. (1995) reports data suggesting that theta in CA3 is a
consequence of theta-related activity in EC. These facts may im-

ply that the processes that cause phase precession may be extra-hippocampal.

Burgess and colleagues (Burgess, Recce, and O'Keefe, 1994; O'Keefe and Burgess, 1996a; Burgess and O'Keefe, 1996) propose a model in which phase precession is a consequence of attention sweeping from landmarks behind the animal to landmarks in front of it. Because, phase precession also occurs in the dark (Weaver et al., 1996), this model cannot be the whole story.

Samsonovich and McNaughton (1996) suggest that phase precession is a consequence of an interaction between path integration mechanism and internal neuronal dynamics. Their hypothesis that the hippocampus is necessary for path integration has been called into question, however, by the recent data from Alyan et al. (1997; see chapter 6). Therefore this model cannot be the whole story either. Although it is unlikely that the hippocampus is the path integrator, this doesn't disprove their phase precession mechanism. It is possible that their mechanism could generate phase precession extra-hippocampally.

Although what produces phase precession is still an open question, the combination of phase precession and asymmetric LTP clearly can produce asymmetric connections that can store routes (Skaggs, 1995; O'Keefe and Burgess, 1996b; Skaggs et al., 1996; Redish and Touretzky, 1998a). One effect of phase precession is that the representation sweeps from behind the animal to in front of it with each theta cycle, seven times a second. This sweep should fire cells in sequence fast enough to produce asymmetric LTP, which in turn should produce asymmetric synaptic weights between the place cells, with cells synapsing most strongly on the cells that follow them on the route.

Off-Route Asymmetries

Imagine an animal somewhere along the route taken. Because place fields cover an extended area, the animal will be inside the place fields of cells whose place field centers are slightly off the route. But because the place field is centered slightly off the route, the cell will not be firing at its maximum rate. Cells whose place fields are closer to the route will have higher firing rates than cells with fields farther from the route. Because LTP is correlational (i.e., it is dependent on the firing rate of both the presynaptic and postsynaptic cells), the synaptic strengths of the outputs of these off-route cells will be biased asymmetrically toward the path traveled.

Data Support

Although no one has been able to show asymmetries in an actual hippocampus (measuring synaptic weight between two cells *in vivo* is not possible with current technologies), experiments by Mehta, Barnes, and McNaughton (1997) strongly suggest that hippocampal recurrent connections do show the hypothesized asymmetries. When they trained a rat to run in a loop on a rectangular elevated maze and recorded place cells in CA1. They found that the place fields shifted backward along well-traversed paths over the course of a single session, confirming a prediction made by Blum and Abbott (1996). In support of the hypothesis that the shift in the place fields is LTP-sensitive, Shen et al. (1997) found that in old animals (which are LTP-deficient; see Barnes, 1998 for a review), the place fields do not shift.

Whatever the mechanism that produces phase precession, the theoretical consequence of the combination of phase precession and asymmetric LTP is clear: it produces asymmetric connections along the route traveled. Blum and Abbott (1996) first suggested that the combination of travel along a route and asymmetric LTP would produce asymmetries in the recurrent connections in CA3 because cells would fire in sequence as the animal travels along the route. However, the time course of LTP is too fast for this to actually work; the representations of location changes too slowly for LTP to create the necessary asymmetries (Redish and Touretzky, unpublished simulations). One effect of phase precession is to sweep the representation of position along the route quickly enough for LTP to produce the asymmetries (Skaggs, 1995; O'Keefe and Burgess, 1996b; Skaggs et al., 1996; Redish and Touretzky, 1998a).

A number of other authors have addressed this question in simulation (Levy, 1996; Levy and Wu, 1996; Shen and McNaughton, 1996; Wu, Baxter, and Levy, 1996). Levy and his colleagues have demonstrated in their simulations that cells with temporally extended effects can store and replay sequences of arbitrary binary vectors. Shen and McNaughton (1996), whose model of attractor dynamics resembles the model presented here, have showne that cells with Gaussian place fields exhibit correlational (Hebbian) learning. When these two effects are combined with random exploration, a local excitation weight matrix is formed (Muller, Kubie, and Saypoff, 1991; Muller, Stead, and Pach, 1996; see also chapter 9). Presented with random input and allowed to settle to a stable state, cells with recently visited place fields are more active than other cells (Shen and McNaughton, 1996), corresponding to data from Pavlides and Winson (1989) and Wilson and McNaughton (1994).

RECALLING ROUTES

If routes have been truly stored in the hippocampus, there must be a mechanism for those routes to be recalled. Due to the symmetric component of the recurrent connections in CA3, the hippocampus will still settle to a coherent activity pattern that represents a valid location even when there is no sensory input into the hippocampal system. Due to the asymmetric component, however, this representation will then drift along the remembered route (Redish and Touretzky, 1998a; see also Tsodyks et al., 1996). Figure 11.2 shows the asymmetries in a hippocampal simulation after the simulated animal traversed four routes to a goal. Figure 11.3 shows the place code settling to a coherent representation of location which then drifts along a recently traveled route.

At this point, let us assume that an animal can, from local view information, self-localize and determine the path it must take to reach the hidden platform in the water maze, The four effects detailed above combine to store routes in the recurrent connections of hippocampus. They produce a vector field pointing toward the path and then leading to the goal. Redish and Touretzky (1998a)

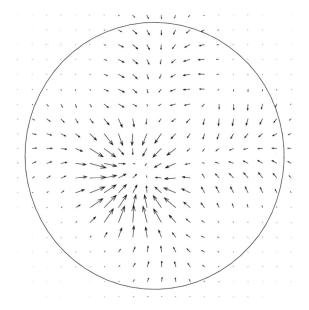

Figure 11.2
Simulation of learned asymmetric connections in hippocampus. For each cell j in the simulated hippocampus, the center of mass of its output connection weights was calculated, and an arrow plotted from the place field center toward that center of mass. Length of arrow is linearly proportional to the distance between the center of cell j's place field and the center of mass of cell j's output connection weights. Arrows outside the environment are for cells with simulated place field centers outside the environment, whose simulated fields overlap the environment. (From Redish and Touretzky, 1998a. Used with permission of the publisher.)

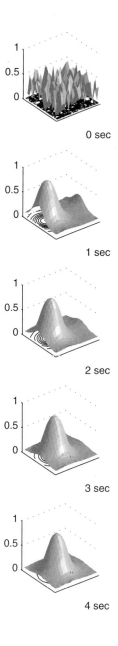

0 sec

1 sec

2 sec

3 sec

4 sec

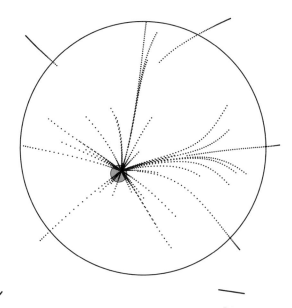

Figure 11.4
Simulated replay of routes during LIA without sensory input. The drifting representations (see figure 11.3) are replaying routes to the goal. Each dot indicates represented location at one time step during one replay sequence. Forty sequences are shown. (From Redish and Touretzky, 1998a. Used with permission of the publisher.)

Figure 11.3
In the absence of sensory input, a simulated hippocampus still settles to a coherent representation of position, which then drifts along the remembered route. Each panel shows the firing rates of all of the simulated CA3 place cells at a single moment in time. The cells are laid out in a two-dimensional sheet with their locations in the sheet corresponding to the centers of their place fields in the environment. (Adapted with permission of the publisher from Redish and Touretzky, 1998a.)

explicitly examined simulations of sequences in the open field, showing (1) that the routes replayed are paths to the goal, and (2) that the self-localization and route storage roles are compatible, even though they seem to require different weight matrices. (Self-localization requires symmetric connections, route storage requires asymmetric connections.)

Redish and Touretzky (1997a) argued that when there is sensory input into the hippocampus and the hippocampus is in LIA mode, sensory cues enter the system via superficial EC, which would make hippocampal place cells that are consistent with the local view more active than place cells that are not. This effect biases the place code to settle to a coherent representation of position, consistent with the local view, as shown in chapter 9.

On the other hand, when there is no sensory input, this bias will be absent, but due to the symmetric component of the recurrent connections in hippocampus, the hippocampus will still settle to a coherent activity pattern that represents a valid location. Due to the asymmetric component, this representation will then drift along the remembered route. Because these drifting representations consist of a coherent representation of location, we can measure the position represented. Figure 11.4 shows the believed position of the simulated rat during forty of these route-replay sequences. This simulation is replaying routes leading to the goal.

TWO INCOMPATIBLE PROCESSES?

The self-localization process described in chapter 9 requires that the synaptic efficacy between two place cells be symmetric with strength proportional to the overlap between their place fields. The route storage process described in this chapter requires that the synaptic efficacy be asymmetric, favoring connections projecting between cells with place fields along recently traveled routes. These two requirements would seem to be incompatible. They are not.

When the animal is self-localizing, sensory input from superficial EC constrains the representation in hippocampus to one of

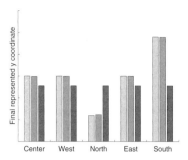

Figure 11.5
The y-coordinates of the final representation of the parallel relaxation process of hippocampal simulations with local view input and symmetric weights only (light bars), local view input and both symmetric and asymmetric weights (medium bars), and both symmetric and asymmetric weights without local view input (dark bars). The x-coordinates (not shown) are similar. (From Redish and Touretzky, 1998a. Used with permission of the publisher.)

the candidate locations and effectively locks the representation in place. Figure 11.5 shows the y-coordinate of the hippocampal representation after a simulated sharp wave occurred under three conditions: (1) when the simulated animal was at five different locations in an environment using only symmetric connection weights (light bars), (2) the same five locations with both symmetric and asymmetric connection weights (medium bars), and (3) in the absence of sensory input, but when the sharp wave began as a representation near each of the five locations (dark bars). There is no difference at all between the simulations shown under conditions 1 and 2 (light and medium bars), indicating that the local view input is sufficient to hold the representation in place. On the other hand, when there is no sensory input to hold the representation in place (condition 3; dark bars); it drifts, reaching the same final value in each case: the goal location (see also figure 11.4). This shows that the recall and replay modes are in fact compatible, at least in simulation.

Neurophysiological evidence suggests that increased experience in an environment increases the overlap along routes (improving route storage) but does not change the centers of place fields (not impairing self-localization). Mehta, Barnes, and McNaughton (1997) recently showed that the place fields of cells shift backward along a much-repeated path as the animal runs along that path. When they trained a rat to run in a loop on a rectangular elevated maze and recorded place cells in CA1, they found that the place fields shifted backward over the course of a single session. This would seem to be a problem for the self-localization process because the location represented by the place cell population changes with time. On the other hand, they also found that whereas the area covered by the place field increased by a factor of almost 2, because of increased firing near the center of the field, the center of mass of the field actually changed very little. This is exactly what we need for the dual-role hippocampus (self-localization and route-storage). Because the number of cells overlapped by the expanded place field increases (due to the increase in area covered), longer routes can be stored, but because the center of mass of the field does not shift much, the self-localization process will not be affected much.

The two roles played by the hippocampus occur by variations of the same mechanism: both are examples of a pWTA network settling to a stable state, only with different boundary conditions. The route replay process occurs when the initial state is uniform noise and no extrinsic input is given; the self-localization process occurs when the initial state includes candidate locations and these candidate locations continue to be input throughout the self-localization process. The candidate locations can be seen as a signal input into the system mixed with noise. Thus the two processes can be seen as opposite extremes of a mathematical continuum: with no signal, the system performs route replay, but with a strong signal, the system performs self-localization.

An interesting (and as yet unanswered) question is how a pWTA network behaves as the signal is increased from 0 (which produces replay) to a very strong signal (which produces recall). Is there partial replay with weak signals? Is there a point at which the system shows a phase change and suddenly shows strong replay instead of strong recall? Although the complex non-linearities of pWTA networks (see, for example, the *resolu-*

tion issue in appendix A) make an analytic solution extremely difficult, simulations would be straight-forward and might show very interesting effects.

We should note, however, that the hypothesis being advanced here is independent of the dynamical behavior of the system at these intermediate parameterizations. The hypothesis here is that the rodent hippocampus plays two roles (recall and replay), which occur at different times, and that these two roles can be accomplished by the same mechanism under these two boundary conditions. I refer to the system as having three modes (storage, recall, and replay) because the dual-role hypothesis implies that the hippocampus does not utilize intermediate states.

12 Consolidation

The concept of consolidation of memories is an old one (Ribot, 1882; Burnham, 1903; Scoville and Milner, 1957; Milner, 1970; Marr, 1970, 1971) and has been extensively studied (Weingart- ner and Parker, 1984; Pavlides and Winson, 1989; Zola-Morgan and Squire, 1990; Squire and Zola-Morgan, 1991; Squire, 1992; Cohen and Eichenbaum, 1993; Wilson and McNaughton, 1994; McClelland, McNaughton, and O'Reilly, 1995; Squire and Al- varez, 1995), as has the idea that memories are stored during theta mode and recalled during large-amplitude irregular activity (LIA; Buzsáki, 1989; Hasselmo and Bower, 1993; Hasselmo and Schnell, 1994; Chrobak and Buzsáki, 1994; Skaggs and McNaughton, 1996; Redish, 1997; Redish and Touretzky, 1998a; see also comments by McNaughton and colleagues in Seifert, 1983). The suggestion that memories are stored during awake states and then replayed dur- ing sleep can be traced back to scientific concepts that preceded even Freud.

In the nineteenth century and earlier, some thought that the events of the previous day provided the raw material for dreams, broken apart and reshuffled (Freud, 1899). In the modern era, Marr (1970, 1971) first suggested that memories were stored in hippocampus during awake states and then replayed into long- term memory in cortex during sleep. Buzsáki (1989) was the first to critcally examine the proposition that memories are written into hippocampus during theta and recalled during sharp waves.

There are two time courses for consolidation that need to be handled separately (Nadel and Moscovitch, 1997; Redish and Touretzky, 1998a): *short-term consolidation* (STC), over the course of hours; and *long-term consolidation* (LTC), over the course of days to years. Although the boundary between STC and LTC is obviously not well defined (Is consolidation that takes three days short- or long-term?), the standard hypotheses are that STC is a consequence of cellular mechanisms while LTC is a consequence of network mechanisms.

The key evidence required for consolidation is that after an experimental manipulation, recent memories are not remembered as well as more remote ones. In other words, retrograde amnesia should be *graded*. This can be shown by experimental manipulations that disrupt acquisition if and only if they occur within a certain time after the training experience.

One example of evidence supporting short-term consolidation is that electroconvulsive shock applied to a structure shortly after an experience can erase that experience (McGaugh, 1966). Another example is that an animal given MK-801 (an NMDA receptor blocker) shortly after training in the water maze shows severe memory deficits (Smith, 1995). Similar effects are seen with REM sleep deprivation (Fishbein and Gutwein, 1977; Karni et al., 1994; Smith, 1995; Hennevin et al., 1995).

STC is most likely to occur as a consequence of the biophysical time course of long-term potentiation (LTP) or other cellular mechanisms. Because LTP has long time constants (days; see Racine, Milgram, and Hafner, 1983, for a review), if it is disrupted, memories could be lost. Indeed, manipulations that disrupt LTP also disrupt memory formation (McNaughton et al., 1986; Castro et al., 1989; Gustafsson and Wigström, 1990; Morris, Davis, and Butcher, 1990; Davis, Butcher, and Morris, 1992; McNaughton, 1993; Reymann, 1993)

On the other hand, the standard model suggests that LTC occurs because memories are stored in a temporary buffer and then written out from that buffer into long-term storage. The hypothesis that the medial temporal lobe (including the hippocampus and adjacent structures) serves as the temporary buffer can be traced back to the original studies on H.M. (Scoville and Milner, 1957; Milner, 1970).

Squire (1992) points out that there are two possible mechanisms of consolidation:

1. Memories may consist of two (or more) components — a quickly fading component and a more slowly fading compo-

nent. Lesions that preferentially affect the quick component would preferentially damage recent memories.

2. Memories may be temporarily stored in a buffer and then written out to a permanent storage facility.

These hypothesized mechanisms can be differentiated because in mechanism 1, no recent memory can be more damaged than remote memories. In contrast, in mechanism 2, experimental manipulations that erase or destroy the buffer will impair more recent memories more than ancient memories.

We should note that some authors (Marr, 1970, 1971; Squire, Cohen, and Nadel, 1984; Nadel, Willner, and Kurz, 1985; Teyler and DiScenna, 1985, 1986; Alvarez and Squire, 1994; McNaughton et al., 1996) have suggested that the medial temporal lobe *indexes* memory. In this formulation, memories, which are stored elsewhere, are initially tied together by the medial temporal lobe and only over time cohere enough to be retrievable without the medial temporal lobe. While the temporal nature of retrograde amnesia predicted by this hypothesis would look like that predicted by the buffer hypothesis (mechanism 2), experiments might be designable which would allow parts of the memory to emerge. Some authors have argued that data showing amnesiacs can recall aspects of events after priming may support the indexing hypothesis (for reviews, see Luria, 1973; Squire, 1987; Weingartner and Parker, 1984).

Memories may consist of multiple components, each of which encompasses a different aspect, and the relation of the aspects may change over time (Nadel and Moscovitch, 1997; Redish and Touretzky, 1998a). A classic example of this is that when one starts a new job and first drives to a new office, one has to concentrate on the route to take — which exits, which streets. Over time, the route becomes automatic. Often it becomes so automatic that one may go to one's office accidentally, without intending to, if the beginning of the route is the same. Are these two proposed mechanisms truly separable? It seems most likely that they are two aspects of a memory, one which is quickly trainable and requires concentration, and one which trains slowly but becomes automatic over time. These two aspects correspond to the *declarative* versus *procedural* distinction often discussed with respect to amnesiac patients (Cohen and Squire, 1980; Squire, 1987; Cohen and Eichenbaum, 1993).

There is also a third mechanism that which must be considered:

3. Memories may gel over time. A memory may need time to set even if it is never written out to another structure.

These three mechanisms can be differentiated by examining the effect of retrograde amnesia. Mechanism 1 predicts that remote memories will never be better remembered than recent memories, while mechanism 2 predicts that there will be a ∧ shape to the memories after the manipulation (Squire, 1992). The third mechansism predicts a difference between experimental manipulations that damage the cohesion (such as perhaps electroshock) and lesions that destroy the structure entirely: the ∧ shape should occur after the nonlesion manipulation, but after the lesion manipulation, there should be a total loss of memory (i.e., complete, ungraded retrograde amnesia). Effects of various manipulations on the three mechanisms are shown in figure 12.1.

EVIDENCE FOR CONSOLIDATION

Rats

Sutherland and Arnold (1987; see also Sutherland and Hoesing, 1993) reported limited retrograde amnesia in rats tested in the Morris water maze. They used colchicine to lesion the dentate gyrus. Colchicine targets DG cells, and tends to leave CA3 and CA1 mostly intact (Goldschmidt and Steward, 1980). If the rats are trained on the task first and then given a hippocampal lesion one week later. If, however, they are given the same lesion twelve weeks after training, they show much smaller deficits (Sutherland and Hoesing, 1993).

More recent experiments have shown that with more complete hippocampal lesions, rats show complete retrograde amnesia even out to thirty-six weeks, almost one-third of a rat's two

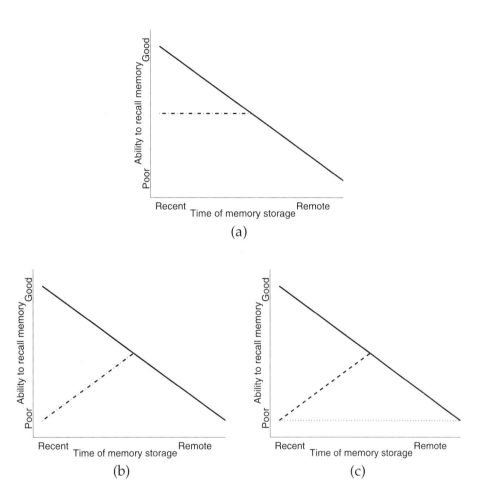

Figure 12.1
Hypothesized differential retrograde amnesia effects under three different assumptions. (a) Memory has multiple components, one of which
is destroyed. (b) Memory is temporarily stored in a buffer, which is
destroyed. (c) Memory takes time to gel, but is never written out of its
immediate storage location. These are theoretical diagrams and do not
show data or simulations. (Panels *a* and *b* after Squire, 1992.)

to three year lifespan (Bohbot et al., 1996; Koerner et al., 1996; Weisend, Astur, and Sutherland, 1996; Koerner et al., 1997).

Bohbot et al. (1996) found that the temporal gradient of retrograde amnesia is better explained as an effect of *time since surgery*: the lateral ventricles expand as time progresses after surgery, compressing nearby structures. Koerner et al. (1996, 1997) explicitly tested the limited nature of retrograde amnesia in the hidden platform water maze by comparing three groups: (1) animals who learned the task and waited 12 weeks, (2) animals who learned the task and received repetitions each week for 12 weeks, and (3) animals who learned 13 different hidden platform water mazes over those 13 weeks. After hippocampal lesions only group 2 showed any performance above chance.

Bolhuis, Stewart, and Forrest (1994) examined animals trained on the water maze with two retention intervals between training and surgery; 2–4 days and 14 weeks. Animals were given either ibotenate hippocampal or subicular lesions. They found no temporal gradient to retrograde amnesia.

On the other hand, Cho, Berracochea, and Jaffard (1993) report definite retrograde amnesia in mice. Animals with bilateral ibotenate entorhinal cortex lesions showed significant impairments of two-choice discriminations (on an eight-arm radial maze) for discriminations learned one-half to two weeks prior to surgery, but no impairment at all for those learned four or eight weeks prior to surgery. In fact, the animals were better at the four- or eight-week old discriminations than at the two-week discriminations. (Normals are better at recently learned discriminations.) This suggests a consolidation time measured in weeks, but with entorhinal not hippocampal lesions.

Winocur (1990) examined social food preference in rats with bilateral electrolytic hippocampal lesions. Normal rats, when paired with a demonstrator rat who has recently eaten a food, prefer that food over other foods. Rats who first acquired the preference (from the demonstrator rat) and then experienced surgery (a dorsal hippocampal lesion) report a significant impairment when less than two days intervened between acquisition and surgery, but were normal when five or ten days intervened.

And Kim and Fanselow (1992) report that rats with current-induced lesions of hippocampus showed retrograde amnesia in context-dependent fear conditioning. (The hippocampus is generally involved in contextual fear conditioning; Good and Honey, 1991; Honey and Good, 1993.) Kim and Fanselow showed a marked number of animals freezing when the animals had been trained one to four weeks prior to the lesion, but no freezing at all in rats trained only one day prior to the lesion. All the lesioned animals, however, showed less freezing than normals with the same delay between training and testing, even out to four weeks. Kim and Fanselow's lesions included dorsal hippocampus but were incomplete — large portions of ventral hippocampus were spared.

Primates

I have not addressed primates previously in this book. However, because most of the findings on consolidation and retrograde amnesia come from the primate (particularly, the human) literature, I will discuss them here. (The rest of the primate hippocampal literature will be left for chapter 14, where I will attempt to reconcile the primate literature with the role hypothesized for the hippocampus in chapter 13.

Zola-Morgan and Squire (1990) report that nonhuman primates trained to discriminate 100 pairs of objects remembered objects learned 12 or 16 weeks before surgery better than they did objects learned 2 or 4 weeks before surgery. However, the effect is small, and the variance between the 8-, 12-, and 16-week memory scores for normal animals is larger than the entire effect.

In humans, retrograde amnesia is usually shown by asking patients questions about time periods 5, 10, 20, 30, or more years before their lesion occured. A number of studies have reported that patients have better memory for early events (forty years before the exam) than for recent events (within the previous ten to twenty years) (Scoville and Milner, 1957; Milner, Corkin, and Teuber, 1968; Zola-Morgan, Squire, and Amaral, 1986; Squire, 1992; Rempel-Clower et al., 1996).

Because many of the patients who show retrograde amnesia have histories of cognitive deficits, it can be difficult to separate retrograde amnesia from unsuccessful storage of the memory in the first place (Squire, 1992). For example, H.M. had minor seizures since the age of 10 and major seizures since the age of 16; this epilepsy was severe enough to justify surgical lesioning of large portions of H.M.'s brain (Scoville and Milner, 1957). For another example, many of the patients who show retrograde amnesia suffer from Korsakoff's syndrome (a consequence of alcholism that entails the destruction of the mammillary bodies and other structures), but Korsakoff's develops over many years (for reviews see Luria, 1973; Squire, 1987, 1992).

Nevertheless, there are patients suffering from retrograde amnesia caused by a single traumatic incident, before which they were normal and after which they are profoundly amnesiac (Zola-Morgan, Squire, and Amaral, 1986; Squire, 1992; Rempel-Clower et al., 1996). The trauma in the cases reported by these authors is an anoxic episode (a cessation of oxygen to the brain). But even in these cases, the gradient nature of retrograde amnesia has been questioned by Nadel and Moscovitch (1997), who pointed out that while the retrograde amnesia in these patients extends back for at least thirty years; it is only in the most remote periods that one finds any remnant of memory.

THE ROLE OF THE HIPPOCAMPUS

Although there is now good evidence that the hippocampus replays recent memories during sleep (Pavlides and Winson, 1989; Wilson and McNaughton, 1994; Skaggs and McNaughton, 1996; Qin et al., 1997; see chapter 11), the evidence that the hippocampus serves as a temporary store for memory is not as strong as it was once thought to be. Nevertheless, even though the hippocampus appears to be required for certain types of very long-term memories in the rodent (Koerner et al., 1996; Weisend, Astur, and Sutherland, 1996; Koerner et al., 1997), it might also serve as a temporary buffer for other types of memory.

Most of the data showing graded retrograde amnesia consists of lesions involving the rhinal cortex and parahippocampal gyrus as well as the hippocampus (Scoville and Milner, 1957; Zola-Morgan and Squire, 1990; Cho, Berracochea, and Jaffard, 1993; Murray, Gaffan, and Mishkin, 1993; Rempel-Clower et al., 1996). If we ask about anatomical requirements, a temporary memory store must, first and foremost, be connected to every other part of the brain (as originally noted by Marr, 1971). Although most authors have suggested the hippocampus for this role, the rhinal cortex is in fact the structure that best meets this requirement (Suzuki, 1996). It is connected to the hippocampus (via the entorhinal cortex), the amygdala, and most of neocortex (Van Hoesen, 1982; Witter et al., 1989; Burwell, Witter, and Amaral, 1995; Suzuki, 1996; Burwell and Amaral, 1998).

If we ask about computational requirements, the main one is that the structure must be able to store memories quickly and then replay them over time (McClelland, McNaughton, and O'Reilly, 1995). Although LTP has been associated with hippocampus (for reviews, see Bliss and Lynch, 1988; Brown et al., 1991; McNaughton, 1993; Malenka, 1995), it is also found in the cortex (Bear and Kirkwood, 1993), as is replay of memories (Qin et al., 1997). Whether rhinal cortex and the parahippocampal gyrus show fast LTP and replay during sleep is still an open question, but it is certainly not outside the realm of possibility.

Lesions of the parahippocampal gyrus and the perirhinal cortices have been implicated in delayed nonmatch-to-sample (DNMS) tasks (Murray and Mishkin, 1984; Zola-Morgan, Squire, and Amaral, 1989; Zola-Morgan et al., 1989; Murray, 1992; Meunier et al., 1993, 1996; Suzuki, 1996), as well as contextual fear conditioning (e.g., Corodimas and LeDoux, 1995; see also Suzuki, 1996). Neurons in the parahippocampal gyrus in monkeys show responses to visual, somatosensory, and auditory stimuli (Suzuki, 1996), while neurons in these areas in rats show responses to olfactory stimuli including maintained encoding during delays (Young et al., 1997).

Whether the parahippocampal gyrus is a temporary memory buffer like that hypothesized by Scoville and Milner (1957) and by

Marr (1971) is still an open question. The evidence is mounting, however, that the hippocampus is not (at least not in certain spatial tasks; Bohbot et al., 1996; Koerner et al., 1996; Weisend, Astur, and Sutherland, 1996; Koerner et al., 1997; see also Nadel and Moscovitch, 1997). Whether the hippocampus replays recent memories, on the other hand, remains an open question.

13 Questions of Hippocampal Function

We have seen how navigation abilities can be understood as an interaction between subsystems: local view, taxon and praxic navigation, head direction, path integration, goal memory, and place code. We have seen how routes are stored and recalled in the place code and how the place code is realized by hippocampal place cells. We have seen how this implies a need for representations of multiple maps in the hippocampus. The interaction of these systems forms a comprehensive, computational theory of navigation.

What does this imply for the role of the hippocampus? It is generally accepted that the hippocampus is involved in spatial navigation, but not that the hippocampus is solely spatial.

Although hippocampal studies have been performed on rodents, rabbits, and both human and nonhuman primates, we have so far considered only rodents, and will continue to do so for the sake of simplicity and because it is not necessarily true that the hippocampus plays the same role across diverse species. I will directly address the relations between the role of the rodent hippocampus and that of the primate in the next chapter.

THE THEORIES

The Hippocampus as Emotional Center

One early theory, taking its cue from strong connections with other parts of the limbic brain, particularly the hypothalamus, proposed suggested that the hippocampus mediates the emotions (Papez, 1937; MacLean, 1973; Isaacson, 1974; MacLean, 1990). The limbic system was believed to control the emotions and feelings beyond our conscious control. Related to ideas of Freud (1923) and the concept of the *triune brain* (in which the limbic system is called the *visceral brain,* MacLean, 1973, 1990; see also Douglas, 1967; Isaacson, 1974), this theory arose mostly from early lesion data and the inability to separate structures that control emotion (such as amygdala and anterior cingulate cortex) from nearby structures (such as hippocampus and posterior cingulate).

Lesion data (particularly the early lesion data) is generally problematic for a number of reasons, most notably that it is nearly impossible for a lesion not to encroach on adjacent structures. Early lesions often affected fibers of passage and other structures that may have been on the way to the intended target. The main problem with this theory is its inadequacy to explain the extensive neurophysiological data that has energized the field over the last twenty years.

Response Inhibition

Another early theory held that the hippocampus served as a basis for Pavlovian inhibition (Douglas, 1967; Kimble, 1968; Altman, Brunner, and Bayer, 1973; Douglas, 1975; Kimble, 1975; Douglas, 1989). The main support for this theory was evidence that hippocampal lesions disrupted spontaneous alternation,[1] and that hippocampal lesions produce hyperactivity (Isaacson, 1974).

However, other plausible explanations for a lack of spontaneous alternation behavior after hippocampal lesions exist (O'Keefe and Nadel, 1978): for example, if an animal is unable to localize itself within an environment, it cannot alternate choices within that environment. Lesions to many other brain structures also impair spontaneous alternation (Douglas, 1989), including the caudate nucleus (which probably plays a role in taxon and praxic navigation; see chapter 4). No one has examined frontal or parietal lesions in relation to spontaneous alternation (according to the review in Douglas, 1989), but in primates parietal lesions cause hemispatial neglect (Bisiach and Vallar, 1988; Stein, 1992) and a wide variety of frontal and parahippocampal structures have been implicated in eight-arm maze (Floresco, Seamans, and Phillips, 1997) and delayed nonmatch-to-sample tasks (Zola-Morgan et al., 1989; Murray, 1992; Otto and Eichenbaum, 1992a; Wiig and Bilkey, 1994; Meunier et al., 1996; Fuster, 1997). Hyperactivity can be partially explained by lack of recognition of an environment leading to exploration (O'Keefe and Nadel, 1978).

In the response-inhibition theory, it is not clear what is being represented or computed by the hippocampus. Therefore the theory is at a complete loss to explain the neurophysiology data (such as the existence of place cells). In addition, the theory depends on a small selection of the lesion results and cannot explain a wide variety of other results (for details see Nadel, O'Keefe, and Black, 1975; O'Keefe and Nadel, 1978).

Hippocampus as Predictive Comparator

Gray (1982a, 1982b) attempted to bring together in one comprehensive theory the disparate findings of research into anxiety (as evidenced by the effects of antianxiety drugs and specific lesions) and the hippocampus (in particular its connections to the septum via the fimbria-fornix). He suggested that a *behavioral inhibition system* (BIS) senses signals of punishments, nonreward, and novel stimuli, sets up conditions of behavioral inhibition, and increases arousal and attention. The effect of antianxiety drugs is hypothesized to reduce anxiety by impairing this BIS.

Gray then took the questionable step of equating the anatomical instantiation of the BIS with the septohippocampal system. The main function of the hippocampus in Gray's theory is as a predictor, sending information to the subiculum, which acts as a comparator: By predicting the future and comparing it to subsequent sensory cues, the animal can decide whether to continue on its current path or to stop and reevaluate the situation.

The main problem with this theory is that it fails to explain much of the navigation data. For example, it tells us nothing about why animals cannot solve the hidden platform water maze after hippocampal lesions (Morris et al., 1982; Sutherland, Whishaw, and Kolb, 1983; Eichenbaum, Stewart, and

Morris, 1990; Morris et al., 1990; Sutherland and Rodriguez, 1990; Packard and McGaugh, 1992).

A more likely anatomical instantiation for the behavioral inhibition system may be the dopamine neurons in the ventral tegmental area recorded by Schultz and colleagues (Schultz et al., 1995b; Schultz, 1997) or the noradrenergic neurons in the locus coeruleus (Sara and Segal, 1991; Aston-Jones, Chiang, and Alexinsky, 1991), which are sensitive to changes in reward and novelty.

Configural Association Theory

As Sutherland and Rudy (1989) see it, the right way to think about the hippocampus is by differentiating between simple and configural associations: a *simple association* relates two elementary stimuli, while a *configural association* combines the stimuli into a unique representation in order to differentiate similar representations, which can then be associated with other stimuli.

Sutherland and Rudy originally proposed their theory as a means of solving the *negative patterning discrimination problem*, which is equivalent to the *XOR* problem: respond in one way to (A) or (B) but in another way to (A and B) or (not A and not B). A linear network cannot solve this problem (Minsky and Papert, 1969), but a multilayer network with simple nonlinearities can (Rumelhart, Hinton, and Williams, 1986; Hertz, Krogh, and Palmer, 1991). In a sense, Sutherland and Rudy are suggesting that the hippocampus is the middle layer of a three-layer network and that the basic learning rule for the rest of cortex is essentially linear. Gluck and Myers (1993, 1996) have made this explicit, simulating the hippocampus as a three-layer autoassociative network trained by backpropagation of error and using the hidden layer representation as an output to inform their model of cortex.

The main problem with this theory is that the environment is always one of the elements of configural associations that rodents have trouble with all. For example, when Alvarado and Rudy (1995a, 1995b) trained rats in the water maze to find a platform indicated by a cue card with a specific marking, animals with hippocampal lesions could learn to find platforms under uniquely marked cards (say vertical stripes), but then could not learn to ignore the vertical striped card and find the platform under an all-black card. Although this dichotomy can be explained as a *transverse patterning* problem, it can also be explained by the spatial theory of hippocampus: finding a platform under uniquely marked stimuli can be solved by taxon navigation. Because it requires recognizing the environment itself, learning to find the platform under a striped cue card when the other choice is all-white, but to find the platform under the black card when the choice is between striped and black requires locale navigation.

Indeed, where the configural association did not involve changing environments, Jarrard (1993) found that animals with ibotenic lesions acquired the association normally (where A was a tone and B was a light). Similar intact configural association abilities after hippocampal lesions have been reported: odor with string size (Whishaw and Tomie, 1991); light with string size (Whishaw and Tomie, 1995); light with a tone (Gallagher and Holland, 1992; Davidson, McKernan, and Jarrard, 1993). As suggested by Nadel (1994, 1995; see also O'Keefe and Nadel, 1978; Nadel and Willner, 1980; Jarrard, 1993, and *Contextual Retrieval* below), it may well be that environmental context is handled specially.

The configural association theory also suggests that there should be no difference between spatial tuning and nonspatial tuning of hippocampal pyramidal cells. As discussed in chapter 10, the correlations to nonspatial aspects shown by hippocampal pyramidal cells must be seen as second-order correlations in that they determine how place field topologies change.

Working Memory

Based on data from a radial maze showing that fimbria-fornix lesioned rats could not remember which arms they had already visited but could remember which arms had never been baited, Olton, Becker, and Handelmann (1979), distinguishing between between memory for within-task information (*working memory*) and between-tasks information (*reference memory*), suggested that the hippocampus mediates working memory but not reference memory. Because the hidden platform water maze, which is strongly hippocampus-dependent (Morris et al., 1982; Sutherland, Whishaw, and Kolb, 1983; Eichenbaum, Stewart, and Morris, 1990; Morris et al., 1990; Sutherland and Rodriguez, 1990; Packard and McGaugh, 1992), requires reference memory, it would appear that the hippocampus is also involved in reference memory.

Jarrard (1993) explicitly tested reference memory and working memory on spatial and cued versions of the radial maze and found that rats with ibotenic hippocampal lesions showed errors of all three kinds in the place version (entries into never-baited arms, repeated entries into once-baited arms, and repeated entries into never-baited arms), implying that the rats were totally lost. In the cued version, however, rats avoided cued arms that were never baited (reference memory) and did eventually learn not to repeat cued arms (working memory) but took much longer to train. Based on Jarrard's results, the hypothesis that the hippocampus mediates working memory and not reference memory must be abandoned, although the concept of working versus reference memory may still be useful for understanding how the hippocampus is involved in the radial maze and certain other tasks. As noted by Olton, Becker, and Handelmann (1979), there is a strong relation between the working memory concept and the general concept of *interference* (for a good description of interference see Hasselmo and Bower, 1993, and Hasselmo, 1993).

WhereOlton, Becker, and Handelmann (1979) lumped together a variety of hippocampal lesions, more recent experiments have brought to light differences between the various components of the hippocampal formation. Fimbria-fornix lesions sever the cholinergic input to the hippocampus, the connections from the subiculum to the nucleus accumbens, and the postsubicular connections to the lateral mammillary nuclei, but do not sever the connections between hippocampus (HC) and entorhinal cortex (EC; that is neither EC → HC nor HC → EC). As noted in chapter 6, ibotenic hippocampal lesions have different effects than fimbria-fornix lesions, for example, fornix lesions impair path integration (Whishaw and Maaswinkel, 1997), while ibotenic hippocampal lesions do not (Alyan et al., 1997).

Cholinergic antagonists (such as scopolomine) have been implicated in impairments of working memory more than reference memory, even on spatial tasks (Eckerman et al., 1980; Wirsching et al., 1984; Buresova, Bolhuis, and Bures, 1986). One possibility is that acetylcholine affects interference (Hasselmo and Bower, 1993; Hasselmo, 1993) and that reference memory is less suceptable to interference than is working memory on the radial maze. This is supported by data from Wirsching et al. (1984) showing that low doses of scopolomine (a cholinergic antagonist) produce working memory errors, but that reference memory errors appear only at higher doses.

An important consideration when looking at anticholinergic effects is that acetylcholine plays a role in a large variety of structures (Cooper, Bloom, and Roth, 1986), for example, as a central neurotransmitter in the basal ganglia (Alexander and Crutcher, 1990; Graybiel, 1990; Afifi, 1994). It is possible that cholinergic antagonists affect downstream structures such as the nucleus accumbens, which may play a role in goal memory (see chapter 7), or the frontal cortex, which may play a role in maintaining memories across delays (Goldman-Rakic, Funahashi, and Bruce, 1990; Goldman-Rakic, 1995; Fuster, 1997). Mizumori et al. (1989) found that septal inactivation did not affect the location specific firing of CA1 cells, but did increase working memory errors. Otto and Eichenbaum (1992a) report that hippocampal cells were better correlated with reward versus nonreward conditions than the animal's behavior, which implies that errors may be occuring downstream from hippocampus.

Other important issues include whether the animals have been pretrained before the lesion. As reviewed by Barnes (1988), most postlesion training methodologies have found strong place dependencies but little or no cue dependence in both reference and working memory aspects. However, the prelesion data reviewed by Barnes (1988) is less clear. Specifics of the training methodology may be as important as the working memory versus reference memory dichotomy proposed by Olton, Becker, and Handelmann

An interesting question is the possible relationship between mislocalization and the working memory versus reference memory distinction. As suggested by the *multiple map* hippocampal hypothesis (see chapter 10), the n-arm radial maze may be encoded by as many as $2n + 1$ maps. Reference memory errors might then consist of between-environment mislocalizations while working memory errors might consist of within-environment mislocalizations. Redish and Touretzky (1997a) suggested that there might be a particular role for cholinergic inputs in the separation of hippocampal maps, particularly in within-environment transitions. The findings by Mizumori et al. (1989) that septal inactivation did not affect CA1 cells but did increase working memory errors on the radial maze would seem to suggest that there is no connection between CA1 place fields and working memory errors. But Mizumori et al. made no specific correlations. Moreover, they also found that CA3 place fields were disrupted during the time period working memory errors were being made. Whether the radial maze is encoded by multiple maps and whether working and reference memory errors correspond to mislocalizations are intriguing hypotheses that remain to be tested.

Cognitive Maps

In contrast to the disproven theories described above, there are three theories that have survived to the present day which I will argue have some strong connection to the actual role of the hippocampus: the *cognitive map theory*; *contextual retrieval*; and *episodic memory*.)

The cognitive map theory proposes that the hippocampus stores a cognitive map (Tolman, 1948) of the environment (O'Keefe and Nadel, 1978, see also O'Keefe and Nadel, 1979). The strongest support for the theory comes from the place cell data (chapter 8; appendix B). Hippocampal lesions have also been shown to have strong effects on spatial navigation abilities of rodents (appendix B). A tremendous number of experiments have been performed based on the hypotheses of this theory, and extensive modeling work has been done, trying to understand what drives place cells to fire the way they do and what role they might play in navigation (see chapter 8).

Indeed, the cognitive map theory has spawned a large number of more specific theories that address the specifics of the role played by the hippocampus in navigation. While many of these address how the hippocampus represents the location of the animal and then how the system can use that representation (e.g., Burgess, Recce, and O'Keefe, 1994; Wan, Touretzky, and Redish, 1994b, 1994c; Brown and Sharp, 1995; Burgess and O'Keefe, 1996; Recce and Harris, 1996; Sharp, Blair, and Brown, 1996; Touretzky and Redish, 1996; see also chapter 8), some theories hypothesize other roles for the hippocampus.

Associative Memory for Reinstantiating Local Views

An early theory of why place cells show place fields was that they were sensitive to combinations of landmarks (see, for example, Zipser, 1985; Leonard and McNaughton, 1990; Sharp, 1991; Hetherington and Shapiro, 1993; Shapiro and Hetherington, 1993; and chapter 8). Because place cells continued to show place fields in the dark (O'Keefe, 1976; McNaughton, Leonard, and Chen, 1989; Quirk, Muller, and Kubie, 1990; Markus et al., 1994), it was recognized that this explanation could not be the whole story (see Chapter 8 for a discussion of this issue). Early hypotheses that the hippocampus might show associative memory properties (Marr, 1971) suggested one possible explanation: some cells were sensitive to remaining landmarks and the rest of the representation was *completed* by the associative memory properties of the hippocampus (McNaughton and Morris, 1987; McNaughton, 1989; Rolls, 1989; Leonard and McNaughton, 1990; Poucet, 1993; Schölkopf and Mallot, 1993; Benhamou, Bovet, and Poucet, 1995; Recce and Harris, 1996).

According to this theory, an animal could also associate local view representations with self-motion information to predict the next expected local view representation in the total absence of cues. This would allow the animal to use a sort of dead reckoning to keep track of its position in the absence of cues. We should note, however, that this hypothesis is not equivalent to the path integration abilities discussed in chapter 6 because an animal must first experience a transition in order for it to be associated with the subsequent local view. This means that rodents would not be able to plan shortcuts or unexperienced paths through an environment. The evidence, however, suggests that they can. For example, rodents can solve the hidden platform water maze, even if they must pass through unexplored areas (Keith and McVety, 1988; Matthews et al., 1995).

Recce and Harris (1996) see the associative memory properties not as performing the path integration function, but as simply filling out a partial local view. They suggest that the path integrator is extrinsic to the hippocampus and that path integration is used to update the local representation outside hippocampus. This has the problem that errors that accumulate will distort the map. A more robust alternative is for the path integration representation (external to the hippocampus) to be input to the hippocampus directly along with the local view (as suggested by O'Keefe, 1976; Wan, Touretzky, and Redish, 1994c; Touretzky and Redish, 1996; Redish and Touretzky, 1997a; see chapter 8).

Fractured Maps

Worden (1992) hypothesized a navigation ability based on the concept of *fragment filters*, each of which represents the animal's location relative to a small number of landmarks (Worden used three). If an animal needs to find a goal in one fragment, but only has access to landmarks in a different fragment, then there must be a mechanism for fitting the two fragments together. It may even be necessary to link more than two fragments in a chain to reach from the currently available landmarks to a distant goal. Worden refers to this as *fragment fitting*. Although he associates certain mathematical operations necessary for his algorithm (such as calculating displacements and rotations necessary for fragment fitting) with anatomical structures (DG and CA3 respectively), he supplies little support for this theory beyond the basic data that hippocampal cells are involved in spatial mapping (e.g., that there are place cells in CA3). The computations required by the processing modules in the Worden (1992) theory do not seem feasible given the details of hippocampal anatomy.

The Cognitive Graph

Muller and colleagues (Muller, Kubie, and Saypoff, 1991; Muller, Stead, and Pach, 1996) point out that correlational (Hebbian) LTP combined with random exploration of an environment will produce a synaptic weight function such that the weight between two place cells is inversely proportional to the overlap between their place fields. The synaptic weight thus represents the distance between the place field centers and the connection matrix the topology of the space. Muller and colleagues suggest the term *cognitive graph* for this structure; evidence that it does exist in the hippocampus after exploration has been reported by Wilson and McNaughton (1994).[2]

Having made this observation, Muller and colleagues then suggest that a *graph-search algorithm* could plan paths using this structure. They propose Dijkstra's shortest-path algorithm (Dijkstra, 1959), discovered independently by Whiting and Hillier (1960; see Bondy and Murty, 1976, pp. 15–21; Cormen, Leiserson, and Rivest, 1990, chapter 25) as a good candidate, but also note the Bellman-Ford algorithm (Bellman, 1958; Ford and Fulkerson, 1962; see also Cormen, Leiserson, and Rivest, 1990, chapter 25) as another possibility. The main problem with this theory is that neither of these algorithms submit to an easy or obvious neural implementation.

Hippocampus as Path Integrator

McNaughton et al. (1996, see also Samsonovich and McNaughton, 1997; Samsonovich, 1997) propose that the hippocampus plays a crucial role as the path integrator (see chapter 6), notably as the *attractor network* that enforces a coherent representation of position. They suggest that the subicular complex is the source of the *offset connections* that allow the system to track self-motion.

In particular, they require that the cognitive graph be prewired into the system before an animal explores an environment. Given that place cells show different place fields in different environments, the actual synaptic weight between two cells should be a function of the minimum distance between their place fields over all environments. They term this extension of the cognitive graph the *multichart* model of hippocampus and each map a *chart*. (We have already reviewed the relationship between the multichart theory and the other multiple map hypotheses in chapter 10.)

Although this theory fits a lot of the data, particularly the place cell data, the multiple charts in the hippocampus require a highly complex connection structure (see chapter 6). While the complexity of the connection structure does not doom the hippocampus as a behavioral path integrator hypothesis, the fact that rats can show path integration abilities after ibotenic hippocampal lesions does (Alyan et al., 1997).

Route Learning as Navigation

As described in chapter 11, the combination of asymmetric LTP and phase precession produces an asymmetric connection matrix in the CA3 recurrent connections that can represent recently traveled routes (Skaggs, 1995; Blum and Abbott, 1996; Skaggs et al., 1996). One effect of these asymmetric connections predicted by Blum and Abbott (that place fields would stretch backward along well-traveled routes) has been confirmed experimentally (Mehta, Barnes, and McNaughton, 1997). Blum and Abbott (1996; see also Gerstner and Abbott, 1997) suggest that these asymmetric connections can be used to guide navigation.

One problem with this hypothesis is its inability to address transfer tasks. By proposing that animals plan shortcuts to a goal by interpolating vector fields, it limits shortcuts to those planned from a location that lies between two previously experienced locations. The transfer experiments of Matthews et al. (1995) in the hidden platform water maze belie this.

Another problem is that the hippocampus is not necessary for online navigation (Alyan et al., 1997): animals can navigate back to a starting point without a hippocampus. As I have argued in chapters 8 and 11, the effect of the asymmetric connections is better understood as a means of *replay* rather than *recall*.

Contextual Retrieval

Hirsh (1974, 1980) suggested that the hippocampus plays the role of supplying context to normal stimulus-response mechanisms. This *contextual retrieval* theory explained the reversal deficit seen in hippocampally ablated animals who acquired a single discrimination at a normal rate, but tended to perseverate which element was chosen when the reward is reversed. It also explained the negative patterning discrimination problem (respond to stimulus A or to stimulus B, but not to the stimulus pair AB) and latent learning (animals learn tasks faster in familiar than unfamiliar environments).

Like the configural association theory, the contextual retrieval theory suggests the role of the hippocampus is to augment a basic stimulus-response learning ability. Like the cognitive map theory, however, it suggests that the augmenting is purely environmental. This theory would seem to draw the same dichotomy between taxon and locale navigation as that drawn by O'Keefe and Nadel (1978; see chapter 2), and that which originally led Tolman and colleagues (Tolman, Ritchie, and Kalish, 1946a, 1946b; Tolman, 1948) to hypothesize the existence of a *cognitive map* in contrast to the stimulus-response theories of the behaviorists (e.g., Hull, 1943). Similar proposals have been made by Nadel and colleagues (Nadel and Willner, 1980; Nadel, 1994, 1995) and Jarrard (1993).

The hippocampus has been implicated in *contextual conditioning*. Honey and Good (Good and Honey, 1991; Honey and

Good, 1993) found that while the association itself was unaffected by hippocampal lesions, hippocampectomized animals,
unlike normals, carried the association between environments.
As pointed out by Jarrard (1993) and Nadel (1994), this suggests that the hippocampus mediates a contextual component
in the association. Conversely, animals with hippocampal lesions cannot learn to make one association in one environment and a different association in another (Selden et al., 1991;
Phillips and Le Doux, 1992).

Temporal Discontiguity

Rawlins (1985) has proposed that the hippocampal lesion data
can be summarized as a problem with spanning delays, as
a problem with *temporal discontiguities*. However, all of the
data cited in support of his theory include contextual transitions within the delay. While he emphasizes the temporal over
the discontiguous, Rawlins' ideas share much with the contextual retrieval points of Hirsh (1974, 1980), Nadel and colleagues (Nadel and Willner, 1980; Nadel, Willner, and Kurz, 1985;
Nadel, 1994, 1995), and Jarrard (1993). His theory also shares
much with that of mislocalization on multiple hippocampal maps
(see chapter 10): a temporal discontiguity implies a necessary *recall* process (see chapters 8 and 9). Errors in the recall process
would produce hippocampally-mediated effects dependent on
temporal discontiguities.

An interesting question becomes what exactly produces a
context-switch. As pointed out by Rawlins, delay learning in
normals is facilitated by removal from the environment during the delay, but it is also facilitated by a salient event occurring soon before the choice. Map transitions can occur within a
single environment in a complex task (Eichenbaum et al., 1987;
Eichenbaum and Cohen, 1988; Quirk, Muller, and Kubie, 1990;
Sharp, 1991; Cohen and Eichenbaum, 1993; Hampson, Heyser,
and Deadwyler, 1993; Markus et al., 1995; Gothard et al., 1996;
Sharp et al., 1995; Barnes et al., 1997). Mislocalizations at these

internal transition points would also produce context-based errors that should probably also be thought of as discontiguities.

Recognition Memory

In his *recognition memory* theory, Gaffan (1972; 1974) proposed that the hippocampus is involved in the detection of familiarity, a position he appears to have abandonded when Gaffan et al. (1984) found that fornix lesions had no effect on stimulus recognition experiments in monkeys. Gaffan's early experiments on rats (Gaffan, 1972, 1974) were based on environmental recognition, while Gaffan et al. (1984) tested stimulus recognition. As discussed above, environmental cues may be handled separately from other aspects.

A mislocalization to an incorrect map might be considered an incorrect recognition of a familiar environment. Barnes et al. (1997) found that old animals (with presumably deficient LTP and hippocampi) do not use the same representation between multiple experiences in an environment. Conversely, Tanila et al. (1997a, 1997b) found that old animals (again with presumably deficient LTP and hippocampi) do not recognize a novel environment and perseverate the use of inappropriate representations.

Episodic Memory

In contrast to the rodent studies, early studies on humans with temporal lobe lesions, such as that of H.M. (Scoville and Milner, 1957), suggested that the hippocampal formation may be involved in memory formation. Hippocampal lesions in humans produce devastating impairments in memory (Scoville and Milner, 1957; Squire and Zola-Morgan, 1988, 1991; Squire, 1992; Cohen and Eichenbaum, 1993; Zola-Morgan and Squire, 1993; Squire and Alvarez, 1995; Rempel-Clower et al., 1996).

Although lesioned patients perform immediate recall tasks normally, their recall is severly impaired at times longer than a few minutes. These patients show a total inability to form new long-term memories, thus demonstrating anterograde amnesia. In addition, they also show a retrograde amnesia (inability to recall things that happened prior to the occurrence of the lesion), although the retrograde amnesia only reaches back a limited time, leaving the earliest memories intact.

Further studies have shown that the hippocampal formation is not involved in all kinds of memory, but only in declarative memory. The distinction between declarative and procedural memory, first made by Cohen and Squire (1980; see also Squire, 1992; Cohen and Eichenbaum, 1993; Eichenbaum, Otto, and Cohen, 1994) is that *declarative memory* stores facts, names, events, and episodes (thus declarative memory is sometimes called *episodic memory*) whereas *procedural memory* stores skills acquired through practice. (I will discuss all of these issues and results in detail in chapter 14.)

Although some authors (e.g., Tulving, 1983; Squire, 1992; Nadel and Moscovitch, 1997) divide declarative memory into *semantic memory* (facts) and *episodic memory* (events), the details of this debate are beyond the scope of this book. Memory theories of hippocampus generally involve the episodic memory components of declarative memory (Squire, 1992; Cohen and Eichenbaum, 1993; Eichenbaum, Otto, and Cohen, 1994; Tulving and Markowitsch, 1997), but the main distinction drawn remains the one between declarative and procedural memory.

This theory has led some researchers to suggest that the hippocampus is the key to declarative memory in the rodent as well (Cohen and Eichenbaum, 1993; Eichenbaum, Otto, and Cohen, 1994). The episodic memory theory proposes that the hippocampus serves as a temporary store for declarative memory (Marr, 1970, 1971; Buzsáki, 1989; Zola-Morgan and Squire, 1990; Squire and Zola-Morgan, 1991; Cohen and Eichenbaum, 1993; Squire, 1992; McClelland, McNaughton, and O'Reilly, 1995; Squire and Alvarez, 1995), but that procedural memory does not require the hippocampus.

Relational Processing

Eichenbaum, Otto, and Cohen (1994) propose that the hippocampus stores *relational representations* in contrast to *individ-*

ual representations. This should not be confused with the configural association theory; Eichenbaum, Otto, and Cohen mean that the hippocampus represents the relations between stimuli; not the compositions of the stimuli. For example, Otto and Eichenbaum (1992a) found cells that fired only when a pair of odors matched independently of the specific odors involved (others fired when the pair did not match). However, this theory suffers from some of the same problems that the configural association theory does in that animals with hippocampal lesions can still solve certain configural association tasks (Whishaw and Tomie, 1991; Gallagher and Holland, 1992; Davidson, McKernan, and Jarrard, 1993; Jarrard, 1993; Whishaw and Tomie, 1995).

Storage and Replay of Sequences

Levy and colleagues (Levy, 1989; Minai and Levy, 1993; Minai, Barrows, and Levy, 1994; Wu and Levy, 1995; Levy, 1996; Levy and Wu, 1996; Wu, Baxter, and Levy, 1996) have proposed that the role of the hippocampus is to store and replay sequences. They show that the recurrent connections in CA3 are well suited for the storage of sequences. The route storage and replay discussed in chapter 11 also stores and replays sequences using similar mechanisms. To store sequences with overlapping codes, Levy and colleagues introduce the concept of *context units* which disambiguate the overlapping codes (Levy, 1996; Levy and Wu, 1996; Wu, Baxter, and Levy, 1996). Essentially, these are hidden units in an autoassociative network (see Kohonen, 1977, 1980; Rumelhart, Hinton, and McClelland, 1986). The concept of multiple hippocampal maps (chapter 10) serves a similar purpose to disambiguate crossing routes (chapter 11).

Replay of Memories during Sleep

In his theory of neocortex, Marr (1970) proposed that the role of the neocortex was classification and long-term memory and that in order for the neocortex to classify two similar pieces of information it would be useful for the system to be trained from another system during sleep. In his theory of archicortex (hippocampus), Marr (1971) suggested that the hippocampus might play this role. The critical question was *where* to store the information, but more recent examinations of this question have addressed other possible reasons for the consolidation of memories through hippocampal function.

McClelland, McNaughton, and O'Reilly (1995) argued that one reason why memories need to be temporarily stored in hippocampus is that connectionist or parallel distributed processing (PDP) networks (in which memories are stored by changes in weight matrices) are subject to *catastrophic interference*, which causes an animal to forget an item when it learns a second item that *interferes* with it. The experiment by Hirsh, Leber, and Gillman (1978) is an example of this: when they tried to train an animal with fimbria-fornix lesions to solve two tasks in a Y-maze alternatively, they found that the rats unlearned one task as they learned the other.

The key to all of these episodic memory theories is the idea that the hippocampus is specially structured to store memories quickly but that neocortex stores memories slowly. McClelland, McNaughton, and O'Reilly (1995) suggested that this allows memories stored in neocortex to be interleaved which would counteract the catastrophic interference problem. As discussed in chapter 11, there is substantial evidence supporting the theory that recent memories are replayed in hippocampus during sleep (Pavlides and Winson, 1989; Wilson and McNaughton, 1994; Skaggs and McNaughton, 1996), whereas the evidence that memories are written out from hippocampus to long-term memory is not so strong (see chapter 12.

WHAT DOES THE HIPPOCAMPUS REALLY DO?

All three of the surviving theories have their problems: The cognitive map theory cannot explain why hippocampal cells are also correlated to nonspatial aspects. The contextual retrieval theory cannot explain the difference between spatial representations (i.e., where on the map the animal is) and nonspatial representations (i.e., on which map the animal is). And the episodic memory theory does not explain how episodes (declarative memories) are represented in the brain.

I have argued that the role of the hippocampus in the navigation domain is twofold:

1. to allow the animal to self-localize on reentering a familiar environment. This allows the animal to reset its path integrator representation from the local view.

2. to replay recently traveled routes during sleep LIA states.

However, hippocampal lesions affect more than just spatial tasks. Eichenbaum (1996a) reviews a collection of nonspatial effects of hippocampal lesions, including social transmission of food preferences (see also Winocur, 1990). When a normal rat exposed to another that has just eaten a food is given a choice, the first animal prefers to eat that food instead of a different food. It turns out that rodents are sensitive to the combination of carbon disulfide (CS_2, a product of digestion) and the food odor. Essentially, if the other rat ate the food and didn't die, the food must be edible. Bunsey and Eichenbaum (1995) showed that the hippocampal lesions only have an effect if a delay is imposed: even with hippocampal lesions, animals showed normal preferences at zero delay.

Hippocampal lesions affect *offline* or *delay* tasks, in other words, tasks that involve a *context-switch*, where the animal has to reinstate the context after the delay. This is exactly what the hippocampus is doing in the navigation domain: on reentry into an environment (read *context*), the animal must self-localize to find its position in that environment (read *determine its current contextual state*).

An important distinction must be drawn between simply bridging a delay by active processes (memories maintained by continuously active reverberating neuronal loops) and a reinstantiation of memory after the delay (James, 1890; Hebb, 1949; Cohen and Eichenbaum, 1993; Eichenbaum, Otto, and Cohen, 1994; see also Squire, 1987; Fuster, 1997). Active processes to bridge delays probably include interactions between prefrontal and other association cortices (Sakurai, 1990a; Otto et al., 1991; Sakurai, 1994; Fuster, 1997).

Bridging a delay by active processes will be disrupted by distractors that require a response (distractors not requiring a response can presumably be ignored). However, reinstantiation may leave the system in the wrong context, as was found for old animals by Barnes et al. (1997).

A very nice dissociation supporting the hypothesis that the hippocampus is involved in reinstantiation while frontal and sensory association cortices are involved in active delay bridging has been shown by Sakurai (1990a, 1990b) and by Otto and Eichenbaum (1992b). Sakurai tested animals in a continuous delayed nonmatch-to-sample auditory task (animals received a sequence of high and low tones and could get reward whenever the sequence changed from high to low or from low to high). Sakurai found sensory and delay correlates in entorhinal cortex and auditory sensory cortex but not in CA1, where he found cells that differentiated reward situations, but did not maintain any noticeable task parameters during the delay (neither sensory cues or reward conditions). When Otto and Eichenbaum examined a delayed nonmatch-to-sample task, this time in the olfactory domain, they found that although many CA1 cells showed delay activity, the activity was unrelated to any parameter in the task. Delay firing did not predict performance, nor was it related to the sensory stimuli. If the animals encode different stages of the task by different reference frames, then we would expect a total decorrelation of cellular activity during the delay with task parameters at the begining or end of the task. On the other hand, when the delay period is over, we should see cells differentiating between the two reward conditions (because different routes need to be taken; see chapters 10 and 11). This is exactly what these experiments found.

The hippocampal reinstantiation theory makes some interesting neurophyioslogical and neurological predictions about hippocampal manipulations in rodents.

1. Hippocampal place cells should have non-navigational correlates and hippocampal lesions should have strong non-navigational effects (in contrast to O'Keefe and Nadel, 1978).

2. Hippocampal lesions should affect both working and reference memory (in contrast to Olton, Becker, and Handelmann, 1980).

3. Hippocampal lesions should affect tasks that involve a context-switch, independent of the absolute delay time (in contrast to Rawlins, 1985).

4. Intramaze context shifts should be hippocampally dependent (in contrast to Hirsh, 1974, 1980, and Nadel, 1994, 1995).

5. An animal with a hippocampal lesion should be able to handle decisions based on multiple cues, as long as the animal does not leave the context (in contrast to Sutherland and Rudy, 1989).

6. An animal should be able to perform path integration, again, as long as the animal does not leave the environment (in contrast to Samsonovich and McNaughton, 1997).

Examples of evidence confirming these assertions have already been discussed:

1. Hippocampal cells show different place field responses when tasks are changed within a single environment (Markus et al., 1995).

2. Rats with hippocampal lesions cannot solve the hidden platform water maze (e.g., Morris et al., 1982; Schenk and Morris, 1985; Eichenbaum, Stewart, and Morris, 1990; Sutherland and Rodriguez, 1990).

3. No delay is necessary to produce map switches (Sharp et al., 1995; Knierim, Kudrimoti, and McNaughton, 1998).

4. Old animals can be driven to change maps by allowing exploration of a novel portion of an environment (Barnes

et al., 1997). A rotation of an environment is sufficient even for young adult animals (Sharp et al., 1995;
Knierim, Kudrimoti, and McNaughton, 1998).

5. Animals with hippocampal lesions can solve configural association problems as long as the components are small
and noncontextual (Whishaw and Tomie, 1991; Gallagher
and Holland, 1992; Jarrard, 1993; Rawlins et al., 1993;
Cassaday and Rawlins, 1995; Whishaw and Tomie, 1995;
Cassaday and Rawlins, 1997).

6. Animals show path integration abilities even with ibotenic
lesions of the hippocampus (Alyan et al., 1997), while those
with fornix lesions show impaired impair path integration
(Whishaw and Maaswinkel, 1997).

We can also predict that rodents with hippocampal lesions
should be able to perform the hidden platform water maze task
if, once the animals reach the goal location, they are carried
smoothly and directly back to the release point. Presumably,
animals in such a situation do not have to relocalize at the wall's
edge. Normally, rodents in the water maze task are carried back
to a home cage to rest or are disoriented by being carried around
the room before being placed at the release point again. If the
prediction is correct, the result would invalidate a number of
hippocampal navigation models, notably, models holding that
the hippocampus is necessary for online navigation (e.g., Dayan,
1991; Blum and Abbott, 1996; Muller, Stead, and Pach, 1996;
Samsonovich and McNaughton, 1997). These models have to be
seriously questioned due to the findings by Alyan et al. (1997).

14 The Primate Hippocampus

Because a homologous brain structure does not necessarily serve the same purpose across diverse orders, we have concentrated thus far on a single order (rodents). The rodent hippocampal literature presents a vast array of experiments from a variety of paradigms; each of these experiments casts a different light on the question under review, allowing us to clearly distinguish possible theories. As discussed in chapter 13, we were able to reject a number of hypotheses and had to modify others to make them consistent with the data. By doing so, we were able to bring the extensive literature of hippocampal data and the variety of theories into a coherent understanding. We can now turn our attention back to primates: *What role does the hippocampus play in the monkey? In the human?*

THE PRIMATE EXPERIMENTAL LITERATURE

The monkey experimental literature is more limited than the rat and the human more limited than the monkey. Historically, both the monkey and human hippocampal literatures have been dominated by lesion experiments.

A few researchers have done single-cell recording experiments of hippocampal cells from awake behaving monkeys (Brown, 1982; Watanabe and Niki, 1985; Miyashita et al., 1989; Rolls et al., 1989; Tamura et al., 1990, Ono et al., 1991; Ono, Tamura, and Nakamura, 1991; Tamura et al., 1992a, 1992b; O'Mara et al., 1994; Eifuku et al., 1995; O'Mara, 1995; Rolls and O'Mara, 1995). However, the monkeys in these experiments were all restrained in a primate chair. In the early experiments, the chair never moved (Brown, 1982; Watanabe and Niki, 1985) although some experimenters did attempt to address the cognitive map theory by measuring differences in position of the cues relative to the monkey (Miyashita et al., 1989; Rolls et al., 1989; Ono et al., 1991; Ono, Tamura, and Nakamura, 1991; Tamura et al., 1992a, 1992b). Even in these tasks, the cues moved relative to the animal, not the animal relative to the cues. The more recent experiments allowed the animal to move around the room in a robotic chair (Ono et al., 1991; Ono, Tamura, and Nakamura, 1991; O'Mara et al., 1994; Eifuku et al., 1995; O'Mara, 1995; Rolls and O'Mara, 1995)).

These experiments should not be taken as equivalent to those with freely-running rats in which place fields are found. Physically restrained rats do not show the same place cell activity that freely behaving rats do (Foster, Castro, and McNaughton, 1989). Rats in similar chairs (in which they ride the chair passively) also do not show normal place fields (Gavrilov, Wiener, and Berthoz, 1996), although rats trained to control the speed of a model train with a lever do (Terrazas et al., 1997).

Single-cell recordings from humans (Halgren, Babb, and Crandall, 1978; Fried, MacDonald, and Wilson, 1997) have been done only on epileptics already selected for surgery. Because the hippocampi of epileptics selected for surgery are clearly abnormal, it remains uncertain how the findings of these experiments bear on normal processing in the human hippocampus. Neither of these studies measured spatial parameters of the neurons, measuring, instead cell firing correlations to pictures and syllables (Halgren, Babb, and Crandall, 1978) or to faces (Fried, MacDonald, and Wilson, 1997). Typical firing rate changes were very small relative to the changes seen in spatial experiments on rats: 1–3 spikes per second, compared to place cells, whose firing rates increase by an order of magnitude within their place fields. These experiments included recordings from both hippocampus proper and surrounding structures such as the parahippocampal cortex, the rest of the hippocampal formation, or amygdala, they found no major differences between them. This suggests that the experimental variables were not as important to the different structures as other variables (such as the location of the subject) might have been.

Recently, nonintrusive techniques such as positron emission tomography (PET) and functional magnetic resonance imaging (fMRI) have become available for examining the human brain (see Orrison et al., 1995). Both of these techniques measure blood flow changes not neuronal firing rates. Most researchers believe that increased blood flow signifies increased neuronal firing (Fox and Raichle, 1986; Ogawa et al., 1992), but debate about its meaning still exists (Kanno et al., 1995; Buxton and Frank, 1997). While the specifics of fMRI and PET are beyond the scope of this book, even if they do measure correlates of neuronal firing, this tells us little if anything about the representations. Many representations vary even as the total number of cells firing at any moment stays constant. For example, in the place cell representation, the number of cells firing at any location is a constant, but each location is represented by a different subset. This would not be detectable with PET or fMRI. Additionally, neither PET nor fMRI can tell us whether the increased firing is in excitatory or inhibitory cells. Nonetheless recent experiments based on PET and fMRI have linked the human hippocampal formation to both spatial and episodic memory tasks (e.g. Squire and Knowlton, 1995; Haxby et al., 1996; Vitte et al., 1996; Nyberg et al., 1996; Schacter et al., 1996; Henke et al., 1997; McGuire et al., 1997; see also Tulving and Markowitsch, 1997).

Even with the availablity of these new techniques, primate hippocampus research has been driven almost entirely by lesion data. Lesion experiments are notoriously problematic as guides for theorizing: (1) Because brain structures work together to accomplish a function (as we have seen throughout the discussion of rodent navigation), interpreting the symptoms produced by a brain lesion can be difficult. (2) Extensive damage to one part of the brain almost always entails damage to other parts. It is extremely difficult to completely destroy a brain structure while completely sparing nearby structures. (3) After a lesion, the brain may reorganize, with other structures changing their function in order to accommodate the damage. (See Luria, 1973 for a discussion of these problems.)

It is often hard to interpret what the effect of a lesion is. That an animal cannot perform a task could mean that the animal has trouble with any number of parameters involved. Traditionally, researchers try to find a pair of tasks that vary along only one variable (for example, the visual and hidden platform water mazes). Even when we find a pair of very similar tasks, one of which the lesioned animal can do, one of which it cannot, there are other hypotheses to consider. The lesioned structure may be critical for the task, while not being directly involved in the representation or computation of the manipulated variable. For example, a structure could provide tonic input that allows another structure to compute the variable.

One example of this problem that will turn out to be critical for our understanding of the role of the primate hippocampus is an experiment by Alvarez and Squire (1994), who tested animals with hippocampal lesions in a delayed nonmatch-to-sample task (DNMS). Animals were presented with an object and then given a delay, after which they were presented with a pair of objects, one from before the delay and the other new. The animal was supposed to pick the new object, which would demonstrates that it remembered the repeated stimulus. Alvarez and Squire found that their hippocampally lesioned animals were impaired at long delays (10 minutes and 40 minutes), but not short delays (8 seconds, 40 seconds, 1 minute). They interpreted this difference as a consequence of the length of the delay. However, they did not use the same experimental paradigm for the short- and long-delay trials: for the longer trials, they removed the monkey from the apparatus, put it back in its home cage during the delay, and returned it to the apparatus after the delay. Thus, as pointed out by Nadel (1995), the long delays entailed a *context change*. This could strongly affect lesioned animals, even if it did not impair normals. We will see later that a recent experiment by Murray and Mishkin (1996) strongly supports this hypothesis.

It is also difficult to guarantee that no other brain structures have been damaged. Early lesion studies used knife cuts to remove the intended structure; this usually produced collateral damage to adjacent brain areas. Although later studies used aspiration or radio frequency techniques, they still damaged axons that passed through the brain structure.[1] More recently, lesions have been made with ibotenic acid which does not damage fibers of passage, although it takes a careful technique to ensure that enough ibotenic acid is injected into the intended brain structure to fully destroy it, but not so much as to damage adjacent structures. Modern techniques use multiple injection sites to alleviate this problem (as many as fourteen, Jarrard, 1989, 1991, 1993).

An example of this second problem relates to an early experiment by Mishkin and Murray (Mishkin, 1978; Murray and Mishkin, 1984) who lesioned hippocampus, amygdala, or both. They found that neither hippocampal nor amygdala lesions affected the DNMS task, but that the combined lesion was devastating. They interpreted this as meaning that the hippocampus and amygdala could both mediate storage and retrieval of the remembered cue, so that one needed to lose both before seeing this impairment. But Mishkin and Murray used aspiration lesions to remove the two brain structures. Both the hippocampus and amygdala reside behind the rhinal cortex. When they lesioned one or the other, they also removed half the rhinal cortex; when they lesioned both, they removed all of rhinal cortex. As it turned out, with complete lesions of rhinal cortex leaving hippocampus and amygdala intact, animals were devastated, but with lesions of hippocampus and amygdala that did not disrupt rhinal cortex, animals were not impaired (Zola-Morgan, Squire, and Amaral, 1989; Zola-Morgan et al., 1989; Murray, 1992; Meunier et al., 1993, 1996).

Human subjects are particularly difficult in regard to the balance between complete lesions of a structure and sparing of adjacent structures because their lesions are not done for scientific study; the lesions are either unintentional, caused by some natural phenomenon (such as a stroke), or are done to alleviate damaged function (as in operations for epilepsy).

Strokes are unlikely to limit themselves to a single brain structure. At one time, it was thought that anoxia (a cessation of oxygen to the brain) produced a limited lesion destroying only the cells in hippocampal area CA1 (Zola-Morgan,

Squire, and Amaral, 1986; Squire and Zola-Morgan, 1991; Squire, 1992). Recent findings, however, have suggested that other areas are damaged soon after the anoxic episode when the CA1 cells die (Bachevalier and Meunier, 1996; Mumby et al., 1996).

Lesions done for medical reasons have one purpose and one purpose only and that is to improve the life of the patient. Because epileptic foci (where epileptic seizures start) tend to be in the temporal lobe, particularly in the hippocampus and adjacent areas, many epileptic patients have undergone such lesions (Scoville and Milner, 1957; Milner, 1970; Smith and Milner, 1989; Bohbot, 1997). To ensure that the lesions do not disrupt too much brain function, they are limited as much as possible. It is therefore very rare to find a human subject with the kind of focused but complete hippocampal lesions made in rats and monkeys. Moreover, an important consideration is whether brains of patients selected for surgical lesions were normal prior to surgery (Milner, 1970; Vanderwolf, 1995; Bohbot, 1997).

Finally, reflecting the coarseness of both lesion and imaging data, experimental papers talk about the *hippocampal formation* or, worse, the *medial temporal lobe*. The term *hippocampal formation* is usually used to include both the dentate gyrus and the CA fields, as well as the subiculum and sometimes even the rest of the subicular complex; the term *medial temporal lobe* refers not only to the hippocampus and its adjacent structures, but the parahippocampal gyrus and rhinal cortex (including both perirhinal and postrhinal cortices), and sometimes even the amygdala. In the rat, each of these structures subserve very different functions. While there is evidence showing a differentiation of function for different medial temporal lobe structures in the primate (e.g. Murray, 1992), most of the primate studies (both monkey and human) continue to lump these areas together. Thus it is unclear whether one should take the primate data as applying to the hippocampus, to one of the adjacent structures, or to some interaction effect between them.

All of these caveats having been noted, we have identified the role of the rodent hippocampus (self-localization in the navigation domain, reinstantiation after a context switch more generally). Therefore, we can now ask, *is this also the role of the primate hippocampus?* In the next section, I will argue that it is.

FROM RODENT TO PRIMATE

Because the rodent data is almost exclusively spatial, the role of the hippocampus in the rodent was originally identified in the navigation domain. Even within the navigation domain, however, it is not sufficient to merely reset the path integrator coordinates. The system also needs to identify the reference frame in which those coordinates will occur. As discussed in chapter 10, this occurs in the rodent hippocampus by a switch in maps (charts, reference frames; McNaughton et al., 1996; Touretzky and Redish, 1996; Redish and Touretzky, 1997a); when one examines the self-localization process in its full-fledged form, it becomes a reinstantiation of context.

People with hippocampal lesions, such as H.M., can hold normal conversations, but they cannot remember facts across different conversations (Scoville, 1968; Milner, Corkin, and Teuber, 1968; Cohen and Eichenbaum, 1993). For example, H.M. can solve difficult crossword puzzles but then forgets them soon afterward (Scoville, 1968). The classic example (told of Jimmie G., a patient with Korsakoff's syndrome[2]) is that of a patient who can talk to someone, address that person by name, and so on, but if the questioner leaves the room and returns, the patient will claim he never met that person before in his life (Sacks, 1985). This effect can be explained because when you leave the room and return, the patient has to reinstantiate the context.

Early reports described patients as being particularly sensitive to interference (Luria, 1973; Squire, 1987), defined as the ability of a subsequent stimulus to disrupt a memory trace. Careful examination of these early interference problems showed that they were really just examples of distractions, that is intervening context-shifts. For example, as reviewed by Luria (1973), these patients could successfully read and repeat a story, but if given intevening arithmetic problems, all traces of the story were forgotten.

From the very earliest case studies of H.M., it was reported that he only had problems remembering across distractions (Milner, 1970): "It was clear that forgetting occurred the instant his focus of attention shifted, but in the absence of distraction, his capacity for sustained attention was remarkable." Milner describes a test in which H.M. was able to remember a number for fifteen minutes by constant rehersal, but as soon as the examiner changed the subject, H.M. forgot the number — in fact, he forgot even that he had been given a number to remember. H.M. is also able to hold verbal material over a longer delay than nonverbal, which suggests that he is using rehearsal to bridge the gap (Milner, 1970).

As discussed in chapter 13, there are at least two ways to bridge a delay: conscious rehersal (sometimes called *short-term active memory* or *active working memory*, Fuster, 1997) and reinstantiation upon returning to a context (Milner, 1970; Eichenbaum, Otto, and Cohen, 1994; Fuster, 1997). Short delays without major distractions can be bridged by rehearsal, but remembering events across context-switches requires a reinstantiation. There is extensive data showing that bridging short delays by rehearsal involves prefrontal cortex, and especially an interaction between prefrontal cortex and sensory or motor cortices (Goldman-Rakic, Funahashi, and Bruce, 1990; Kolb, 1990b; Goldman-Rakic, 1995; Fuster, 1997).

In the nonhuman primate also, there is growing evidence that the role of the hippocampus is in bridging context-switches. As mentioned before, when Alvarez and Squire (1994) tested rhesus macaques with hippocampal lesions in a standard DNMS task, they found much worse deficits after 10- and 40-minute delays than after delays of 1 minute or less. They attributed the effect to the length of the delay, but during the 10- and 40-minute delays, they removed the animals from the experimental situation, which they did not do for the short delays. Although this does not affect normals, it might have a severe effect on lesioned animals if the hippocampus is involved in retrieving the context where the task was done (Nadel, 1995; Redish, 1997). In support of this hypothesis, Murray and Mishkin (1996) showed that hippocampal-lesioned rhesus macaques are not impaired on a continuous nonmatch-to-sample (CNMS) task at 10 or 40 minutes. The CNMS task is similar to the DNMS task, except that animals are shown a sequence of example objects and then shown novel pairs in reverse order. This means that although there is a delay between the time animals see the first object and the corresponding last pair, they never leave the experimental situation. If the animals do not leave the context, they can perform the task well even without a hippocampus.

15   Coda

Taking note at the outset that how we store and recall episodic memories was too complicated a question to address directly, and that computational models of episodic memory did not generally address real tasks, we began by examining the role of the hippocampus in navigation. On our journey through navigation, we looked at what needed to be represented, how that was represented, and how those representations were maintained and computed.

By carefully reviewing a large corpus of experiments across a variety of paradigms, a synthesis of the theoretical literature into a consistent picture was possible, rejecting some theories, accepting some, and modifying others (see chapter 13).

Adding to and extending O'Keefe and Nadel's (1978) taxonomy the synthesized theory divided the navigation system into functional subsystems: local view (chapter 3), taxon and praxic navigation (chapter 4), a head direction system (chapter 5), path integration system (chapter 6), a goal memory (chapter 7), and a place code (chapter 8). It proposed that the hippocampus plays the role of the place code, operating in three different modes: storage, recall, and replay (see chapters 8, 9, and 11).

However, a number of aspects of the theory remain unresolved at this time. For example, there are two possible mechanisms that can separate reference frames in novel environments: orthogonalization in the dentate gyrus, and prewired maps in CA3 (see chapter 10). Although chapter 8 favors the DG hypothesis, there is no data disproving the CA3 hypothesis, and the two hypotheses are not incompatible. Whether one, both, or neither mechanism occurs in the rodent brain will have to be left for the future.

For another example, which mechanism produces phase precession in the hippocampus remains an open question (see chapter 11). A number of proposals have been made about phase precession (O'Keefe and Recce, 1993; Burgess, Recce, and O'Keefe, 1994; Samsonovich and McNaughton, 1996; Tsodyks et al., 1996), but none of them fit all of the available data.

Nevertheless, by looking at the big picture and examining interaction effects between systems, we were able to make certain novel predictions. For one, we predicted that although strongly involved in navigation, and necessary for both self-localization after significant context switches and for replaying routes during sleep to allow for memory consolidation, the hippocampus is *not* necessary for online navigation. This prediction, which was originally made in Redish and Touretzky (1997a), follows from the hypothesis that the path integrator is extra-hippocampal. It has recently been confirmed by Alyan et al. (1997), who showed that rats continue to show path integration abilities during online navigation even after cytotoxic hippocampal lesions.

WHERE TO FROM HERE?

This book represents a snapshot of the interrelated fields of rodent navigation and hippocampal function, a look back over the last century to take stock of where we are (or were as of January 1998) before moving on. Although this book brings together a comprehensive theory of rodent navigation, it also leaves a number of questions open (see appendix C).

Of these, two important general questions that require exploratory experimental work before major theoretical work can be undertaken are

- *What is the representation of local view in the rodent?* Although important work has been done in the primate (for reviews, see Andersen et al., 1993, and Colby, Duhamel, and Goldberg, 1995), only preliminary work has been done in the rodent (Chen et al., 1994a, 1994b; McNaughton et al., 1994). An important consideration is that the primate parietal cortex consists of a host of subareas (Colby and Duhamel, 1991; Stein, 1992). Preliminary anatomical evidence suggests that this is also true of the rodent (Zilles, 1990).

• *How do rodents plan complex routes and avoid obstacles?* Animals are generally very successful at planning complex trajectories around obstacles, but it is not currently known how
this planning occurs, nor even how obstacles are represented
in the rodent brain. Until the neurophysiology is done to
find the neural correlates of obstacles, specific theoretical
work understanding the representation is very difficult.

Two important specific questions that are ready for theoretical
or simulation work are

• *Can the proposed path integration mechanism be made to track
actual trajectories of real animals?* How accurate can the mechanism described in chapter 6 be? What is required to make
it accurate? By simulating the head direction system accurately, unexpected complexities were found (for example,
the deformation of the tuning curve) that were not obvious
from the theoretical model (see chapter 5). No one has yet
reported an accurate simulation of two-dimensional path
integration based on the moving hill hypothesis.

• *What is the effect of changing the ratio of signal-to-noise in
the boundary conditions for the pseudo-winner-take-all (pWTA)
mechanism?* The two extremes show qualitatively different modes and can solve qualitatively different navigational
problems (self-localization and route replay; see chapter 11).
However, it is still unknown how a pWTA network behaves
as the sensory input signal is increased from zero (which
produces replay) to a strong signal (which produces recall).
Is there partial replay with weak signals? Is there a point
at which the system shows a phase change and suddenly
shows strong recall? Although the complex nonlinearities
of pWTA networks (see, for example, appendix A) make an
analytic solution extremely difficult, simulations would be
straightforward and might show very interesting effects.

In addition, there are a number of strong predictions we can
take from the specific hypotheses presented here, notably:

• *If it is true that the self-localization process occurs during awake
sharp waves and is a pseudo-winner-take-all (pWTA) process,*

then it should be possible to observe the self-localization process neurophysiologically. First, one needs to determine the place fields of each cell. This can be found by recording during an experience within an environment. Second, one needs to record the spikes of a cell population simultaneously during a self-localization process. The position represented by the population can be displayed at each moment by plotting the weighted sum of place fields (i.e., the sum of all fields of all cells that fired a spike at a moment in time). The representation should begin as a very broad (essentially uniform) distribution and then tighten up over the course of the self-localization process. In the end, it should be a coherent representation of the animal's position.

- *The hypothesized self-localization process should exhibit averaging of nearby candidate locations, but competition among distant candidate locations.* This can be tested behaviorally by examining the search time of animals (such as gerbils) in a two-landmark task. If the animals are trained to find food at the center of a pair of landmarks and then tested with the landmarks at varied distances, the distance between candidate locations can be experimentally controlled. At large distances, animals should alternate search between two locations, but at small distances, animals should search once in the center of the pair. Although gerbils have been shown to search at two locations when faced with a stretched pair of landmarks, and at the center of the pair when faced with the same pair as training (Collett, Cartwright, and Smith, 1986; Saksida et al., 1995; Redish, 1997), where this transition occurs has not been tested.

This synthesis of data and hypotheses of the rodent navigation domain offers an example of one way that systems-level theoretical neuroscience might be done. Taking a single, well-defined domain, we built up a comprehensive theory based on experimental and theoretical work done by many researchers. I believe that there are a number of other domains in systems-level neuroscience that are ripe for this kind of synthesis. These domains must (1) be well defined, (2) have extensive experimental results from a variety of paradigms, and (3) have extensive theoretical work on components of the system. Two examples that fit these criteria are procedural learning in the basal ganglia (see Houk, Davis, and Beiser, 1995, for a starting point) and the representation of egocentric space in primate parietal cortex (see Colby and Duhamel, 1991; Stein, 1992; Andersen et al., 1993; Pouget and Sejnowski, 1995).

FROM PLACE CELLS TO EPISODIC MEMORY

I began this book by saying that there were two major theories of hippocampal function, locale navigation (O'Keefe and Nadel, 1978) and episodic memory (Cohen and Eichenbaum, 1993). I then claimed that the episodic memory theory was not computational enough to pull together into a comprehensive, computational theory that made very specific predictions about specific tasks. I promised that when I had synthesized a theory of the role of the hippocampus in navigation, I would return to the question of the role of the hippocampus in episodic memory.

The key experimental results that have driven the episodic memory theory are (1) that hippocampal pyramidal cells show firing rates correlated to aspects of tasks beyond the location of the animal (O'Keefe and Conway, 1978; Kubie and Ranck, 1983; McNaughton, Barnes, and O'Keefe, 1983; Eichenbaum et al., 1987; Muller and Kubie, 1987; Thompson and Best, 1989; Otto and Eichenbaum, 1992b; Cohen and Eichenbaum, 1993; Hampson, Heyser, and Deadwyler, 1993; Markus et al., 1995; Gothard, Skaggs, and McNaughton, 1996; Gothard et al., 1996), (2) that after hippocampal lesions, patients have trouble remembering the events that happen in their lives (i.e., they show anterograde amnesia; Scoville and Milner, 1957; Milner, 1970; Luria, 1973; Cohen and Squire, 1980; Squire, 1992; Cohen and Eichenbaum, 1993), (3) that after hippocampal lesions, patients show a limited retrograde amnesia for events that happened prior to the lesions (Squire, 1992; Cohen and Eichenbaum, 1993; Rempel-Clower et al., 1996), and (4) that their learning of procedural tasks is close to normal (Scoville, 1968; Milner, 1970; Cohen and Eichenbaum, 1993; Squire and Knowlton, 1995). Additionally, many episodic memory theories hypothesize that the role of the hippocampus is to serve as a temporary memory buffer (Scoville and Milner, 1957; Milner, 1970; Marr, 1971; Squire, 1992; Cohen and Eichenbaum, 1993), in which memories are replayed during sleep (Marr, 1970, 1971; Buzsáki, 1989; McClelland, McNaughton, and O'Reilly, 1995; Shen and McNaughton, 1996; Skaggs and McNaughton, 1996; see also discussion in Seifert, 1983).

In examining the role of the hippocampus in navigation, we have addressed each of these components:

1. *Place cells are correlated to task parameters beyond the location of the animal.* In the navigation domain, place cells must be correlated to certain nonspatial parameters because the hippocampus represents space by multiple maps (chapter 10). As noted in chapter 10, this explains the difference between hippocampal cell responses to spatial parameters and to nonspatial. Cell responses to nonspatial parameters appear as a change in place field topologies across that nonspatial parameter.

2. *Hippocampal lesions produce anterograde amnesia in certain tasks.* Many spatial tasks are affected by hippocampal lesions. For example, animals with hippocampal lesions cannot learn the hidden platform water maze (Morris et al., 1982; Sutherland, Whishaw, and Kolb, 1983; Eichenbaum, Stewart, and Morris, 1990; Morris et al., 1990; Sutherland and Rodriguez, 1990). This is a form of anterograde amnesia. On the other hand, hippocampal lesions also affect nonspatial tasks (Cohen and Eichenbaum, 1993; Bunsey and Eichenbaum, 1995; Eichenbaum, 1996a). The nonspatial tasks affected by hippocampal lesions all entail a *context-switch* (i.e., they are all *offline* tasks; see chapters 8 and 13). Animals with hippocampal lesions are unable to recognize that they are being returned to a familiar context. In an animal with language, the animal would likely be un-

able to remember any specific events that happened within that context.

3. *Hippocampal lesions produce retrograde amnesia.* Whether hippocampal lesions produce retrograde amnesia in rodents has recently been questioned (Sutherland and Hoesing, 1993; Bohbot et al., 1996; Koerner et al., 1996; Weisend, Astur, and Sutherland, 1996; Koerner et al., 1997; see discussion in chapter 12), as has whether such lesions produce retrograde amnesia in primates (Nadel and Moscovitch, 1997; see discussion in chapter 12).

4. *Hippocampal lesions do not affect procedural learning.* The spatial analogue to procedural learning is taxon and praxic (route) navigation. As described in chapter 4 (see also chapter 2), the route navigation system is probably formed from subcortical structures optimized to learn stimulus-response mechanisms and to handle motor sequences. This sequence learning is exactly what the episodic memory theory identifies as procedural learning.

5. *Memories are replayed in the hippocampus.* The evidence that spatial memories are at least replayed in hippocampus is now quite strong (Pavlides and Winson, 1989; Wilson and McNaughton, 1994; Skaggs and McNaughton, 1996), and by looking at the navigation domain, we now have ideas about the possible mechanisms that might produce such replay (Shen and McNaughton, 1996; Redish and Touretzky, 1998a; see chapter 11).

The Role of the Hippocampus

In chapter 13, I argued that the role of the hippocampus in the navigation domain is twofold: (1) to reset an internal coordinate system, and (2) to replay recently traveled routes during sleep states (see chapter 13 for a discussion of the relation between these hypothesized roles and previous theories). Both of these functions, necessary for navigation, are also keys to episodic memory.

1. *Reinstantiation of Context.* The primary role of the hippocampus in the navigation domain seems to be to allow an animal to reset its internal coordinate system from external cues
   when it returns to a familiar environment (see chapters 8,
   9, and 13). The hippocampus must not only reset the path
   integrator coordinates; it must also recognize the external
   context in which navigation occurs. This is why hippocampal cells show different place field topologies under different conditions (see chapter 10). Thus the self-localization
   process described in chapter 9 is actually *recognizing* or *rein-
   stantiating the context.*

   An inability to successfully reinstantiate a context is one of
   the key problems that patients with hippocampal lesions
   have. They can hold a conversation, they can perform a
   task, but as soon as they are distracted, as soon as they have
   to leave a context and then return to it, they forget that they
   ever held that conversation, did the task, or experienced
   the context (Scoville and Milner, 1957; Milner, 1970; Squire,
   1992; Cohen and Eichenbaum, 1993). While monkeys with
   hippocampal lesions cannot perform a delayed nonmatch-
   to-sample (DNMS) task if they are removed from the context
   (Alvarez and Squire, 1994), they can if they are not (Murray
   and Mishkin, 1996).

2. *Replay of Recent Memories.* The secondary role of the hippocampus in the navigation domain seems to be to replay
   recently traveled routes (see chapters 8, 11, and 13). As
   discussed in chapter 12, the role of this replay is still not
   proved, but one likely role is to facilitate consolidation of
   memory from the hippocampal (locale navigation) system
   into long-term (route) memory.

   Because the hippocampus represents, not just location, but
   location within a reference frame, it represents the general
   context an animal has experienced as well as the sequence
   of locations. Thus when route sequences are replayed, the
   map within which the sequences occurred is also replayed.
   This means that the hippocampus is in fact replaying the

general context. This contextual replay would be exactly what the episodic memory theory would require.

It is not yet clear whether all memories are consolidated out of the hippocampus, nor is it clear exactly what the role of the hippocampus is in this consolidation. As discussed in chapter 12, the evidence for consolidation has recently been shown to be far weaker than previously thought. For example, certain memories do not seem to be consolidated out of the hippocampus (Koerner et al., 1996; Weisend, Astur, and Sutherland, 1996; Koerner et al., 1997). Also, many of the primate lesions believed to affect solely the hippocampus have been shown to actually affect adjacent structures (Scoville and Milner, 1957; Zola-Morgan and Squire, 1990; Murray, Gaffan, and Mishkin, 1993; Bachevalier and Meunier, 1996; Mumby et al., 1996; Rempel-Clower et al., 1996; Nadel and Moscovitch, 1997). The existence, extent, and exact dynamics of the role of the hippocampus in consolidation of memory thus remains an open question.

From Place Cells to Episodic Memory

While this book does not lay out a complete answer to the episodic memory question, it may be useful as a starting point. We have come from place cells to episodic memory. In our journey through the rodent navigation domain, we have seen examples of episodic memory in real tasks. We have seen how hippocampal cells show activity correlated to aspects beyond the location of the animal (multiple maps within the hippocampus; chapter 10), how an animal reinstantiates its context after certain kinds of delays (self-localization; chapter 9; see also chapter 14), and how memories are stored and replayed in the hippocampus (chapter 11). Even if we have not answered the episodic memory question completely, by understanding the navigation domain in depth and detail, we can begin to address episodic memory in a concrete way, with models of specific experiments that make explicit predictions in specific tasks.

Appendix A: Attractor Networks

Attractor networks play important roles in the theories explaining the various components described in this book. There are two important cases: one- and two-dimensions. In the one-dimensional case, cells are assumed to be located along a ring (as head direction cells are; see chapter 5); and, in the two-dimensional case, to be located around a torus. This appendix will review only the one-dimensional case. The two-dimensional analogy is straightforward.

Imagine a population of cells. Let each cell be associated with a direction (0°–360°). If cells with nearby preferred directions are more strongly interconnected (i.e., have a higher synaptic weight) than cells with distant preferred directions and there is global inhibition, then this system will have dynamics such that a stable state is a hill of activation. No matter what state the system starts in, as long as there is some activity in the system and no external input, the system will settle to a single hill of activation (see figure A.1). This local excitation, global inhibition connection structure has been studied by a number of researchers in one-dimension (Wilson and Cowan, 1973; Amari, 1977; Ermentrout and Cowan, 1979; Kishimoto and Amari, 1979; Kohonen, 1982, 1984; Skaggs et al., 1995; Redish, Elga, and Touretzky, 1996; Zhang, 1996; Redish and Touretzky, 1997b; Redish, 1997; Skaggs, 1997) and in two dimensions (Kohonen, 1982, 1984; Droulez and Berthoz, 1991; Munoz, Pélisson, and Guitton, 1991; Arai, Keller, and Edelman, 1994; McNaughton et al., 1996; Shen and McNaughton, 1996; Zhang, 1996; Redish and Touretzky, 1997b; Redish, 1997; Redish and Touretzky, 1998a; Samsonovich and McNaughton, 1997; Samsonovich, 1997).

Note that any direction is a stable attractor state and a coherent representation of direction. That is, the ring in figure 5.2 can

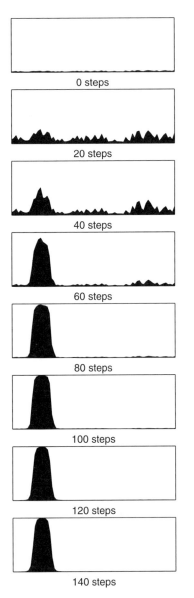

0 steps

20 steps

40 steps

60 steps

80 steps

100 steps

120 steps

140 steps

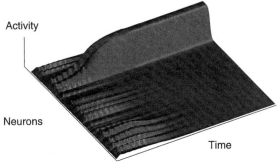

Figure A.1
Simulation of an attractor network settling to a coherent representation from noise. Each panel (*left*) shows the population activity of the excitatory neurons in a simulation of a one-dimensional attractor. The activity of each neuron at each moment in time is plotted at its preferred direction. Three-dimensional plot of activity of each neuron by time (*above*). The left panels plot slices of the right taken at different times. Similar simulations have been reported by Kohonen (1982, 1984), Redish, Elga, and Touretzky (1996), Zhang (1996), Redish (1997), Samsonovich and McNaughton (1997), and Samsonovich (1997).

be rotated to any direction. Although there is no "global north," indeed no correspondence to north or south at all, the system knows that when the population peak is at the top of the ring, the animal is facing 180° from when the population peak is at the bottom of the ring. While the system can represent any direction and differentiate the different directions, the correspondence between represented direction and environment is not hard-wired — it must be inferred by observation.

EXTERNAL EXCITATORY INPUT

What is the effect of excitatory input onto this attractor network? There are four possible cases, depending on the location and magnitude of the extrapopulation input. (I assume input only synapses on excitatory neurons.)

1. If an attractor network is in a stable state and receives input (synapsing on excitatory cells) that is peaked at the same direction as is currently being represented, then nothing will change. The attractor network will still be in a stable state representing the same direction. The overall activity in the attractor network may change slightly, but the represented direction will not change.

2. On the other hand, if the input is offset slightly, then the attractor network will precess until the new representation is centered at the input direction (Skaggs et al., 1995; Redish, Elga, and Touretzky, 1996; Zhang, 1996; Samsonovich and McNaughton, 1997). figure A.2 shows an attractor network with offset input, which quickly precesses from its current representation to a new representation compatible with the input.

3. If input is weak and offset by a large angle, the current representation will not change (Redish and Touretzky, 1997b; Redish, 1997). figure A.3 shows an attractor network with offset input that does not change the current representation.

4. Finally, if input is strong enough and offset by a large angle, the representation of the current direction will disappear and the activity will reappear at the offset location (Zhang, 1996; Redish and Touretzky, 1997b; Redish, 1997; Samsonovich and McNaughton, 1997; see figure A.4).

The two simulations shown in figures A.2 and A.3 used the same input strengths. When weak excitatory drive is input near the peak of a coherent representation, the peak precesses to align itself with the offset drive. But if weak excitatory drive is offset substantially from the peak, then the peak does not move.

This makes a prediction in cue conflict situations where external cues conflict with internal representations. If the external cues suggest a candidate location near the currently represented location, the representation will shift to match the cues. If all candidates are distant from the current representation, the representation will not change. Near and distant can be quantitatively defined as twice the breadth of the tuning curve of the component cells.

Figure A.5 demonstrates this effect. It shows the final represented direction when a small extra excitation is input offset from the center of the bump. When the extra excitation is input near to the center of the bump, the bump precesses (figure A.2), but when the excitation is input far from the center, there is no effect (see also figure A.3). Note that the effect of the external input is linear out to approximately $\pm 60°$, but vanishes very quickly beyond that.

SETTLING FROM NOISE

Figure A.1 shows a system settling from random noise. In chapter 9, it was argued that a two-dimensional attractor network settling from noise with biases provided by local view inputs could be used for self-localization. But what happens in cue-conflict situations where the biases do not all suggest the same location?

Even if an attractor network is initialized with a uniform random noise and two candidate biases are input the network will

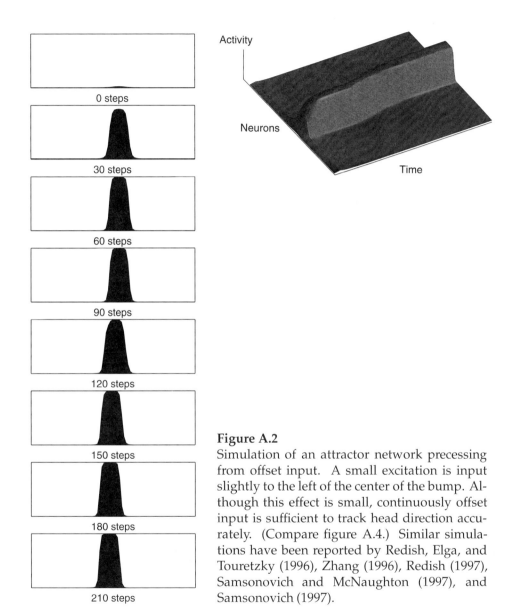

0 steps

30 steps

60 steps

90 steps

120 steps

150 steps

180 steps

210 steps

Activity

Neurons

Time

Figure A.2
Simulation of an attractor network precessing from offset input. A small excitation is input slightly to the left of the center of the bump. Although this effect is small, continuously offset input is sufficient to track head direction accurately. (Compare figure A.4.) Similar simulations have been reported by Redish, Elga, and Touretzky (1996), Zhang (1996), Redish (1997), Samsonovich and McNaughton (1997), and Samsonovich (1997).

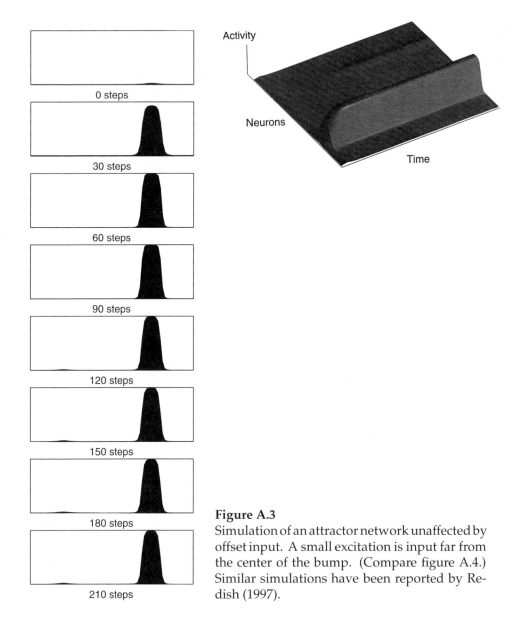

Figure A.3
Simulation of an attractor network unaffected by offset input. A small excitation is input far from the center of the bump. (Compare figure A.4.) Similar simulations have been reported by Redish (1997).

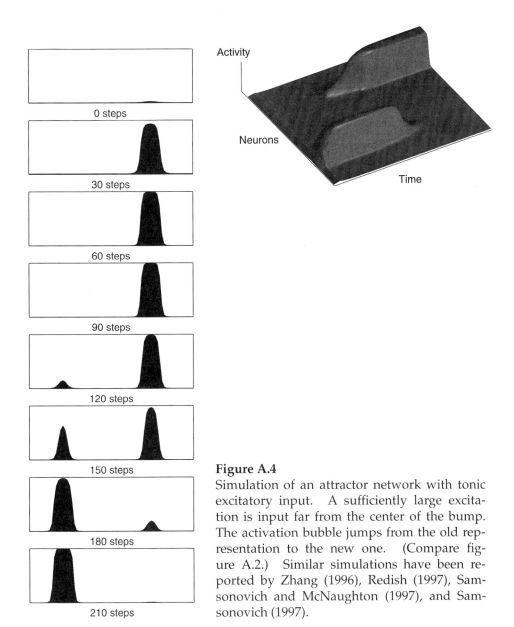

0 steps

30 steps

60 steps

90 steps

120 steps

150 steps

180 steps

210 steps

Activity

Neurons

Time

Figure A.4
Simulation of an attractor network with tonic excitatory input. A sufficiently large excitation is input far from the center of the bump. The activation bubble jumps from the old representation to the new one. (Compare figure A.2.) Similar simulations have been reported by Zhang (1996), Redish (1997), Samsonovich and McNaughton (1997), and Samsonovich (1997).

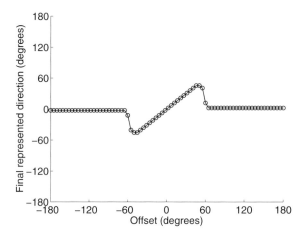

Figure A.5
Simulation of the influence of offset excitatory drive on final represented
direction of an attractor network.

still settle to a single hill of activation. However, where this hill
ends up depends on the separation of the locations of the two
biases. If the biases are near each other, then the hill will be at the
average of the two. If the biases are distant, then the hill will be
at the location of one or the other. In other words, nearby biases
average, but distal ones compete. This can be seen in figures A.6
and A.7.

   Although no one has yet shown averaging (the experiment
has not been done), an example of competition has been reported
by Collett, Cartwright, and Smith (1986) and replicated by Saksida et al. (1995, see also Redish, 1997), in which gerbils were
trained to dig for food at a point halfway between two landmarks. When the gerbils were tested (without food) with the
space between the landmarks doubled, they did not search at the
center; instead, they searched at two locations, each the correct
bearing and distance from one landmark.

   This suggests an interesting experimental prediction, one that
can be seen in either one dimension or two. For simplicity, I
will present the prediction in one dimension. Train an animal to
expect a small cue card (e.g. 5° width) in a standard cylindrical

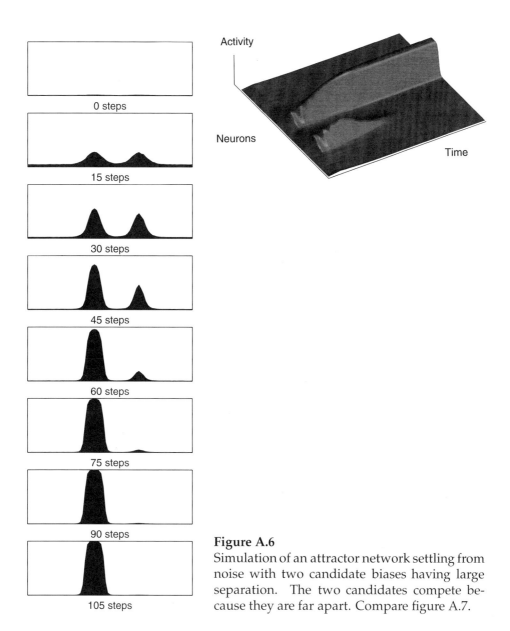

0 steps

15 steps

30 steps

45 steps

60 steps

75 steps

90 steps

105 steps

Activity

Neurons

Time

Figure A.6
Simulation of an attractor network settling from noise with two candidate biases having large separation. The two candidates compete because they are far apart. Compare figure A.7.

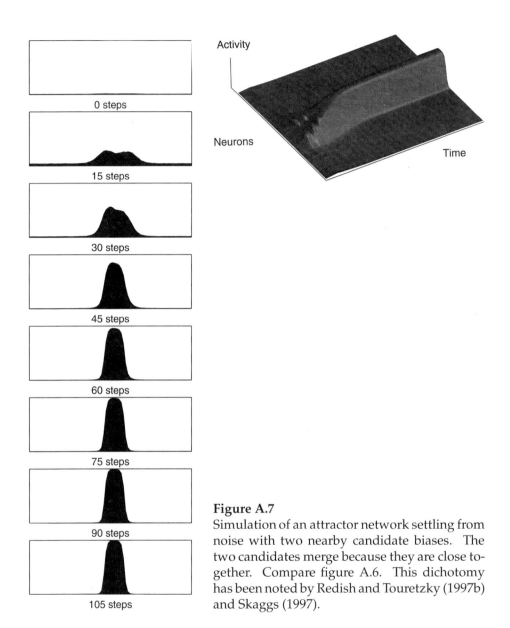

0 steps

15 steps

30 steps

45 steps

60 steps

75 steps

90 steps

105 steps

Figure A.7
Simulation of an attractor network settling from noise with two nearby candidate biases. The two candidates merge because they are close together. Compare figure A.6. This dichotomy has been noted by Redish and Touretzky (1997b) and Skaggs (1997).

environment. Then, while recording from head direction cells (chapter 5), place the animal in the environment in the dark. Spin the environment quickly until the animal is dizzy. Then turn the lights on and allow the animal to see two cue cards separated by an angle θ. When θ is small, the head direction tuning curves should follow the average of the two cue cards, but when θ is large, the tuning curves should follow one or the other (the cards should compete). This prediction is a consequence of the hypothesis that the head direction system is an attractor network (see chapter 5).

EXAMPLE CODE

To complete this appendix, I include the `Matlab` 5.0 program used to generate the examples above. It simulates 75 excitatory neurons and one inhibitory interneuron using a neuronal model based on a variant of the Wilson-Cowan equations (Wilson and Cowan, 1973; see also Pinto et al., 1996). The figures in this appendix were generated by varying the `IN` array.

```
function RESULTS = Attractor(figure_to_show)
%
% Attractor
%
% One dimensional attractor sample code
% Written for Matlab 5.0
%
% Written by A. David Redish, 1998,
% for the book _Beyond the Cognitive Map_,
% published by MIT Press, 1999.

global dt
global W_EI W_IE W_II W_EE
global tauE gammaE tauI gammaI

%-----------------------------
% set random seed
%-----------------------------

rand('state', 0)
```

```
%----------------------------
% PARAMETERS
%----------------------------

NE = 75;          % Number of excitatory neurons

dt = 0.001;       % time step, in ms

tauE = 0.01;      % time constant, excitatory neurons
gammaE = -1.5;    % tonic inhibition, excitatory neurons

tauI = 0.002;     % time constant, inhibitory neuron
gammaI = -7.5;    % tonic inhibition, inhibitory neuron

E = zeros(NE,1);  % allocate space for NE excitatory neurons
I = 0;            % one inhibitory neuron

W_EI = -8.0 * ones(NE,1);      % I -> E weights
W_IE = 0.880 * ones(1,NE);     % E -> I weights
W_II = -4.0;                   % I -> I weights
W_EE = BuildWeightMatrix(NE);  % E -> E weights

%----------------------------
% Input functions
%----------------------------

switch figure_to_show

 case 1,              % figure A.1

  IN = cat(1, ones(100,1) * rand(1,NE), zeros(100,NE))';

 case 2,              % figure A.2

  IN0 = exp(-(((1:75) - 35).^2)/25);
  IN1 = ones(100,1) * IN0;
  IN0 = 2 * exp(-(((1:75) - 40).^2)/25);
  IN2 = ones(200,1) * IN0;
  IN = cat(1,IN1,IN2)';

 case 3,              % figure A.3

  IN0 = exp(-(((1:75) - 20).^2)/25);
  IN1 = ones(100,1) * IN0;
  IN0 = exp(-(((1:75) - 60).^2)/25);
  IN2 = ones(200,1) * IN0;
  IN = cat(1,IN1,IN2)';

 case 4,               % figure A.4
```

```
   IN0 = exp(-(((1:75) - 20).^2)/25);
   IN1 = ones(100,1) * IN0;
   IN0 = 2 * exp(-(((1:75) - 60).^2)/25);
   IN2 = ones(200,1) * IN0;
   IN = cat(1,IN1,IN2)';

 case 6,              % figure A.6

  IN0 = 0.5 * (0.1 * rand(1,75) + exp(-(((1:75) - 25).^2)/40));
  IN1 = 0.5 * (0.1 * rand(1,75) + exp(-(((1:75) - 45).^2)/40));
  IN = (ones(150,1) * (IN0 + IN1))';

 case 7,              % figure A.7

  IN0 = 0.5 * (0.1 * rand(1,75) + exp(-(((1:75) - 29).^2)/40));
  IN1 = 0.5 * (0.1 * rand(1,75) + exp(-(((1:75) - 41).^2)/40));
  IN = (ones(150,1) * (IN0 + IN1))';

 otherwise, disp('Unknown input set')

end

%---------------------------
% CYCLE
%---------------------------

steps = size(IN,2);

RESULTS = zeros(NE,steps);

for t=1:steps

 VE = W_EI * I + W_EE * E + gammaE + IN(:,t);
 VI = W_II * I + W_IE * E + gammaI;

 FE = 0.5 + 0.5 * tanh(VE);
 FI = 0.5 + 0.5 * tanh(VI);

 E = E + dt/tauE * (-E + FE);
 I = I + dt/tauI * (-I + FI);

 RESULTS(:,t) = E;

end
```

```
%----------------------------
% DRAW
%----------------------------

figure(1)
clf
surfl(RESULTS);
shading interp
view([-30 75])
colormap(bone)
xlabel('time')
ylabel('neurons')
zlabel('activity')
set(gca,'Xtick',[])
set(gca,'Ytick',[])
set(gca,'Ztick',[])

figure(2)
clf
timeslices = 1:(steps/10):steps;
for i=1:8
 subplot(8,1,i);

 fill([1 1:NE NE],[0 RESULTS(:,timeslices(i))' 0],'k');
 axis([1 NE 0 1]);
 xlabel([num2str(timeslices(i)-1) ' steps'])
 set(gca,'Xtick',[]);
 set(gca,'Ytick',[]);

end

%----------------------------
% Build Weight Matrix
%----------------------------
function W = BuildWeightMatrix(NE)

stddevConst = 15;       % degrees
Wconst = 6.0;           % weight constant

variance = stddevConst^2 / (360^2) * NE ^2;

i = ones(NE,1) * (1:NE);
j = (1:NE)' * ones(1,NE);

d_choices = cat(3,abs(j + NE - i), abs(i + NE - j), abs(j - i));
d = min(d_choices, [], 3);

W = exp(-d .* d / variance);
W = Wconst * W./(ones(75,1) * sum(W));
```

Appendix **B**: Selective Experimental Review

One of the advantages of rodent navigation as a domain for studying information processing in the brain is that there is a vast literature of experimental results in a variety of paradigms, including anatomical, behavioral, neurophysiological, and neuropharmacological. This literature ranges back over most of the twentieth century. In this appendix, I review the key experimental results that have informed this book.

A comprehensive experimental review of the rodent navigation data would add hundreds of pages to an already long book. This review will concentrate on data from the last twenty years. For a review of the hippocampal data prior to 1978, I refer the reader to O'Keefe and Nadel (1978). Gallistel (1990) also contains a good review of the early literature, particularly the behavioral literature. For a review of the primate data (both human and nonhuman), I refer the reader to Cohen and Eichenbaum (1993). Finally, for an experiment-by-experiment review (with each experiment detailed separately), I refer the reader to chapter 2 of my Ph.D. dissertation (Redish, 1997).

ANATOMY

The existence of an anatomical connection does not imply that it must be required for proper function of the navigational system, although the lack of an anatomical connection can be troubling for a theoretical hypothesis. Because the anatomy of the navigation system is extremely complex and not completely known, and because the relation of anatomical data to theory may be complex, I reviewed the anatomy of each structure as it was required and will not review it again here.

BEHAVIORAL AND LESION DATA

The Water Maze

The water maze, first introduced by Morris (1981); see figure 2.1, consists of a large pool of water mixed with milk, chalk, or paint so as to make the water opaque. Somewhere in the pool, there is a platform on which the rodent can stand and be out of the water. Sometimes the platform is submerged just below the surface; this is called the *hidden platform water maze*. Other times, the platform sticks out above the surface; this is called the *visible water maze*. Sometimes the location of the platform is indicated by a colocalized cue (such as a light bulb hanging directly over the platform). Even when hidden, this colocalized cue indicates the location of the platform. This version is called the *cued water maze* and is similar to the visible water maze.

Morris (1981) found that normal rodents placed in the pool quickly learn to swim to a consistently located platform, even if it is hidden. If the platform is then removed from the pool, the animals spend most of their time near the location the platform used to be, which shows that the animals know the location of the platform and have an expectation of its location.

The water maze has been used to examine effects of lesions (Morris et al., 1982; Milner and Lines, 1983; Sutherland, Whishaw, and Kolb, 1983; Schenk and Morris, 1985; Kolb and Walkey, 1987; Sutherland, Whishaw, and Kolb, 1988; DiMattia and Kesner, 1988; Annett, McGregor, and Robbins, 1989; Dean, 1990; Eichenbaum, Stewart, and Morris, 1990; Morris et al., 1990; Sutherland and Rodriguez, 1990; Packard and McGaugh, 1992; Taube, Klesslak, and Cotman, 1992; McDonald and White, 1993; Sutherland and Hoesing, 1993; McDonald and White, 1994; Alvarado and Rudy, 1995a, 1995b; Nagahara, Otto, and Gallagher, 1995; Whishaw, Cassel, and Jarrard, 1995; Whishaw and Jarrard, 1996; Schallert et al., 1996); neuropharmacological manipulations (Schallert, De Ryck, and Teitelbaum, 1980; Sutherland, Whishaw, and Regehr, 1982; DeVietti et al., 1985; Whishaw, 1985; Packard and White, 1991; Day and Schallert, 1996); grafts (Nilsson et al., 1987; Bjorklund, Nilsson, and Kalen,

1990); genetic mutants (Silva et al., 1992; Tsien, Huerta, and Tonegawa, 1996; Wilson and Tonegawa, 1997); and aging (Gallagher and Burwell, 1989; Gallagher, Burwell, and Burchinal, 1993; Gallagher and Nicole, 1993; Gallagher and Colombo, 1995; Gallagher, Nagahara, and Burwell, 1995; Barnes et al., 1997; Barnes, 1998). I will review each of these effects in turn.

Lesions

Hippocampal or fimbria-fornix lesions impair navigation to hidden but not visible or cued platforms (Morris et al., 1982; Sutherland, Whishaw, and Kolb, 1983; Eichenbaum, Stewart, and Morris, 1990; Morris et al., 1990; Sutherland and Rodriguez, 1990; Packard and McGaugh, 1992). Morris et al. (1982, 1990) found that hippocampally lesioned rats swam in stereotyped circles the correct distance from the wall. Rats with ibotenic hippocampal lesions show a complete inability to remember learned water mazes out to thirty-six weeks (i.e., they show retrograde amnesia; Koerner et al., 1996; Weisend, Astur, and Sutherland, 1996; Koerner et al., 1997.

A number of authors have lesioned the fimbria-fornix as a simpler hippocampal lesion (Eichenbaum, Stewart, and Morris, 1990; Sutherland and Rodriguez, 1990; Packard and McGaugh, 1992; Whishaw, Cassel, and Jarrard, 1995). Most authors suggest that fornix lesions are similar to hippocampal lesions: they impair acquisition of a hidden but not a visible platform (Sutherland and Rodriguez, 1990; Packard and McGaugh, 1992) . Eichenbaum, Stewart, and Morris (1990) and Whishaw, Cassel, and Jarrard (1995) both report that fornix-lesioned animals cannot learn the water maze with a variable start, but that they can learn the task if they are always started from the same place or if there is a cue identifying the path to take.

An important consideration is that while a fimbria-fornix lesion severs the cholinergic input to the hippocampus, the connections from the subiculum to the nucleus accumbens, and the postsubicular connections to the lateral mammillary nuclei, it does not sever the hippocampus–entorhinal cortex connections (neither EC → HC nor HC → EC). Therefore fimbria-fornix lesions are not equivalent to hippocampal lesions.

Rats with hippocampal or fimbria-fornix lesions can learn to perform the hidden platform water maze under certain conditions (Morris et al., 1990; Whishaw, Cassel, and Jarrard, 1995; Schallert et al., 1996; Whishaw and Jarrard, 1996). When Whishaw, Cassel, and Jarrard (1995) trained animals with fimbria-fornix lesions to find a visible platform and then removed the visible platform, the animals concentrated their search where the platform had been. Whishaw and Jarrard (1996) have shown the same effect with cytotoxic hippocampal lesions. Schallert et al. (1996) used animals with kainate-colchicine hippocampal lesions (destroying both DG and the CA3/CA1 fields). The animals were first trained with a large platform that filled almost the entire maze. Once the animals could reach the platform reliably, it was shrunk trial by trial until it was the same size as a typical platform in a water maze task. With this training regimen, the animals could learn to solve the water maze without a hippocampus.

Morris et al. (1990) reported a similar result when they trained their animals on forty-eight trials with interspersed hidden and cued platforms. Neither hippocampal nor subicular lesions alone were sufficient to produce deficits, but combined hippocampal and subicular lesions still produced deficits.

Rats with colchicine lesions (destroying DG but leaving CA3 and CA1 intact; Goldschmidt and Steward, 1980) show impairments in hidden platform water maze tasks if given the lesion one week after training, but not if given the lesion twelve weeks after training (Sutherland and Hoesing, 1993). When McNaughton et al. (1989) also examined the effect of colchicine lesions on acquisition (but not retention) of the water maze, they found that colchicine lesions produced severe deficits.

Whereas hippocampal lesions/inactivation impair navigation to hidden platforms, caudate nucleus lesions/inactivation impair navigation to visible platforms. In the water maze, lesions of the caudate nucleus disrupt navigation to cued platforms, such as visible platforms or platforms with a large black card marking the quadrant containing the goal, but not to hidden platforms (Packard and McGaugh, 1992; McDonald and White, 1994).

McDonald and White (1994) trained rats in the water maze for twelve days, on the first three days with a visible platform, but on the fourth day with a hidden platform at the same location. This four-day sequence was repeated three times. After these twelve days, the animals were tested with a visible platform in a new location. Half of the animals went to the new visible platform, half went to the location where the old platform had been. With hippocampal inactivation (by lidocaine), all of the animals went to the new platform, whereas with caudate inactivation, all of the animals went to the old location.

Packard and McGaugh (1992) compared caudate and fornix lesions on a water maze with two platforms, one stable, one unstable. If the animals tried to climb up on the unstable platform, they fell back into the water. Both platforms were hidden. Packard and McGaugh ran two versions of the experiment. In the first version, the stable platform was always in one quadrant, while the other was always in the opposite, so location of the platform denoted its stability; in the second version, the platforms alternated quadrants randomly from trial to trial, but a visual cue demarcated which of the two was stable. They found that fornix lesions impaired acquisition of the location-stable platform, but caudate lesions did not affect the performance on the location-stable platform. On the other hand, caudate lesions impaired acquisition of the cue-stable platform, but fornix lesions did not affect the ability to find the cue-stable platform.

Rats with subiculum lesions appeared to search randomly as if they had never seen the environment before (Morris et al., 1990). While hippocampal animals circle the environment at the correct distance from the wall (implying that they may know some information about the location of the hidden platform), subicular animals wander the environment seemingly at random.

The effects of entorhinal lesions (Schenk and Morris, 1985; Nagahara, Otto, and Gallagher, 1995) are much less consistent, sparing certain abilities (such as crossing the actual platform location) while producing deficits in other abilities (such as spending time in the correct quadrant). Nagahara, Otto, and Gallagher (1995) found that rats with entorhinal lesions were more impaired after a 5-minute delay relative to a 30-second delay. In contrast, Schenk and Morris (1985) found extensive spatial deficits with both acquisition and retention, but Schenk and Morris admit that their "entorhinal" lesions encroached on presubiculum, parasubiculum, and subiculum proper, any or all of which may have had strong effects.

Nucleus accumbens lesions also produce deficits in naive rats on the hidden platform version, but not on the visible platform or in pretrained rats (Annett, McGregor, and Robbins, 1989; Sutherland and Rodriguez, 1990). Annett, McGregor, and Robbins (1989) report that their rats did eventually learn the task, although they were never as good as normals. We should note, however, that the lesions were incomplete.

Anterior cingulate lesions have no effect on learning the water maze, but animals with posterior cingulate lesions can not learn to go directly to a hidden platform (Sutherland, Whishaw, and Kolb, 1988; Sutherland and Hoesing, 1993). Sutherland and Hoesing report that when unilateral hippocampal lesions are combined with contralateral posterior cingulate lesions the deficits are as severe as bilateral hippocampal or bilateral cingulate lesions — in other words, devastating. These effects occur even if the cingulate lesions are made twelve weeks after training.

Lesions to the anterior thalamic nuclei (ATN) produce severe deficits in the water maze (Sutherland and Rodriguez, 1990), as do postsubicular (PoS) lesions (Taube, Klesslak, and Cotman, 1992). Taube, Klesslak, and Cotman found that although performance in the water maze was impaired relative to normals, performance did improve over time. Neither study found errors in the cued water maze.

Lesions to the parietal cortex produce severe deficits in cued water maze tasks (Kolb and Walkey, 1987; DiMattia and Kesner, 1988; Kolb, 1990a). Animals with parietal lesions show poor initial heading errors even with cued platforms (Kolb and Walkey, 1987). Kolb (1990a) reports that the animals never improve their initial trajectory, even with visual cues indicating the location of the platform; DiMattia and Kesner (1988) suggest that animals are reduced to random search strategies with parietal lesions.

Lesions to superior colliculus impair navigation to visible, cued and hidden platforms in the water maze (Milner and Lines, 1983). Even giving the animals time on the platform does not improve performance.

Te2-lesioned rats[1] are unable to learn a visual match to sample, even with no delay, but they can learn the hidden platform water maze (Kolb, 1990a). In contrast to posterior parietal lesions, Te2 lesioned rats are poor at visual pattern discriminations, but not at spatial orientation discriminations (Kolb, 1990a). They are unable to learn to perform a visual match to sample, even with no delay (Kolb, 1990a). But they can learn the hidden-platform water maze normally.

Neuropharmacological Manipulations

One consequence of fimbria-fornix lesions is to remove the cholinergic input into the hippocampus. Rats treated with atropine sulfate show no improvement in finding platforms that remain in a single location over animals shown random platform locations (Sutherland, Whishaw, and Regehr, 1982), although, given enough training, they can learn the location of a single hidden platform (Whishaw, 1985). Sutherland, Whishaw, and Regehr also report that the number of times the atropine-infused animals reared when on the platform did not decrease from trial to trial. Whishaw found that the treated rats could not learn a set of places, although normals could, if, for example, the platform was moved through a regular sequence of locations. When rats that had acquired a learning set were treated with atropine, their performance was totally disrupted.

Acetylcholine (ACh) may be involved in resolving interference (Hasselmo and Bower, 1993; Hasselmo and Schnell, 1994) or in the separation of hippocampal maps (Redish and Touretzky, 1997a; see chapter 10). ACh may also affect other structures downstream from hippocampus (such as nucleus accumbens; see also discussion in review of *Radial Arm Maze*, below).

Using a large platform, which they slowly shrank, Day and Schallert (1996) were able to train animals to find a hidden platform. This procedure, which can also be used to train animals with hippocampal lesions (Schallert et al., 1996), may allow the training of route navigation strategies (see chapter 2).

Grafts

If the main effect of fimbria-fornix lesions is to remove the cholinergic input from the hippocampus, then it may be possible to graft fetal tissue into the septal areas, and, by reinnervating the hippocampus, to restore hippocampal function. Nilsson et al. (1987) have done just that. When they lesioned fimbria, fornix, and corpus callosum and then grafted fetal septal tissue into the third ventricle near the dorsal hippocampus, they found (1) fimbria-fornix transection disrupted spatial learning; (2) animals with grafts were able to use spatial cues, although they were impaired relative to normals both in learning time and in spatial accuracy; and (3) atropine sulfate disrupted the spatial ability of animals with grafts.

Bjorklund, Nilsson, and Kalen (1990) showed that the fetal septal grafts reinnervated the hippocampus with a similar layering to that seen in normal animals. They also reviewed data that rats with combined septal and raphe (supplying serotonin) lesions required both septal and raphe grafts to see improvements in the water maze, and that the raphe transplants showed similar afferentations to that of normal animals.

Genetic Mutants

The technology now exists to produce animals with deficits in specific areas, specific neurotransmitters, even specific receptors. While I do not have the room to review the recent genetics advances here, I want to note two recent studies examining genetic mutants in the water maze.

Silva et al. (1992) developed a mouse with a malfunctioning NMDA receptor, and found that it could not learn the water maze. Tsien et al. (1996) developed a mouse with malfunctioning

NMDA receptors only in CA1. NMDA receptors are involved in long-term potentiation. These mice also could not learn the water maze (Tsien, Huerta, and Tonegawa, 1996; Wilson and Tonegawa, 1997).

Aging

Although normal old rats generally show deficits in all standard measures on the hidden platform water maze, they do not on the cued or visible platform version (Gallagher, Burwell, and Burchinal, 1993; Barnes et al., 1997; see Barnes, 1998, for a review). Barnes et al. (1997) report that both young and old animals show a distinct bimodality in their ability to solve the hidden platform water maze — on some trials, they take relatively direct paths to the goal; on others they are severely impaired. In normal young animals, the short trials soon dominate, but in old animals, the long trials continue to perseverate even after extensive training.

Latent Learning

To examine latent learning in the hidden platform water maze, Sutherland et al. (1987) placed a barrier across the middle of the tank so that the animals could only experience half of the maze when searching for the platform. They then removed the barrier and allowed the animals to start from the other half (in which they had no experience) and found that animals were severely impaired in finding the hidden platform. However, Matthews et al. (1995) point out that the Sutherland et al. (1987) task is confounded by the existence (and then absence) of a very salient cue — the barrier. Matthews et al. repeated the experiment, but moved the barrier slowly away from the animal, so that on one trial it allowed access to half the arena and on the next it allowed access to a little more than half, and on the next, more than that, and so on. At first, the animals went to examine the barrier, but they quickly learned to ignore it. After they had learned to ignore it, the animals were tested starting from a part of the maze in which they had never been; they went directly to the platform. In another experiment in the water maze, Keith and

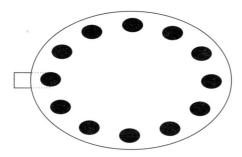

Figure B.1
Hole board circular platform. Black circles indicate holes in the board. One hole leads to a hidden nest. The arena is bathed in bright light. In order to escape the bright light, rats try to find the hole with the nest where they can hide.

McVety (1988) also showed that animals could learn to navigate to a platform through a part of the environment in which they had no experience.

The Hole Board Circular Platform

The hole board arena, introduced by Barnes (1979; see figure B.1) consists of a large open platform, bathed in bright light. Around the edge of the platform are holes, one of which allows access to an escape tunnel. Like the water maze, the hole board forces animals to use distal cues to find an escape route from an aversive stimulus (in this case, bright light). It differs in that the animals have to choose among discrete holes rather than find a hidden platform in a continuum of open water. Because the holes are all around the edge of the platform, it would be sufficient to know the orientation of the escape hole.

Old animals show deficits in finding a hidden location in the hole board circular platform (Barnes, 1979). Young animals show better retention of the location of the escape hole even after a week's delay (Barnes, Nadel, and Honig, 1980). Barnes (1979) found that both old and young animals showed three basic behavioral patterns: (1) they examined many holes with many center-crossings; (2) they systematically explored the holes, going from one hole to the next; and (3) they took a direct path to the escape hole. Early on, rats showed the first pattern, followed eventually by the second, and finally (after enough trials) the third. Although old animals were impaired on this task, they did show a spatial strategy in that when the tunnel was moved, their latency to goal increased significantly. Like rats on the water maze, even after the location of the escape tunnel is changed, animals with a nonspatial strategy (such as check all holes randomly) will not increase the latency to reach the goal, while animals who prefer to keep trying to use a spatial strategy will (Barnes, 1979).

As reviewed in *Water Maze Lesions* above, colchicine destroys the dentate granule fields while sparing the CA3 and CA1 hippocampal fields (Goldschmidt and Steward, 1980). McNaughton et al. (1989) report that animals with colchicine lesions showed many more errors than controls and were relatively less impaired when the escape hole was changed, implying they were using a nonspatial strategy to find the escape tunnel.

Bach et al. (1995) tried to train mice who had been genetically engineered to be deficient in long-term potentiation under certain conditions. LTP was ineffective *in vitro* when shocks were given at a frequency of 5–10 Hz, but LTP was still normal when the stimulus was in the 100 Hz range. Bach et al. found that animals could not learn the location of the escape hole based on the distal cues.

Small, Enclosed Arenas

Although small, enclosed arenas (see figure B.2) have generally been used to examine the effects of environmental manipulations on place cells (see *NEUROPHYSIOLOGY*, below), some important behavioral experiments performed in these apparati. When Otto et al. (1996) examined a task that paired an odor with a location (given a specific odor, go to a specific location), they found that lateral entorhinal cortex lesions produced occasional odor

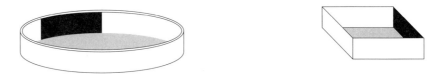

Figure B.2
Small, enclosed arenas. Food is scattered on the floor of a small cylinder
or rectangle. Typical cylinder diameters are 50–100 cm.

discrimination errors (animal went to the location indicated by
the wrong odor). When the lesions encroached on medial entorhinal cortex, the animals also occasionally made spatial errors
(animal went to a location not associated with any odor).

Disoriented rats cannot learn to differentiate two geometrically similar but identifiably different corners (Cheng, 1986);
nondisoriented rats have no trouble differentiating these two corners (Margules and Gallistel, 1988). Cheng tried to train rats to
find food at one corner of a rectangular arena (figure B.2). To
make the corners as distinct as possible, he placed a panel at each
one, covered with a different type of material. In addition, the
panels had different numbers of pinholes through which light
was visible, and two of the panels had unique odorants behind
them. Cheng disoriented the rats before placing them in the arena
at a random location, and found that although the rats were able
to distinguish one pair of diagonally opposed corners from the
other, they could not distinguish the two corners in each pair.
The animals chose the correct corner in approximately 50 percent
of the trials, and the corner opposite it in the other 50 percent.
This suggests that the rats are sensitive to the geometric structure of the environment, and were ignoring other cues that could
distinguish between the two corners.[2] Margules and Gallistel
replicated the experiment without disorientation and found that
most animals had no difficulty selecting the correct corner more

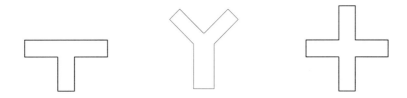

Figure B.3
T, Y, and plus mazes. Typical arm lengths are 50 cm.

than 75 percent of the time; some achieved better than 90 percent success rates.

These results are consistent with the disorientation results of (Knierim, Kudrimoti, and McNaughton, 1995; see chapter 5) in which head direction cells no longer respond to a cue card after enough trials begun with disorientation.

T-, Y-, and Plus Mazes

Tolman, Ritchie, and Kalish (1946b) found that rats can be more easily trained to go to a place than to engage in a response. They tested rats on a plus maze (see figure B.3), training one group to always turn left, whether started from the north or south arm of the plus, and training the other group to go to a place (e.g., turn left from the north arm and right from the south, always going east). Place-learning rats took from 11 to 18 trials to reach a criterion of 10 perfect trials. In contrast, the response-learning rats took 25 or more trials, and four of seven never reached criterion in 72 trials.

Barnes, Nadel, and Honig (1980) tested old and young animals on a T-maze (see figure B.3) with differing textures on the floor of the two goal arms. Animals were trained to always make a right turn with the T always in the same orientation. This allows the animals to use three strategies (see chapter 2): a cue strategy (taxon navigation; turn based on floor texture), a response strategy (praxic navigation; always turn right), or a spatial strategy (locale navigation; go to a place). These can be differentiated by flipping the textures, rotating the T, and moving the distal cues.

Both young and old animals were most likely to use response strategies, but young animals used place strategies much more than old. One problem with this experiment is that animals may switch strategies depending on the amount of training received. This was explicitly explored by Packard and McGaugh (1996), who tested rats on a plus maze: rats were always started on the south arm and trained to turn left (to the west arm). The animals were given four trials per day for seven days. On the eighth day, they were placed on the north arm. They all turned right (to the west arm). This demonstrates that they were using a place or locale strategy (see chapter 2). The animals were then trained for seven more days to turn left from the south arm to the west arm. Then, on the sixteenth day, they were again placed on the north arm. They all turned left (to the east arm), demonstrating a response or praxic strategy (see chapter 2). Packard and McGaugh then inactivated the caudate nucleus (with lidocaine) and tested the animals on the north arm. All of the animals turned right, indicating the place strategy again.

The Y-maze (see figure B.3) has been used to demonstrate latent learning (see Tolman, 1948, for a review). This maze includes a food reward at the end of one arm of the Y and a water reward at the other. Animals were allowed to explore this environment but were neither hungry or thirsty. Half of the animals were then made hungry and the other half thirsty. The hungry animals immediately ran to the food source and thirsty animals to the water source. This demonstrates that animals do not have to be strongly rewarded for them to learn goal locations.

Hirsh, Leber, and Gillman (1978) also ran rats on the Y-maze with food at one end and water at the other. Animals were hungry or thirsty on alternate days. Normal animals learned this task easily, going to the food source when hungry and to the water source when thirsty, while animals with fornix-lesions could not learn both tasks, learning one task completely and then unlearning it as they learned the other. In other words, they could learn to go to one of the arms, but could not remember two rewards on two arms.

The Y-maze has also been used to examine delayed non-match-to-sample tasks, where at the ends of the arms are goal boxes with different local cues inside them. Animals are trained to alternate between them. This task is strongly related to spontaneous alternation behavior (Dember and Richman, 1989). This task is only hippocampally dependent when the goal boxes are large enough to become *contexts* (Rawlins et al., 1993; Cassaday and Rawlins, 1995, 1997).

Radial Arm Maze

The radial arm maze, shown in figure B.4, consists of a central platform with thin arms radiating out from it. A four-arm radial maze is essentially equivalent to the plus maze (figure B.3). This task has been studied under a number of different conditions, including after cue manipulations (Olton and Samuelson, 1976; Suzuki, Augerinos, and Black, 1980), while recording extracellularly (McNaughton, Barnes, and O'Keefe, 1983; Mizumori and Williams, 1993; Chen et al., 1994a, 1994b; McNaughton, Knierim, and Wilson, 1994; Lavoie and Mizumori, 1994; Young, Fox, and Eichenbaum, 1994; Markus et al., 1995; Mizumori and Cooper, 1995; Dudchenko and Taube, 1997); after neuropharmacological manipulations (Decker and McGaugh, 1991; Ohta, Matsumoto, and Watanabe, 1993; Shen et al., 1996); after lesions (Olton, Becker, and Handelmann, 1980; Taube, Klesslak, and Cotman, 1992; Jarrard, 1993; Floresco, Seamans, and Phillips, 1997); after grafts (Shapiro et al., 1989; Hodges et al., 1991a, 1991b); and in aged animals (Barnes, Nadel, and Honig, 1980; Barnes, 1988; Mizumori, Lavoie, and Kalyani, 1996; Mizumori and Kalyani, 1997; see Barnes, 1998, for a review).

Olton and Samuelson (1976) first introduced the radial maze as a spatial *working memory* task: Each arm of the maze was baited; after the reward was taken from the end of an arm, the arm was not rebaited. This meant that if an animal returned to an arm it had already visited, it did not receive any additional reward. Returning to an unbaited arm was scored as a *working memory error*. In the *delayed working memory* version of this task,

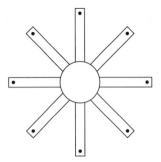

Figure B.4
Radial arm maze. Black ovals indicate food locations. Each arm is baited only once. Some mazes also include gates at the entrances to each arm. In some paradigms, some arms are never baited. Typical arm lengths are 50–100 cm.

the animals are allowed to enter three of the arms, then a delay is imposed, after which the rats can enter any arm. In the *reference memory version*, some of the arms are never baited (Olton, Becker, and Handelmann, 1979), which forces the animals to remember those arms across all trials.

Olton and Samuelson (1976) found that rats chose an average of more than seven different arms in their first eight choices. This suggests that the animals are able to recognize the different arms. Although they don't use an easily recognizable search pattern, they are still able to differentiate the arms. By interchanging arms, Olton and Samuelson were able to show that animals were going to spatial locations not to some local cue identified with the arms of the maze.

Rats could also be trained to use a cued version of the task in which the arms had distinctive floor textures and the arms were rotated after each choice (Olton, Becker, and Handelmann, 1979). Unfortunately, this task includes a strong delay component after each choice as the arms are rotated, and there is no way to remove that delay component from the cued version of the task.

Olton and Samuelson (1976) showed that even in the delayed version, rats skip the previously visited arms and only choose the remaining arms once. Accuracy is not dependent on time of delay but only on the number of choices experienced before the delay.

The behavior of rats is sensitive to the constellation of external cues, not to individual ones. Suzuki, Augerinos, and Black (1980) tested rats on the eight-arm radial maze: they allowed the animals to retrieve food from three of the eight arms and then gave the rats a delay. During the delay the landmarks were rotated as a group by 180°. When the animals were returned to the maze, they looked for food in the 180° rotational equivalent of the arms they had not been in before. In contrast, when landmarks were permuted rather than rotated, the rats behaved as if the environment were unfamiliar. This implies that rats are sensitive to combinations of distal landmarks.

Jarrard (1993) found that rats with hippocampal and fimbria-fornix lesions show both reference memory and working memory place errors. Using two different tasks, a place task in which never-baited arms depended on extramaze cues and a cue task in which the never-baited arms depended on intramaze cues, Jarrard found that animals with ibotenic hippocampal lesions made both reference memory and working memory errors on the place task but not on the cue task. On the other hand, he also found that animals trained on the place task before surgery did not show the same errors.

Floresco, Seamans, and Phillips (1997) tested both nondelayed and delayed versions of the radial maze with bilateral infusions of lidocaine into the ventral aspects of CA1 and subiculum. They found no effect when the lidocaine was injected before training but found a significant effect when it was injected after training, in particular, rats with lesions made more across-delay errors. They also tested disconnection lesions of ventral CA1 and subiculum with nucleus accumbens and ventral CA1 and subiculum with prelimbic frontal cortex. They found no effect of crossed subiculum/prelimbic lesions on the nondelayed version, but found a strong effect on the delayed version. Conversely, they found no effect of crossed subiculum/nucleus accumbens lesions on the delayed version, but found a strong effect on the nondelayed version.

Seamans and Phillips (1994) tested a delayed version of the radial maze and found that lidocaine injected into nucleus accumbens affected the abilities of animals when infused during the delay and when infused prior to the predelay phase, though less so. When they tested a cued version where animals had to find food on the same four arms of an eight-arm maze before and after the delay, they found that lidocaine in nucleus accumbens had no effect on this second task.

Potegal (1982) showed that caudate lesions impair certain navigation tasks on radial mazes. Animals were trained on a twelve-arm radial maze in which the food was located on a single arm at a constant angle from the starting arm. This meant that the only viable strategy to find the food was to go to the center of the maze and make a turn at that angle. Caudate lesions impaired the animals' ability to find the food.

To test reference memory, McNaughton et al. (1989) trained animals on an eight-arm radial maze. They baited one arm of the maze; a different arm each day, but the same arm all that day. Animals with colchicine infusions (which destroys the dentate gyrus granule cells) made more errors than normals.

To examine working memory and reference memory across the cue-spatial axis, Rasmussen, Barnes, and McNaughton (1989) examined rats on a collection of tasks on the radial maze. For nonspatial reference memory, one floor-texture-cued arm was baited; for spatial reference memory, one externally-cued arm was baited. For nonspatial working memory, four arms of the eight were baited and rearranged after each choice (forcing this to be a delayed version); for spatial working memory, rats were allowed to visit four arms, and, after a delay was imposed, allowed to visit any of the eight arms. Rats with entorhinal lesions took longer to reach criterion on the spatial reference memory and working memory tasks, but not on the nonspatial tasks.

Taube, Klesslak, and Cotman (1992) found that postsubicular lesions affected performance on the radial maze. Although lesioned animals did improve with additional training, they never reached the levels of normals even with fifteen days of training.

Old animals make many working memory errors on the radial maze (Barnes, Nadel, and Honig, 1980; Mizumori, Lavoie, and Kalyani, 1996). Barnes, Nadel, and Honig (1980) found that old animals repeated 30 percent more sequences than young animals. Mizumori, Lavoie, and Kalyani (1996) found that old animals make almost three times as many errors as young animals on the radial maze.

Scopolomine infusions also impair performance on the radial maze (Eckerman et al., 1980; Wirsching et al., 1984; Buresova, Bolhuis, and Bures, 1986; Hodges et al., 1991a, 1991b). Buresova, Bolhuis, and Bures (1986) tested rats in a water tank modification of the radial maze: each arm was an underwater track in which the animals could swim; goals were small platforms at the ends of each arm, which could be dropped to the bottom as a means of de-baiting the arm. Animals infused with scopolomine (a cholinergic antagonist) repeated more arms. Not surprisingly, the proportion of errors increased with the number of arms already visited. When Buresova, Bolhuis, and Bures (1986) tested a delayed version of this task (rats were allowed to wait for forty minutes on a central platform), they found that (1) normal rats made about twice as many errors in the delayed version than in the uninterrupted version, (2) scopolomine produced a dramatic increase in the number of errors (four times as many on the delayed as on the uninterrupted version). Other researchers (Eckerman et al., 1980; Wirsching et al., 1984; Hodges et al., 1991b) also found that cholinergic antagonists disrupted working memory on the radial maze. Both Wirsching et al. and Hodges et al. reported that working memory ws much more impaired than reference memory, although Wirsching et al. (1984) found that reference memory errors tended to increase at higher doses.

Open Field Navigation

Collett, Cartwright, and Smith (1986) examined a task similar to the water maze, but in a dry open field. A large arena was filled with gravel, and a sunflower seed buried in the arena; gerbils were trained to run to a point relative to a local landmark array and to dig for the seed. Open field navigation has also been studied by Biegler and Morris (1993, 1996), Gothard, Skaggs, and McNaughton (1996), and Touretzky and colleagues (Saksida et al., 1995; Redish, 1997). Biegler and Morris examined the effects of landmark stability relative to the wall of the environment, while Gothard, Skaggs, and McNaughton recorded from hippocampal place cells as the animals performed a simplified version of one of these tasks (see discussion of neurophysiological recordings in *NEUROPHYSIOLOGY*, below). Touretzky and colleagues replicated many of Collett, Cartwright, and Smith's results and applied statistical tests to separate theoretical possibilities. In addition, a number of investigators exploring cache behavior in rodents have found that the animals used constellations of landmarks (Vander Wall, 1990; Jacobs and Liman, 1991; Jacobs, 1992; Sherry and Duff, 1996). Collett, Cartwright, and Smith used female gerbils; Biegler and Morris used male hooded rats; and Gothard, Skaggs, and McNaughton used male albino rats. Touretzky and colleagues used both male and female gerbils.

In Collett, Cartwright, and Smith (1986), both the gerbils' starting location and the location of the landmark array varied randomly for every trial, but the food reward was always located at the same position relative to the array and the start box always had the same orientation. The arena was surrounded by walls painted black and was illuminated by a single incandescent bulb above its center, which left the walls in shadow. The floor was covered by black granite chips. Probe trials were run without a food reward, and the time spent at each location was histogrammed.

Gothard, Skaggs, and McNaughton (1996) used a more limited task in which the start box was always along the southern wall and the landmarks were always placed to the north. They

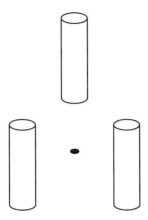

Figure B.5
Typical open field navigation task. Small white cylinders arranged in
an array form the local landmarks. Cylinders are translated from trial
to trial within the arena, but the array configuration is not changed.
Orientation of the array is also kept constant. Animals are trained to
find food at a constant relation to the landmark configuration and are
then tested with the landmark configuration in a novel location and no
food.

also did not cover the floor; it was bare black tile. They used
chocolate sprinkles for food reward, which were presumably not
visible on the black floor. This technique, however, has a distinct disadvantage in that the animals do not have to commit
to a goal location: they can sweep over the sprinkles and vac-
uum up the reward in passing, which means that, unlike those
of Collett, Cartwright, and Smith, histograms of position by time
do not produce strong peaks at the goal. Gothard, Skaggs, and
McNaughton did include nonreinforced trials during which the
animals would be expected to spend time searching near the goal,

although if an animal were very accurate in its search, it might quickly recognize that there was no reward.

Biegler and Morris (1993, 1996) trained their rats to find food at one of a small number of feeders placed in their environment, which included a polarizing wall cue. In these experiments, however, the rats were disoriented before each trial (unlike the experiments of Collett, Cartwright, and Smith; Gothard, Skaggs, and McNaughton; or Touretzky and colleagues). This may have disrupted the landmark–head direction association (see chapter 5).

Touretzky and colleagues (Saksida et al., 1995; Redish, 1997) followed the training technique of Collett, Cartwright, and Smith (1986), with a few exceptions. They used both male and female gerbils. The environment was cue-rich; no attempt was made to control the external landmarks in the surrounding room. The gerbils were started from one of eight locations around the arena and they were always started facing the wall. The floor of the arena was covered with wood chips instead of gravel.

All four research teams report that animals can learn to search at a single location relative to local landmarks. With two or more landmarks, the array can be manipulated during probe trials (i.e., rare trials with no food available, included only after complete training to determine where the animals believe the food is).

Both Collett, Cartwright, and Smith (1986) and Touretzky and colleagues (Saksida et al., 1995; Redish, 1997) found that when the animals are trained to search at the midpoint of a pair of landmarks, but are given only a single landmark, they search at two points, as if they alternately believed the landmark was one or the other of the original pair. Similarly, when faced with the two landmarks more separated than during training, the animals do not search at the midpoint of the array; instead, they search at the two interior locations the correct distance and bearing from the landmarks.

When trained with three landmarks, and faced with only two, the animals search at the correct distance and bearing to the two remaining landmarks (Collett, Cartwright, and Smith, 1986), although Touretzky and colleagues (Saksida et al., 1995;

Redish, 1997) found that a proportion of the time was also spent at the correct distance, but the opposite bearing (i.e., as if the animals were searching the reflected triangle). If the animals are shown a "stretched" triangle (two landmarks in the same spatial relationship to each other, the third landmark displaced), they search at the correct distance and bearing to the nondisplaced landmarks (Collett, Cartwright, and Smith, 1986). They do not search at the center of mass of the stretched triangle (Saksida et al., 1995; Redish, 1997). Finally, when the animals are faced with a triangle rotated by 180°, they search at the center of the triangle, but also spend time at three exterior points defined by reflecting the rotated triangle around each pair of landmarks (Collett, Cartwright, and Smith, 1986; Saksida et al., 1995; Redish, 1997). It is not known whether the animals are actually searching at these three exterior points or if they are simply passing through on their way to the center of the rotated triangle.

Path Integration

The open field has also been a critical place for studying path integration (see chapter 6 for a discussion of path integration and its related computational and theoretical issues). Mittelstaedt and Mittelstaedt (1980) showed that a female gerbil searching for a missing pup via an apparent random walk could execute a straight-line return to the nest once the pup was found. The experiment was performed in the dark to rule out visual homing. Displacement of the animal during its search at speeds below the vestibular detection threshold caused its return path to be offset by a comparable amount, eliminating the possibility that auditory or olfactory cues guided the trajectory.

Etienne (1987) showed a similar results: golden hamsters trained to find food at the center of a circular arena used path integration to return to the nest. When the environment was rotated 90° or 180° while the animal was at the center of the arena, the animal returned to where the nest had been originally, ignoring the rotation of the arena (Etienne et al., 1986; Etienne, 1987; Etienne, Maurer, and Saucy, 1988).

Müller and Wehner (1988) found that desert ants (*Cataglyphis fortis*) made systematic errors in path integration. Following on this work, Seguinot, Maurer, and Etienne (1993) tested hamsters on simple 1- to 5-stage paths. When they measured the direction the animals started home, they also found systematic errors, depending on specifics of the path taken. Other species make similar errors (Maurer and Seguinot, 1995).

Alyan et al. (1997) tested rats in two tasks. In the first task, rats were lured via a circuitous route to a location in the arena, from which they were allowed to return to the nest. They went directly back. In probe trials, animals were lured to the center. A rotation of the arena (with no corresponding rotation of the animals) ruled out intramaze cues driving the return journey. In the second task, rats were trained to take an L-shaped path, which then was blocked, forcing them to try another route back. Rats started back along the shortest path, turning directly toward the other end of the L. Both tasks were performed in the dark to rule out visual homing. In both cases, there were no significant differences between normals and lesioned animals, implying that even the lesioned animals had intact path integration abilities.

Whishaw and Maaswinkel (1997) trained rats on a large platform to leave a hole, find a food pellet and return to a specific hole. After training, blinders were placed on some rats and they were released from a different hole. Rats without blinders returned to the original hole they had been trained from (indicating that they were using some sort of visually guided navigation). Rats with blinders returned to the new hole (indicating that they were using some sort of path integration). With fornix lesions, rats without blinders were normal, but with blinders they were lost.

Local Landmarks and Exploration

Although, in general, less studied than the goal-directed tasks previously reviewed (Renner, 1990), exploration is an important spatial behavior (Archer and Birke, 1983; Renner, 1990). It is a critical component of latent learning (Blodget, 1921; Tolman, 1948; Hirsh, 1974, 1980), and does seem to be hippocampally dependent (O'Keefe and Nadel, 1978). From the earliest examinations of exploration, it was clear that animals exploring an environment spent large portions of their time in specific locations, called *home bases* (Chance and Mead, 1955). A similar behavior has been reported by Leonard and McNaughton (1990), who report that animals begin exploration by making small excursions from the initial entry point. More recently, Golani and colleagues (Eilam and Golani, 1989; Golani, Benjamini, and Eilam, 1993) have shown that not only do animals spend more time at these home bases, but they also visit the home base more than any other site in the environment. In addition, animals rear more and spend more time grooming themselves at these home bases then elsewhere in the environment (Eilam and Golani, 1989; Golani, Benjamini, and Eilam, 1993). Similar results have been reported by Touretzky et al. (1996; see also Redish, 1997).

The most extensive work done on determining the role of local landmarks and exploration is that of Poucet, Thinus-Blanc, and their colleagues (Poucet et al., 1986; Thinus-Blanc et al., 1987, 1991; Thinus-Blanc, Durup, and Poucet, 1992). When they tested hamsters in a cylinder with a striped cue card subtending 90° and three or four objects placed in a regular arrangement around the environment, they found that moving a landmark into or out of the array produced additional exploration. But they also found that expanding or contracting the square formed by the four landmarks did not produce additional exploration, whereas removing a landmark entirely produced extensive exploration.

More complex mazes

Many of the early experiments in rodent navigation were done in extremely complex mazes (Watson, 1907; Carr and Watson, 1908; Carr, 1917; Dennis, 1932; Honzik, 1936; Tolman, 1948; see figure 2.2): Although the environments in which rodents are tested have become simplified over recent years (allowing better control of the variables involved), there is still important data to be gleaned from these early experiments.

A key early result is that well-trained rats can navigate complex mazes under extreme sensory deprivation (Watson, 1907; Carr and Watson, 1908; Carr, 1917; Honzik, 1936). For example, Honzik (1936) found that rats could navigate complex mazes even with strong sensory deficits (i.e. after being blinded or made anosmic). Watson (1907) found that animals could navigate a Hampton-Court maze without ever touching the walls, even when blind, deaf, anosmic, and lacking vibrissae.

Carr and Watson (Watson, 1907; Carr and Watson, 1908; Carr, 1917) report that well-trained rats run the maze very fast and "with confidence." They note that the rats do not seem to be using external sensory cues to guide them. When placed in the maze at a point along the route (i.e., not the start), the rats seems confused at first, but once they "get their cue," (to use Carr and Watson's words) they run at top speed to the goal (Carr and Watson, 1908). Unfortunately, this means that if a corridor is shortened or lengthened the rats ran full tilt into the wall (Carr and Watson, 1908). Analogously, Dennis (1932) reports that when dead ends on an elevated maze are changed, rats run right off the edge, sometimes barely catching themselves with their hind claws.

NEUROPHYSIOLOGY

Hippocampal EEG

The hippocampus shows two major modes of activity differentiated by characteristic EEG signals (Vanderwolf, 1971; O'Keefe and Nadel, 1978; Vanderwolf and Leung, 1983; Buzsáki, 1989; Stewart and Fox, 1990; Vanderwolf, 1990). During motion and REM sleep, in the presence of acetylcholine and serotonin, the hippocampal EEG shows a 7–12 Hz rhythm called theta; during rest and slow-wave sleep, the hippocampal EEG shows Large-amplitude Irregular Activity (LIA), characterized by short-duration sharp waves. During LIA, hippocampal pyramidal cells tend to fire during sharp waves, but are then mostly all silent (Buzsáki, 1989; Ylinen et al., 1995). During theta, each cell fires only when the animal is in the corresponding place field. Because each cell has a different place field, cells fire a few at a time (see *Place Cells*, below).

Many of the EEG navigation experiments relating to navigation were done in the 1970s. These experiments were reviewed in depth by O'Keefe and Nadel (1978), including an extensive appendix categorizing them by their relation to task and structure, so I will not review them here. A few recent results, however, do need to be noted.

First, there is the discovery of high-frequency oscillations that ride on top of the slower theta and sharp-wave oscillations: gamma oscillations (40–100 Hz) during theta (Bragin et al., 1995; Chrobak and Buzsáki, 1996) and ripples (200 Hz) during sharp waves (Ylinen et al., 1995; Chrobak and Buzsáki, 1996). These oscillations are synchronized throughout the hippocampal axis and show interesting relations to inhibitory interneurons (Bragin et al., 1995; Ylinen et al., 1995; Chrobak and Buzsáki, 1996). Second, both theta and gamma oscillations can be found in entorhinal cortex (Chrobak and Buzsáki, 1994, 1996, 1998). Chrobak and Buzsáki (1994) have shown that during theta, cells in superficial layers of EC fire in a pattern correlated to the theta rhythm, whereas cells in deep layers of EC do not. In contrast, during LIA, cells in deep layers of EC fire in a pattern correlated to the sharp waves, while cells in superficial EC do not. Finally, the place fields of hippocampal pyramidal cells precess which each theta cycle (see discussion of *precession*, below).

Hippocampal Place Cells

For spatial tasks, the first-order correlate of spikes fired by hippocampal CA3 and CA1 pyramidal cells is the location of the rat: each cell fires when the animal is in a specific place (called the *place field* of the cell) (O'Keefe and Dostrovsky, 1971).

The typical place field (shown in figure B.6) is a continuous, compact field with a single peak that falls off smoothly in all di-

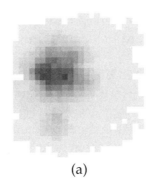

(a)

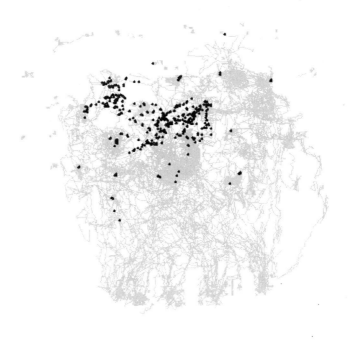

(b)

rections. Because place cells show such a clear correlate between firing rate and a spatial variable, many experiments have been done to explore how they react to environmental manipulations. Place fields have been recorded from

- small enclosed arenas (figure B.2) (Muller, Kubie, and Ranck, 1987; Muller and Kubie, 1987; Sharp, Kubie, and Muller, 1990; Wilson and McNaughton, 1993; Knierim, Kudrimoti, and McNaughton, 1995; Markus et al., 1995; O'Keefe and Burgess, 1996a),

- T- and plus mazes (figure B.3) (O'Keefe, 1976; O'Keefe and Conway, 1978; Pico et al., 1985; O'Keefe and Speakman, 1987; Young, Fox, and Eichenbaum, 1994; Markus et al., 1995),

- radial mazes (figure B.4) (Miller and Best, 1980; Olton, Branch, and Best, 1978; McNaughton, Barnes, and O'Keefe, 1983; Pavlides and Winson, 1989; Thompson and Best, 1989, 1990; Markus et al., 1994, 1995; Mizumori, Lavoie, and Kalyani, 1996),

- open fields (figure B.5) (Gothard et al., 1996),

- linear tracks (O'Keefe and Recce, 1993; Markus et al., 1994; Gothard, Skaggs, and McNaughton, 1996),

Figure B.6
(a) Place field in a small, enclosed arena. Animals randomly forage for food in the environment. Darker shading indicates areas in which a higher mean firing rate was seen. (Data courtesy D. Nitz, C. Barnes, and B. McNaughton.) (b) Place field in a large open arena. Animals are trained to find food relative to landmarks that move every trial. Dots indicate location of the animal when a spike was fired. Gray lines indicate trajectory of the animal. (Data courtesy K. Gothard, B. Skaggs, K. Moore, C. Barnes and B. McNaughton.)

- elevated tracks, such as triangular (Skaggs et al., 1996; Skaggs and McNaughton, 1996) or rectangular loops (Mehta, Barnes, and McNaughton, 1997; Barnes et al., 1997),

Place fields have also been recorded under a number of manipulations, including

- in the dark (O'Keefe, 1976; McNaughton, Leonard, and Chen, 1989; Quirk, Muller, and Kubie, 1990; Markus et al., 1994),

- during multiple and complex tasks (Eichenbaum et al., 1987; Eichenbaum and Cohen, 1988; Wiener, Paul, and Eichenbaum, 1989; Cohen and Eichenbaum, 1993; Hampson, Heyser, and Deadwyler, 1993; Markus et al., 1995),

- with environmental manipulations (O'Keefe and Conway, 1978; O'Keefe and Speakman, 1987; Kubie and Ranck, 1983; Muller and Kubie, 1987; Sharp, Kubie, and Muller, 1990; Bostock, Muller, and Kubie, 1991; Sharp et al., 1995; Sharp, 1997).

- in old rats (Barnes, McNaughton, and O'Keefe, 1983; Markus et al., 1994; Mizumori, Lavoie, and Kalyani, 1996; Shen et al., 1996; Barnes et al., 1997; Mizumori and Kalyani, 1997; Tanila et al., 1997a, 1997b),

- after sensory deprivations (Hill and Best, 1981; Save et al., 1998), lesions (Miller and Best, 1980; McNaughton et al., 1989; Shapiro et al., 1989; Mizumori et al., 1989, 1994; Dudchenko and Taube, 1997), grafts (Shapiro et al., 1989), and genetic manipulations (Rotenberg et al., 1996; McHugh et al., 1996; Wilson and Tonegawa, 1997).

Over the following pages, I will review the major results from the place cell experiments. This list is as complete as I could make it, but it is organized by topic rather than by experiment. For details of each experiment, please refer to the original papers.

Place fields are seen on initial entry into an environment.

Hill (1978) reports that place cells show relatively strong place fields the first time an animal passes through the field, whereas later studies have found that place cells can require 10–30 minutes (Wilson and McNaughton, 1993) or even as much as 4 hours (Austin, White, and Shapiro, 1993) to "tune up" their place fields, which become more reliable and more stable over that initial exploration period (Austin, White, and Shapiro, 1993; Wilson and McNaughton, 1993). Tanila et al. (1997b) report that some cells showed strong place fields in the first few minutes, while others took more than thirty minutes to build up their fields, during which time the mean selectivity increased.

Place cells are directional when an animal traverses repeated paths, but not when wandering randomly over open arenas.

When the animal traverses repeated paths, such as back and forth on a linear track, (Gothard, Skaggs, and McNaughton, 1996), along the arms of a radial arm maze, (McNaughton, Barnes, and O'Keefe, 1983), or in a fixed trajectory on an open field maze, (Markus et al., 1995)), place fields tend to be directionally dependent. In open environments, however, the firing rate of place cells is independent of head direction (Muller et al., 1994).

Markus et al. (1995) examined the question along two complementary axes: whether the environment produces limited trajectories (thin arms of the plus maze versus the two-dimensional space of the open field) and whether the food distribution is uniform or not. They found that cells in the plus maze were very directional, but that some place cells in the open field were more directional than others. They found a higher proportion of directional cells when food was sequentially placed at the four corners of a square on an open field than when it was uniformly distributed at random over the same field, suggesting that the trajectories taken may determine directionality.

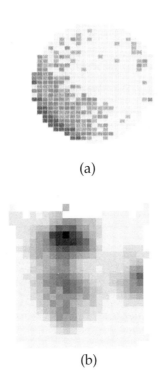

(a)

(b)

Figure B.7
(a) Place field that hugs the wall. From Muller et al. (1991). Used
with permission of author and publisher. Original in color. (b) Place
field with two subfields. (Data courtesy B. Skaggs, C. Barnes, and
B. McNaughton.)

Not all cells show simple place fields with Gaussian fall-off as distance from the center increases.

Some place fields are crescent-shaped, hugging the arena walls in the cylinder (Muller, Kubie, and Ranck, 1987). Some place cells show multiple subfields within a single environment (see figure B.7). Although many early reports of place fields suggested that cells had multiple subfields (e.g., O'Keefe and Conway, 1978; O'Keefe and Speakman, 1987), it should be noted that place cells recorded with a stereotrode (McNaughton, O'Keefe, and Barnes, 1983) show fewer subfields than those recorded with a single-wire electrode, and that place cells recorded with a tetrode (Wilson and McNaughton, 1993) show even fewer.

Moving distal landmarks produces corresponding movements in place fields.

Many early experiments used T-, plus, or radial mazes with cues available on the walls of the surrounding room (e.g. O'Keefe and Conway, 1978; Miller and Best, 1980; O'Keefe and Speakman, 1987; Shapiro et al., 1989; Young, Fox, and Eichenbaum, 1994). Even if there were no differing textures on each arm of the maze, one would expect some sort of local intramaze cues. The local and distal cues can then be separated by rotating the maze. Place cells generally followed the distal cues (Miller and Best, 1980; Shapiro et al., 1989).

Similar results have been found by Cressant, Muller, and Poucet (1997), who showed that place fields rotate with landmarks inside a small circular arena only if the landmarks are pushed all the way against the wall, that is, only if they are *orienting* or *distal* stimuli. If the landmarks (three colored cylinders) were clumped together and on the interior of the arena, the place fields were not tied to the landmarks, whereas if the landmarks were pushed to the walls of the arena, the place fields followed them. The task used by Cressant, Muller, and Poucet (1997) was independent of the actual locations of the landmarks. In tasks where the animals must attend to the landmarks in order to find reward, they can learn to do so (Collett, Cartwright, and Smith, 1986; Biegler and Morris, 1993;

Saksida et al., 1995; Biegler and Morris, 1996; Gothard et al., 1996; Redish, 1997). The place fields are then tied to the landmarks when the animal is near them (within 70 cm; Gothard et al., 1996).

Place cells can also be controlled by nonvisual landmarks (Hill and Best, 1981; Save et al., 1998). When Hill and Best examined place fields in blind and deaf rats on a six-arm maze, they found that cells continued to show place fields, but most of the cells followed local cues when the maze was rotated. Save et al. showed that even rats who had been blinded one week after birth continued to show normal place fields as adults. Their place fields were sensitive to the rotation of prominent somatosensory landmarks. The landmarks were placed at the edge of a circular arena; to determine their location, the rats first went to the wall and then made a loop around the circumference of the arena. When the landmarks were rotated, the place fields also rotated.

Place cells continue to show place fields when landmarks are removed.

As mentioned above, place fields can change when landmarks are moved. Hippocampal cells continue to show compact place fields when visual landmarks are removed (Muller and Kubie, 1987; O'Keefe and Speakman, 1987). When the cue card was removed from the cylindrical environment shown in figure B.2, the place fields sometimes rotated around the center of the arena, but they did not change shape (Muller and Kubie, 1987), suggesting that the cue card serves mainly as an orienting stimulus. O'Keefe and Speakman (1987) trained rats on a plus maze and then removed the landmarks. Both O'Keefe and Conway (1978) and Pico et al. (1985) found that, when animals were not placed in the environment with the cues present, removing some of the visual cues did not disrupt place fields, removing all of the cues did.

Place cells continue to show compact fields in the dark.

Quirk, Muller, and Kubie (1990) found that when animals are placed into the arena in the light and the light extinguished, the place fields rarely change. Even when they do, they continue to show the same shape and distance from the arena wall; it is only their orientation that varies. Markus et al. (1994) found that more cells had fields and that place fields were more reliable in the light than in the dark. In particular, if the first trial in a session occurred in the light, then cells were much more likely to be stable (measured by the correlation to the mean place field in the light) than when sessions started with a dark trial.

Place fields show interactions between consistent entry locations and external landmarks.

Sharp, Kubie, and Muller (1990) examined rats in a small cylindrical arena with a cue card subtending 90° (see figure B.2). During training the animals were not disoriented before entering the arena and always entered at the same location (the northwest corner). They then tested the animals with (1) the original configuration, (2) the cue card on the opposite side from its original location, (3) both cue cards from the previous configurations, and (4) two cue cards rotated by ±30°. They tested each of these cases in two conditions: with the animals entering the arena at the northwest corner and with the animals entering the arena at the southeast corner.

When a second cue card was added opposite the first, most place fields did not double. Instead, the cells continued to fire at their original locations. However, when the animals were introduced into the double-card environment at the *southeast* corner, the place fields rotated by 180°, although rotation did not occur in probe trials with the original configuration and a southeast entry point. When the animals were tested with cue cards rotated by ±30°, Sharp, Kubie, and Muller observed that place field locations were controlled by an interaction of the choice of entry point with the cue card positions. Five of the eighteen cells recorded changed their place fields over the various recording sessions, including three that showed doubled (symmetric) place fields at one time or another.

The specific timing of spikes fired by place cells as an animal traverses a place field precesses along the theta rhythm.

O'Keefe and Recce (1993) and Skaggs et al. (1996) have shown that as the animal then moves through the place field, the cell generally fires its spikes earlier and earlier in the theta cycle. Although this effect is most easily seen on linear tracks, it also occurs in two dimensions (Skaggs et al., 1996).

Place fields shift with experience.

Mehta, Barnes, and McNaughton (1997) have shown that the place fields shift backward along a much-repeated path as the animal runs along that path. When rats run in a loop on a rectangular elevated maze, CA1 place fields shift backward over the course of a single session. Shen et al. (1997) found that old animals do not show this shift, even though both phase precession and the theta rhythm were not significantly changed.

Place cells disrupted by fimbria-fornix lesions are restored by septal grafts.

Shapiro et al. (1989) studied place cells in normal rats, in rats with lesions to the fimbria-fornix (thus lacking acetylcholine) and in rats with fetal basal forebrain tissue grafted in (with acetylcholine restored). Recording from place cells in a radial arm maze and then rotating the maze, they found that place cells in fimbria-fornix-lesioned rats followed local cues, but were partially influenced by distal cues, as evidenced by the lower reliability of place fields in lesioned rats during rotated trials (but not during nonrotated trials). In rats with grafts, place fields followed distal cues, as they do in normal rats (Miller and Best, 1980; Shapiro et al., 1989).

Septal inactivation produces significant reduction in location specific firing of CA3 but not CA1 cells on a radial maze.

> When Mizumori et al. (1989) tested medial septal inactivation (with tetracaine) while recording from place cells in both CA3 and CA1. They found that the CA3 fields were disrupted, whereas the CA1 fields were not. They also found a significant increase in working memory errors on the radial maze during the septal inactivation.

Place cells are sensitive to more than place.

> The firing rates of hippocampal pyramidal ("place") cells are also correlated with information other than location of the animal: speed, direction, and turning angle (McNaughton, Barnes, and O'Keefe, 1983; Wiener, Paul, and Eichenbaum, 1989; Markus et al., 1994); texture underfoot (Young, Fox, and Eichenbaum, 1994); odor (Eichenbaum et al., 1987; Eichenbaum and Cohen, 1988); task (Markus et al., 1995); match/non-match of samples (Otto and Eichenbaum, 1992b); and stage of task (Eichenbaum et al., 1987; Otto and Eichenbaum, 1992b; Hampson, Heyser, and Deadwyler, 1993).
>
> If a cell has a place field under one condition, it may or may not show a place field under the other, and if two cells both show place fields under both conditions, then the spatial relationships between them may change drastically from one condition to the other. Thus many of these effects can be said to be second-order effects because they determine how the place fields change. Essentially, a cell's place field (or whether it has a place field at all) is independent from one condition to another.

The spatial relationship between place cells changes from environment to environment.

> Kubie and Ranck (1983) recorded from place cells in rats in three different environments (a radial maze, an operant-conditioning chamber, and a home cage). They found that when cells have fields in multiple environments, the topologies of the fields under

any two environments are unrelated. Thompson and Best (1989) also recorded from place cells in three environments (a radial maze, a circular drum, and a small box). They first identified cells during barbiturate anesthesia (when hippocampal cells are much more active) and then measured them in each of the environments. They found that the numbers of cells that showed place fields in each environment was compatible with the hypothesis that 10–25 percent of the CA1 cells[3] show a place field in any environment, and that, for any specific environment, the subpopulation of cells with place fields is random and independent of that seen in any other environment.

All of these experiments show that when an animal is returned to an environment, the place fields return to the representation encoding that environment. In other words, place fields are stable from session to session (Muller, Kubie, and Ranck, 1987). Thompson and Best (1990) report recording a place fields that were stable for months.

Changing the cue card from white to black eventually produces change in place field topology.

Bostock, Muller, and Kubie (1991) recorded from place cells in a cylindrical arena (figure B.2), first with a white cue card, and then with a black cue card. Sometimes the place fields were similar and sometimes they were unrelated (as if the two situations were encoded as different environments). Once a place field changed with the cue card then all other place fields recorded subsequently from the same animal changed with the cue cards, but when the white cue card was returned, the place field returned to its original configuration.

A single environmental manipulation halfway through a recording session eventually produces a change in place field topology.

Sharp et al. (1995) saw a similar effect in their experiment examining the effects of vestibular cues on place cells. By rotating the environment (or part of the environment) 20 minutes into a 40 minute recording session, they found that in some sessions the fields rotated with the manipulation, but in others, the field changed location dramatically or disappeared completely when the manipulation occurred. The probability of a radical change or disappearance increased over the sessions.

Old animals do not show place field transitions with environmental manipulations that produce novel transitions in young animals.

Using a plus maze and rotating it relative to the external world, Tanila et al. (1997b) found that old and young animals reacted differently to this manipulation. Young rats tended to create a new map, while old rats did not. Both young and old animals had extensive experience with the original environment.

Older animals show unstable representations of the environment.

Barnes et al. (1997) recorded a few dozen cells simultaneously, while animals ran a rectangular loop track for 25 minutes. The animals were then removed from the track for one hour, after which they were returned to the track for another 25 minutes. For young animals, the ensemble correlation between the place fields seen during the first and second 25-minute experiences showed a unimodal distribution (around 0.7, indicative of a similar representation between experiences). But for older animals, the ensemble correlation was bimodal (around 0, indicative of a complete remapping, and around 0.7, indicative of a similar representation between experiences). Within a single 25-minute run, the ensemble correlation (taken between two halves of the run) was always high (around 0.8).

Mice that have been genetically engineered to have long-term potentiation deficits in CA1 show instability in their place fields between sessions.

Rotenberg et al. (1996) measured place fields in mice that were genetically engineered to be deficient in LTP when stimulation was in the 5–10 Hz range. Such mice show severe spatial deficits (Bach et al., 1995). Like Barnes et al. (1997; see previous reviewed result), Rotenberg et al. found that place fields in the mice were stable within a single session but unstable across sessions.

Place cells are sensitive to task within a single environment.

When Markus et al. (1995) trained rats to search for food on a large elevated platform either randomly or at the corners of a diamond, they found that different subsets of place cells were active for each task, and that some cells that were active for both tasks had different place fields, as if the animals were encoding the tasks as different environments. When the animals switched between these two tasks, the change between representations was rapid, suggesting a shift in a property encompassing the entire system.

Place cells are sensitive to odor cues in certain tasks.

In more complex tasks than simply finding food scattered on the floor of the arena, place cells do not always fire when the animal is in the place field. Eichenbaum and colleagues (Eichenbaum et al., 1987; Eichenbaum and Cohen, 1988) tested rats in an odor-detection task and found some place cells dependent on whether the rat was going to the reward location. In a similar task, Eichenbaum and colleagues (Otto and Eichenbaum, 1992b; Cohen and Eichenbaum, 1993) found that cells responded when two odors matched in a delayed match-to-sample task, but not when they did not. Animals in the Eichenbaum et al. (1987) task had been trained to go to a reward location given one set of odors (S^+) but not given another (S^-). This meant that the animals were learning to take two different paths to reward depending on whether the odor was in the S^+ or S^- set. Eichenbaum et al. report that hippocampal pyramidal cells ("place" cells) are odor sensitive. However, they are sensitive not to different odors, but different reward conditions, indicated in this experiment by different *odor sets*. Equivalently, the Otto and Eichenbaum (1992b) experiment showed place cells sensitive to matching versus non-matching pairs. Similar results were found by Sakurai (1990b) in an auditory matching task: cells were sensitive to matching versus nonmatching tones.

Place cells are sensitive to stages of complex tasks.

In addition to sensitivity to reward availability, Eichenbaum and colleagues (Eichenbaum et al., 1987; Eichenbaum and Cohen, 1988; Otto and Eichenbaum, 1992a; see also Sakurai, 1990b) found that some cells are correlated with location during different stages of the task. For example, one cell might show a place field when an animal is approaching a sniff port to sample the odor (to determine whether it is an S^+ or an S^- odor), but not when the animal leaves the sniff port to go either to the reward location or back to the starting point.

Hampson, Heyser, and Deadwyler (1993) trained rats to do a multiple lever-pressing delayed match-to-sample task. They found place cells dependent on whether a lever had already been pressed. They also found cells sensitive to which lever had been pressed (and therefore which lever had to be pressed to receive reward). When an animal made a mistake, the place code indicated the incorrect lever.

Gothard et al. (1996) found place cells sensitive to components (or stages) of a open field landmark task. They trained animals to leave a start box when a door was opened and proceed across an open floor to a pair of landmarks. Forming a triangle with the pair of landmarks was a small food reward. After an animal found the goal location, it was to return to the start box for another trial. They found cells correlated (within this task) to leaving the start box, to passing through the open room, to the goal location itself, and to returning to the start box.

Hippocampal representations are replayed during sleep.

Pavlides and Winson (1989) showed that cells with recently visited place fields were more active during REM sleep than other cells whose place fields had not been recently visited. Wilson and McNaughton (1994) found that, during slow-wave sleep (SWS), cells showing correlated firing during a session in an environment (because their place fields overlapped) also showed a stronger correlation during sleep immediately after the session relative to sleep before the session. When Skaggs and McNaughton (1996) explicitly examined the temporal nature of replay during sharp waves in slow-wave sleep, they found that the temporal bias during sleep after running on a linear track is strongly correlated with the temporal bias seen while the animal was running.

There are differences between place fields in dorsal and ventral hippocampus.

All of the cells previously described in this section were recorded from dorsal hippocampus. Jung, Wiener, and McNaughton (1994) found that among hippocampal pyramidal cells, place fields were fewer and the average spatial selectivity lower for ventral cells than for dorsal cells. Although Poucet, Thinus-Blanc, and Muller (1994) did not find any differences between dorsal and ventral place cells, their methodology preselects cells showing place fields that look similar to those in figure B.6, so their result can only be taken as proving that place cells exist in ventral hippocampus.

Extrahippocampal place cells

Place cells have also been found in dentate gyrus (Jung and McNaughton, 1993), medial entorhinal cortex (Barnes et al., 1990; Mizumori, Ward, and Lavoie, 1992; Quirk et al., 1992), subiculum (Barnes et al., 1990; Muller, Kubie, and Saypoff, 1991; Sharp and Green, 1994; Sharp, 1997), and parasubiculum (Taube, 1995b). Jung and McNaughton (1993) found that granule cells also showed clear place fields on a radial maze. Like CA3 and CA1 place fields, these cells showed a strong directionality on the radial maze.

Quirk et al. (1992) found that MEC place fields were larger and more noisy than hippocampal place fields, although they did show strong spatial signals reminiscent of hippocampal place fields. MEC place fields rotated with a cue card, but the cells continued to show place fields when the card was removed. Nor did they change their topology between two similar environments, a cylinder and a rectangle in both of which a cue card subtended 90° (see figure B.2). MEC place fields stretched topologically between the environments. All cells that had place fields in one environment had a corresponding place field in the other. These two environments produce dramatic changes in hippocampal place field topologies. Mizumori, Ward, and Lavoie (1992), recording from a radial maze (see figure B.4), also found broad place fields in medial entorhinal cortex but noted a weak directional component to the place fields.

Like entorhinal place cells, but unlike hippocampal place cells, dorsal subicular place cells show similar place fields across different environments (Sharp, 1997). When Sharp tested dorsal subicular cells in four variations each of the cylinder and square environments (see figure B.2). She found that (allowing for translation and rotation) subicular cells always showed similar place fields between the two environments. Unlike entorhinal or hippocampal cells, subicular cells do show a (weak) directional signal, even in the open environment (Sharp and Green, 1994). Phillips, Tanila, and Eichenbaum (1996) report that ventral subicular cells do not show place fields in complex environments. It is not known whether there is a difference between dorsal and ventral subicular cells as there seems to be between dorsal and ventral hippocampal cells (Jung, Wiener, and McNaughton, 1994) or whether there is a difference between simple and complex environments.

Although Taube (1995b) found parasubicular cells with place fields in a cylinder, because of the methodology used (prescreening for spatial signals), the percentage of cells with fields is not known. Because Taube tested these cells in only one environment, it is also not known whether parasubicular place cells show the same preservation of topology between environments — like medial entorhinal place cells (Quirk et al., 1992), and like subicular place cells (Sharp, 1997), but unlike hippocampal place cells (Kubie and Ranck, 1983; Muller and Kubie, 1987; Thompson and Best, 1989). Taube notes that the fields in parasubiculum are larger and qualitatively more like subicular place fields than like hippocampal.

Head Direction Cells

Certain cells in the rodent brain show firing rates correlated with the orientation of the animal. These head direction cells are found in a variety of structures, including the postsubiculum (PoS: Ranck, 1984; Taube, Muller, and Ranck, 1990a, 1990b), the anterior dorsal nucleus of the thalamus (AD nucleus of the ATN; Blair and Sharp, 1995; Knierim, Kudrimoti, and McNaughton, 1995; Taube, 1995a; Blair, Lipscomb, and Sharp, 1997), the lateral mammillary nuclei (LMN; Leonhard, Stackman, and Taube, 1996) as well as the lateral dorsal thalamus (LDN; Mizumori and Williams, 1993), the caudate nucleus (Wiener, 1993; Mizumori, Lavoie, and Kalyani, 1996), and the parietal and cingulate cortices (Chen et al., 1990; Chen, 1991; Chen et al., 1994a, 1994b; McNaughton et al., 1994). (For more detail on the different properties of each of these areas and a discussion of how these firing properties are maintained, see chapter 5.)

Whenever multiple head direction cells have been recorded from ATN, PoS, or LMN the difference between their preferred directions is a constant across all recording sessions in all environments (Taube, Muller, and Ranck, 1990b; Goodridge and Taube, 1995; Taube and Burton, 1995; see figure 5.1).

Postsubicular, lateral mammillary, and anterior dorsal thalamic head direction cells are sensitive to rotation of distal cues (Ranck, 1984; Taube, Muller, and Ranck, 1990b; Taube, 1995a; Goodridge and Taube, 1995; Knierim, Kudrimoti, and McNaughton, 1995; Leonhard, Stackman, and Taube, 1996). In all of these cases, head direction cells were recorded from a small cylinder with a cue card subtending 90° (see figure B.2). When an animal was returned to the arena, the head direction tuning curve was oriented identically relative to the cue card (Taube, Muller, and Ranck, 1990b; Taube, 1995a; Goodridge and Taube, 1995; Leonhard, Stackman, and Taube, 1996).

However, Knierim, Kudrimoti, and McNaughton (1995) found that when animals were disoriented prior to each experience, the tuning curves in anterior dorsal thalamus (AD nucleus of the ATN) no longer followed the cue card as strongly. Even in rats who had been first disoriented before a number of sessions, then allowed sessions without disorientation, the cue card had no effect on the initial tuning curve of the cell (Knierim, Kudrimoti, and McNaughton, 1995).

Examining a similar issue, Taube and Burton (1995) allowed rats to explore a cylinder and rectangle connected by a U-shaped passage. After exploration, the animals were removed from the environment and the cue card in the cylinder rotated by 90°. When the animals were returned to the cylinder, the head direction tuning curves rotated proportionally. When the animals traversed the U-shaped passage, they encountered a cue-conflict situation: the internal cues (from the self-motion via the passage from the cylinder) and the external cues (from the cue card in the rectangular arena) were conflicting. Taube and Burton found that in some animals the tuning curves rotated and in others they did not. The shift was generally constant within each animal, even though it differed between animals.

Postsubicular and anterior thalamic head direction cells do not require visual input to show a strong directional signal (see Taube et al., 1996 for a review). If a rat is brought into a maze in the dark, the head direction is carried over from its previous environment, most likely by vestibular input, but probably also by motor efferent information if available (Ranck, 1984; Goodridge and Taube, 1995; Taube et al., 1996).

(Mizumori, Ward, and Lavoie, 1992) found that, in contrast, neurons in the lateral dorsal nucleus (LDN) of the thalamus that are sensitive to head direction require exposure to the environment in the light in order to show directional sensitivity. With a 30-second exposure, that saw directionality about 47 percent of the time, but with a 60-second exposure, they always saw directionality, and the directionality was consistent with prior exposures to the environment. Moreover, when the lights were turned off, directionality was maintained for approximately two to three minutes, after which it began to rotate regularly left or right.

In addition to the correlations to head direction, lateral mammillary nuclei (LMN) cell activity is strongly correlated with angular velocity as well as direction (Leonhard, Stackman, and Taube, 1996). McNaughton, Chen, and Markus (1991) have reported that some cells in parietal cortex are correlated with both head direction and angular velocity. Taube, Muller, and Ranck (1990b) and Sharp (1996) have also reported that some PoS cells are correlated with both as well. But these cells are rare, while most of the cells in LMN seem to be strongly correlated with both head direction and angular velocity (Leonhard, Stackman, and Taube, 1996).

PoS head direction cells are best correlated with current head direction, whereas AD cell activity is best correlated with head direction approximately 20–40 ms in the future (Blair and Sharp, 1995; Taube and Muller, 1995). ATN cell activity is best correlated not with current head direction, but with head direction approximately 20–40 ms in the future (Blair and Sharp, 1995; Taube and Muller, 1995). Both Blair and Sharp and Taube and Muller report an optimal correlation of ATN activity with future head direction and of PoS activity with current head direction, but both have recently revised their estimates (Taube et al., 1996; Blair, Lipscomb, and Sharp, 1997), suggesting that although ATN activity still anticipates future head directions (by 25 ms), PoS activity may lag behind the current head direction (by 15 ms).

Leonhard, Stackman, and Taube also report that LMN cells are correlated with future direction (by as much as 83 ms), at least in one direction, but it is not yet clear whether this anticipation occurs for both clockwise and counterclockwise turns. Because LMN activity is also correlated with angular velocity, it might seem to anticipate future head direction with angular velocity in one direction but not the other.

Blair, Lipscomb, and Sharp (1997) have recently reported that the tuning curves of ATN cells change during rotations. Figure 5.3 shows an AD cell recorded during left, right, and nonrotations. During rotations one of the peaks increases while the other decreases.

Lesions to the anterior thalamus cause a disruption of directional selectivity in the postsubicular head direction population (Goodridge and Taube, 1994). In contrast, postsubiculum lesions do not seem to disrupt the directional selectivity of anterior thalamic cells (Goodridge and Taube, 1994; Taube et al., 1996), however, after postsubiculum lesions, anterior thalamic cells are not sensitive to external sensory cues, they are only driven by vestibular cues (Goodridge et al., 1998). Lesions of the lateral dorsal thalamus (LDN) do not affect the directional selectivity of PoS head direction cells (Golob and Taube, 1994).

After vestibular lesions, anterior thalamic head direction cells are no longer correlated with head direction (Stackman and Taube, 1997). Because Stackman and Taube only record from one neuron at a time, it is not clear whether these results show a population whose coherent representation of head direction has been decoupled from the real world, or whether the representation itself is disrupted. Multiunit recordings could distinguish between these two possibilities.

Appendix C: Open Questions

This appendix lays out what I consider to be some of the most important open questions in rodent navigation. I have been careful in the main text to present both sides of the debate when each issue arose; here, I attempt to clarify those open questions. Where possible, I suggest experiments that might be able to help resolve the debate.

Some of the open questions require extensive exploratory experimental and theoretical work; answering them will take a major research effort. Other open questions relate more directly to specific components discussed in the book; often these questions can be answered by a few well-designed experiments. Finally, sometimes explicit predictions can be made following specific hypotheses.

LOCAL VIEW

How is the local view actually represented?

Chapter 3 identified some of the key variables that have to be represented in the local view (e.g., distance, egocentric and allocentric bearing) and some of the cortical areas that seem to be involved (e.g., lateral dorsal nucleus of the thalamus, posterior parietal cortex). Exactly how those variables are represented, however, is still an unresolved question. Tremendous work has been done in the primate (for reviews, see Andersen et al., 1993; Colby, Duhamel, and Goldberg, 1995), but I know of little equivalent work in the rodent. Additionally, primate parietal cortex has been shown to be anatomically and functionally divided into a host of subareas (Colby and Duhamel, 1991; Stein, 1992). Although preliminary anatomical evidence suggests that such subareas may also exist in rodent (Zilles, 1990), no neurophysiological work has been done to establish separate functionally for these subareas.

Does the rodent visual system also separate into two streams?

There is extensive evidence suggesting that the primate visual system consists of two dissociable streams, the dorsal stream, passing through parietal cortex, supporting spatial aspects, and the ventral stream, passing through inferotemporal cortex, supporting identity aspects (for reviews, see Mishkin, Ungerleider, and Macko, 1983; Ungerleider and Haxby, 1994; Goodale et al., 1994). There is some preliminary evidence that this is also true of the rodent (Kolb, 1990a; Kolb et al., 1994), but more work could be done on this issue. An interesting corollary to this question is whether nonvisual rodent sensory representations also divide into these two streams.

TAXON AND PRAXIC NAVIGATION

Is the caudate nucleus a monolithic structure or should it be considered a conglomeration of separately acting substructures?

The basal ganglia in general have a diverse internal anatomical structure (*patch* and *matrix*; Graybiel, 1990; Groves et al., 1995; White, 1997; White and Hiroi, 1998), but these do seem to interact with each other (Groves et al., 1995). A number of authors have hypothesized that different aspects of the caudate nucleus are critical for different tasks (Winocur, 1974; White, 1989; Beiser, Hua, and Houk, 1997; White and Hiroi, 1998). Others have hypothesized that the basal ganglia in general maintain their separate inputs through the entire structure (Alexander and Crutcher, 1990), while still others have emphasized the convergence of different inputs (Finch, 1996). It is not currently clear whether the basal ganglia funnel input from much of cortex to perform a single function (e.g., Mishkin and Appenzeller, 1987), perform a single function on diverse input (e.g., Alexander and Crutcher, 1990; Barto, 1995; Connolly and Burns, 1995), or are functionally diverse (e.g., White, 1989).

What is the role of cingulate cortex in navigation?

Recordings by McNaughton and colleagues (McNaughton, Chen, and Markus, 1991; Chen et al., 1994a, 1994b; McNaughton et al., 1994) from posterior cingulate cortex show cells tuned to behavioral and directional aspects of certain tasks. These recordings, however, are preliminary; more extensive experimental work examining the role of posterior cingulate cortex is necessary before its role can be truly elucidated. Lesions of posterior cingulate cortex have been implicated in navigational tasks (Sutherland and Hoesing, 1993; Bussey, Everitt, and Robbins, 1997; Bussey et al., 1997), but Neave and colleagues (Neave et al., 1994; Neave, Nagle, and Aggleton, 1997) have suggested that these lesions disrupted the cingulum bundle (connecting the anterior thalamic nuclei and postsubiclum) rather than the posterior cingulate cortex itself.

What is the anatomical underpinning of praxic navigation?

As discussed in chapter 4, the caudate nucleus seems to play a strong role in praxic strategies (Potegal, 1972; Abraham and Potegal, 1979; Potegal, 1982; Abraham, Potegal, and Miller, 1983; Kesner, Bolland, and Dakis, 1993; Packard and McGaugh, 1996). Some researchers have hypthesized that it is involved in sequencing movements (West et al., 1990; Berridge and Whishaw, 1992; Pellis et al., 1993; Schultz et al., 1995a). Exactly what role the caudate nucleus plays, however, and what other structures are involved in taxon and praxic navigation are still unknown.

HEAD DIRECTION

Does the head direction system include attractor dynamics?

A key component of the head direction system described in chapter 5 is the attractor dynamics hypothesized to occur as a consequence of the pseudo-winner-take-all network structure. This can be explicitly tested by multi-unit recording. If one records from multiple head direction cells simultaneously (twenty cells, say), then the population encoding can be directly observed. If noise is injected into the system by microstimulation, then the representation should be transiently disrupted. Because nearby postsubicular cells encode different directions (Sharp, 1996), microstimulation should effectively add noise into the system by firing a set of cells with unrelated preferred directions. If the system includes attractor dynamics, then even in darkness, without external or self-motion cues, the population's firing rates should return to a well-formed representation of head direction.

Is the head direction representation maintained in the absence of angular velocity input?

Stackman and Taube (1997) lesioned the vestibular system using intratympanic injections of sodium arsanilate. After the surgery, Stackman and Taube could not find any head direction cells in the anterior thalamic nuclei. However, there are two possible explanations for this: (1) the population activity may have been a valid representation of head direction, but simply uncoupled from motor action, or (2) the representation itself may have been disrupted. This question is important because it bears on the attractor nature of the system: is the neural mechanism underlying head direction specifically constructed so as to produce a coherent representation of head direction, or is the coherent representation an epiphenomenon occurring as a consequence of the cells showing head direction tuning curves? Although the single-unit recording procedure used by Stackman and Taube could not differentiate these two possibilities, multi-unit recording could.

How can the theory explain the findings that postsubicular lesions do not affect anterior thalamic nuclei head direction tuning curves?

Postsubicular lesions do not disrupt ATN head direction cells (Goodridge and Taube, 1994; see also Taube et al., 1996). Whereas the theory in chapter 5 predicts that postsubicular lesions should devastate them. There are three possible explanations: (1) the postsubiculum may be part of a larger structure, (2) other areas may be able to play similar roles to that played by the postsubiculum, (3) there may be problems with the theory (or the experiment). Additional theoretical and experimental work is needed to bring the theory into alignment with the findings of Taube and colleagues.

Can the head direction system be reset from local cues? If so, how does this happen?

Head direction can be reset from distal cues directly because distal cues do not change their allocentric bearing over the environment (Gallistel, 1990; McNaughton, Chen, and Markus, 1991; Skaggs et al., 1995). To reset head direction from local cues, however, the system requires a representation of the animal's position such as is provided by the place code (Wan, Touretzky, and Redish, 1994c; Redish and Touretzky, 1996; Touretzky and Redish, 1996). Experiments examining head direction tuning curves in tasks that require reorientation to local cues, such as finding food relative to a rotating pair of landmarks (Collett, Cartwright, and Smith, 1986; Biegler and Morris, 1993, 1996), would help answer this question.

Do cues at similar orientations average while widely separated cues compete?

A prediction can be made following the hypothesis that the head direction system (chapter 5) is based on attractor networks such as those described in appendix A. Train an animal to expect a small cue card (e.g., 5° width) in a standard cylindrical environment. Then, while recording from head direction cells, place the animal in the environment in the dark. Spin the environment quickly until the animal is dizzy. Then turn the lights on and allow the animal to see two cue cards separated by an angle θ. When θ is small, the head direction tuning curves should follow the average of the two cue cards, but when θ is large, the tuning curves should follow one or the other (the cards should compete).

PATH INTEGRATION

What is the anatomical locus of path integration?

A number of hypotheses for the anatomical locus of path integration were discussed in chapter 6: hippocampus (McNaughton et al., 1996), subiculum (Sharp, 1997), and a three-stage loop of subiculum, parasubiculum, and superficial entorhinal cortex (Redish and Touretzky, 1997a). While the experiments of Alyan et al. (1997) imply that the hippocampus is not the critical component, they do not prove that these other structures are involved. Nor can the experiment by Whishaw and Maaswinkel (1997) showing that fornix lesions impair path integration be taken as proof that subiculum is involved in path integration. A fornix lesion also disrupts connection between postsubiculum and the anterior thalamic nuclei, which almost certainly would disrupt the head direction system, making it impossible for the system path integrate correctly.

A number of experiments can be performed to test these hypotheses more directly. We can predict that lesions made to any structures invovled should impair the path integration ability of rodents. Neurophysiologically, place cells in all involved structures should show normal activity in the dark. I know of no recordings from any nonhippocampal structures in the absence of sensory cues during spatial tasks, although Quirk et al. (1992) report that cells in the superficial layers of entorhinal cortex continued to show normal place fields after the cue card was removed.

If the anatomical hypothesis and mechanism discussed in chapter 6 are correct, then two additional neurophysiological predictions can be made. First, one of the three structures should anticipate future position, the way that ATN cells anticipate future head direction (Blair, Lipscomb, and Sharp, 1997; see chapter 5). Although Taube (1995b) reports that parasubicular place cells are optimally tuned to a slight anticipation (by ~100 ms) of position, more work needs to be done to show that this anticipation is a consequence of the moving hill mechanism discussed in chapter 6.

Second, the topology of fields in the involved structures should not change from environment to environment. If one measures a path integrator place cell in one environment, nothing can be predicted about the location of its place field in another environment except that it must exist, but if one measures the place fields of two cells, the distance between their place fields must be identical in the two environments. Finally, if one records fields from three place cells, one cannot predict where the center of the triangle formed by their centers will be, but the triangle in the second environment must be *geometrically similar*[1] to the first.

Can the proposed path integration mechanism be made to track actual trajectories of real animals?

How accurate can the mechanism described in chapter 6 be? What is required to make it accurate? By simulating the head direction system accurately, Redish, Elga, and Touretzky (1996) found complexities (for example the deformation of the tuning curve) that were not obvious from the theoretical model. No one has yet reported an accurate simulation of two-dimensional path integration based on the moving hill hypothesis.

GOAL MEMORY

What is the anatomy of the goal memory?

As discussed in chapter 7, there is evidence that the nucleus accumbens is a key component of the goal memory, first hypothesized by Mogenson (1984), although animals with fimbria-fornix lesions and septal grafts can still learn navigation tasks such as the water maze (Nilsson et al., 1987). This means that there must be alternate pathways from the hippocampus to motor structures. One candidate may be the posterior cingulate cortex (Sutherland and Hoesing, 1993). Further work needs to be done to fully determine the role played by the nucleus accumbens in the navigation system, as well as the role played by other structures such as the posterior cingulate cortex.

How do rodents plan paths and avoid obstacles?

An important role of the goal memory is to plan a trajectory from
the animal's current position to a goal. If there are obstacles
in the way, or if the animal must take a complex path to reach
the goal, the goal memory should be able to plan these kinds
of complex trajectories. Animals are generally very successful
at planning complex trajectories and avoiding obstacles (for examples, see Watson, 1907; Carr and Watson, 1908; Honzik, 1936;
Chapuis and Scardigli, 1993). It is not currently known how obstacles are represented in the rodent brain or how the planning is
done to avoid them. Although a number of robotics algorithms
have been developed to avoid obstacles or plan complex paths,
they do not lend themselves to neural implementations: potential
field navigation (Khatib, 1986; Connolly, Burns, and Weiss, 1990;
Tarassenko and Blake, 1991; Connolly and Grupen, 1992), occupancy grids (Moravec, 1988), sinusoidal transforms (Pratt,
1991a, 1991b), graph search (Muller, Kubie, and Saypoff, 1991;
Muller, Stead, and Pach, 1996), see Trullier et al. (1997) for a review of additional algorithms. More theoretical and experimental
work is needed to understand how rodents plan paths and avoid
obstacles.

PLACE CODE

**Why are place cells directional when rodents traverse limited paths, but
not when they search open fields randomly?**

There are two important issues here: (1) why do cells show directional place fields when traversing repeated paths; and (2) why do
cells not show directional place fields when wandering randomly
over open fields?

In chapter 8 (see also chapter 10), I argued that a different
reference frame is used for each direction on the linear track,
but that a single reference frame is used on the open field (Wan,
Touretzky, and Redish, 1994b; Touretzky and Redish, 1996; Redish
and Touretzky, 1997a; Redish, 1997). A similar proposal has been

put forward by McNaughton and colleagues (McNaughton et al., 1996; Samsonovich and McNaughton, 1997; Samsonovich, 1997).

Although I have argued that this last proposal is the most parsimonious with the data, it has not been proven. Among other things, it predicts that there will be a *map-transition* at the ends of the linear track and that place cells will be equally reliable in both directions, and in both environments (the linear track and the open field).

What produces crescent-shaped fields?

As discussed in chapter 8, three hypotheses have been advanced to explain this result. (1) Cells with crescent-shaped place fields might be sensitive to distal landmarks, such that the center of the place field is external to the maze and only a small edge of the place field is accessible to the animal (Sharp, 1991). (2) Place fields could be small, compact (Gaussian-shaped) fields, but they could drift in orientation (due to drift in the head direction system; B. McNaughton, personal communication). (3) Place cells could be sensitive to the surface orientation of the wall (Touretzky and Redish, 1996).

Although the first hypothesis can be rejected (these fields have concave sides, not convex), the other two cannot. At least, not yet. I have argued that the third is most likely to be correct, although the second does still fit the current data. Hypothesis 2 predicts that the place fields should appear as small, compact, convex fields when the time over which the measurements are integrated is small, and that simultaneously recorded place fields with locations near the wall should all stretch in synchrony. In contrast, hypothesis 3 predicts that certain cells should stretch along the walls, independently of other place fields recorded simultaneously.

How do the three major components driving hippocampal pyramidal cell activity — local view, path integration, and auto-associative properties — interact?

The model in chapter 8 describes place cell activity as a consequence of local view input, path integrator input, and autoassociative properties. We can imagine each cell receiving some proportion of these three inputs ($a_1 \cdot \text{LV} + a_2 \cdot \text{PI} + a_3 \cdot \text{AA}$). Different cells presumably receive different proportions of each of these inputs. Although various researchers have examined theoretical models that use specific proportions of these inputs (e.g., Burgess, Recce, and O'Keefe, 1994; Tsodyks and Sejnowski, 1995; McNaughton et al., 1996; O'Keefe and Burgess, 1996a; Recce and Harris, 1996; Tsodyks et al., 1996; Redish, 1997; Samsonovich and McNaughton, 1997; Samsonovich, 1997; Redish and Touretzky, 1998a), large portions of the parameter space are still unexplored.

SELF-LOCALIZATION

Is the self-localization process directly observable?

If self-localization occurs as a consequence of pWTA dynamics in the hippocampus, then the self-localization process should be observable from multiunit recording. If the place fields of a population of cells are recorded during an experience in an environment and then the spikes fired by all of the cells are recorded (simultaneously), the position represented by the population can be displayed at each moment in time by plotting the weighted sum of place fields (i.e. the sum of the place fields of all the cells that fired a spike at a moment in time). The representation should begin as a very broad (essentially uniform) distribution and then tighten up over the course of the self-localization process.

When does the self-localization process occur?

The self-localization process discussed in chapters 8 and 9 is clearly necessary on returning to a familiar environment. Redish and Touretzky (1998a; see also Redish, 1997) proposed that self-localization occurs during a single sharp wave. This predicts that one should see sharp waves on entry into a familiar environment. Even if one doesn't see sharp waves, as long as the animal is using the place code to self-localize, one should still see the tightening of the representation on entry.

It is not known whether the self-localization process occurs during motion within an environment. For example, does self-localization occur when an animal turns around at the end of an arm of a linear track or at the end of the arms of a radial maze? If we assume that different directions along a linear track are represented by different maps (Wan, Touretzky, and Redish, 1994c; McNaughton et al., 1996; Touretzky and Redish, 1996; Redish and Touretzky, 1997a; Redish, 1997; Samsonovich and McNaughton, 1997; Samsonovich, 1997), and that self-localization occurs during map transitions (Redish and Touretzky, 1997a; Redish, 1997), we would expect self-localization at the ends of the arms of a linear track.

Similarly, does self-localization occur along a well-travelled path? Gothard, Skaggs, and McNaughton (1996) found realignment to occur at intermediate points along the journey. One explanation for their findings is that the animals were realigning their representations to successive reference frames along their journey from the box to the room to the landmarks.

Do nearby candidate locations average while distant candidate locations compete?

The hypothesis that the self-localization process is realized by psuedo-winner-take-all network settling to a stable state predicts that nearby candidate locations will average together, while distant candidate locations will compete. This prediction can be tested behaviorally by examining search time of animals (such as gerbils) in a two-landmark task. If the animals are trained to find food at the center of a pair of landmarks and then tested with the landmarks at varied distances, the distance between candidate locations can be experimentally controlled. At large distances, the animal should alternate between two goal locations (Collett, Cartwright, and Smith, 1986; Saksida et al., 1995; Redish, 1997), but at small distances, the animal should search at one location at the center of the pair.

What is the relationship between hippocampal mislocalization errors and behavioral errors?

If the radial maze is encoded by multiple maps, then there might be a relationship between reference memory errors, working memory errors and mislocalizations. Reference memory errors might consist of mislocalizations between environments while working memory errors might consist of mislocalizations within an environment. Data from Mizumori et al. (1989) suggests that CA1 place fields did not change even though working memory errors were made, but that CA3 fields were disrupted. More experiments explicitly designed to test this hypothesis might produce interesting results.

MULTIPLE MAPS IN THE HIPPOCAMPUS

How are new reference frames separated in novel environments?

As described in chapter 10, there are two possible mechanisms for separating reference frames between two similar environments: (1) CA3 could be prewired into a number of charts (Samsonovich and McNaughton, 1997); or (2) the dentate gyrus could orthogonalize the input ((McNaughton and Morris, 1987); see also Marr, 1969; McNaughton, 1989; Rolls, 1989; O'Reilly and McClelland, 1994; Rolls, 1996; Redish, 1997). These two mechanisms are not incompatible, and both may be correct. More experimental work is needed to understand which mechanisms occur in the rodent brain and more theoretical work is needed to understand the interaction between these two mechanisms.

Do the spatial and contextual input enter the hippocampus through separate structures?

There is some preliminary evidence that location information (such as landmark spatial aspects) and reference frame selection information (such as object identity and olfactory information) enter the hippocampal formation through different pathways. Otto et al. (1996) found a difference between lateral and medial entorhinal cortex (LEC and MEC) lesions. Quirk et al. (1992) found broad sensitivities in MEC to location but no sensitivity to environment; to my knowledge, no one has recorded from LEC.

There is also room for modeling work on this issue. Is it possible for both the spatial and contextual input to enter through the same pathway? How does this affect the path integrator input into the hippocampal formation? Is it necessary for the two inputs to be anatomically separated?

Are maps truly independent or does the system ever remap only a subset of the place fields?

The multiple-map theory advanced in chapter 10 describes multiple maps as if they were complete — as if every map were truly independent of every other. However, Markus et al. (1995) found that some fields did not remap between the two tasks studied. It is not yet known whether this is a between-animals or within-animal phenomenon, nor whether certain portions of the local view/path integrator/autoassociator parameter space can accommodate partial remapping while still producing accurate self-localization and route-replay.

ROUTE REPLAY

What mechanism drives phase precession in the hippocampus? Is the mechanism internal or external to the hippocampus?

Place cells in the hippocampus show *phase precession* (O'Keefe and Recce, 1993; Skaggs et al., 1996), that is, the position represented by the place code sweeps across the actual position of the animal with each theta cycle (Tsodyks et al., 1996). As reviewed in chapter 11, there have been a number of proposals put forward to explain this effect, including that it is an intrinsic process formed by an interaction of two rhythms with similar frequencies just different enough to produce beats (O'Keefe and Recce, 1993), that it can be generated by asymmetric connections (Tsodyks et al., 1996), that it is a consequence of attention sweeping from back to front with each theta cycle (Burgess, Recce, and O'Keefe, 1994; O'Keefe and Burgess, 1996a; Burgess and O'Keefe, 1996), and that it is a consequence of an interaction between the mechanism that drives path integration and internal neuronal dynamics (Samsonovich and McNaughton, 1996). Most of these hypotheses fail to fit one finding or another. There is room here for theoretical work showing a simulation of phase precession that fits all of the currently available data and quantitatively matches the recordings from Skaggs et al. (1996). One possibility that should be addressed is whether phase precession is generated extrahippocampally. Bragin et al. (1995) have shown that the theta rhythm is partially driven from entorhinal cortex, but this would also require that EC place cells show phase precession, which has not yet been tested.

Is replay specific to the hippocampus or do most cortical structures replay memories during sleep states? Is the hippocampus necessary for replay to occur?

Qin et al. (1997) report that certain neocortical areas also replay recent memories during sleep. One hypothesis is that replay is a general property of the mammalian brain. Another is that neocortical replay is a consequence of hippocampal replay. Measuring neocortical replay after hippocampal lesions might be able to distinguish these hypotheses.

MEMORY CONSOLIDATION

Can retrograde amnesia really be limited?

The role of the hippocampus in consolidation has been hotly debated (Nadel, 1991; Squire, 1992; Cohen and Eichenbaum, 1993; Nadel and Moscovitch, 1997), in particular, whether the hippocampus is only a temporary memory store or whether it is always necessary for navigation (Bolhuis, Stewart, and Forrest, 1994; Bohbot et al., 1996; Koerner et al., 1996; Weisend, Astur, and Sutherland, 1996; Koerner et al., 1997). Although Sutherland and Hoesing (1993) would seem to conclusively lay the question to rest (at least for a specific spatial task in rodents), but the lesion was made with colchicine (Sutherland, personal communication), which selectively targets dentate gyrus granule cells, and tends to spare the CA3 and CA1 fields. Koerner et al. (1996, 1997) have repeated this experiment with more complete hippocampal lesions (being very careful not to damage adjacent structures); they found complete retrograde amnesia (i.e., no retrograde gradient) even out to thirty-six weeks. People have reported definite consolidation effects in rodents (Winocur, 1990; Cho, Berracochea, and Jaffard, 1993; Sutherland and Hoesing, 1993), but none of these lesions were purely or completely hippocampal. On the other hand, ischemic lesions produce clear limited retrograde amnesias in humans (Squire, 1992; Rempel-Clower et al., 1996) and the only observable damage is to the CA1 hippocampal field, although there may be covert damage beyond the hippocampus producing the limited retrograde effect (Bachevalier and Meunier, 1996; Mumby et al., 1996).

What is the role of sleep states in memory consolidation?

As discussed in chapter 11, the different roles of REM and slow-wave sleep states in consolidation is still an open question. While disruption experiments and multiunit recording experiments have implicated both states in various aspects of consolidation, the specifics roles played by the two have not been resolved.

What is the relationship between replay and consolidation? Are memories actually written out of the hippocampus?

The evidence that the hippocampus replays recently traveled routes does not imply that those routes are written out to cortex. Evidence is mounting that the hippocampus itself does not play the role of temporary buffer (Bachevalier and Meunier, 1996; Bohbot et al., 1996; Koerner et al., 1996; Mumby et al., 1996; Weisend, Astur, and Sutherland, 1996; Koerner et al., 1997; Nadel and Moscovitch, 1997). But at the same time, there is strong evidence that the hippocampus replays memories during subsequent sleep states (Pavlides and Winson, 1989; Wilson and McNaughton, 1994; Skaggs and McNaughton, 1996). The relation between these two findings and the question of consolidation were discussed in depth in chapter 12, but must be identified as a very important open question.

Are nonspatial memories consolidated out of hippocampus?

Recent evidence has suggested that spatial memories are not consolidated out of the hippocampus (Koerner et al., 1996; Weisend, Astur, and Sutherland, 1996; Koerner et al., 1997), although it is still possible that nonspatial memories are. For example, spatial cues could be used as the indices in memory indexing (O'Keefe and Nadel, 1978; Nadel, Willner, and Kurz, 1985; McNaughton et al., 1996; see also Marr, 1970, 1971; Squire, Cohen, and Nadel, 1984; Teyler and DiScenna, 1985, 1986). This would suggest that while spatial memories would also require the hippocampus, certain nonspatial ones would only require the hippocampus until they were consolidated out. This question, like the previous one, must be considered still open.

NEUROPHARMACOLOGY

What are the roles of the neuromodulators in hippocampal function?

One of the most intriguing current issues in rodent navigation is the question of the roles of neuromodulators such as acetylcholine, norepinephrine, serotonin, and dopamine. These neuromodulators may be involved in changing the state of the navigational system (for example, from storage to recall or replay). Although there has been some remarkable progress in correlating behavioral variables to dopaminergic (Schultz et al., 1995b; Schultz, 1997) and noradrenergic (Sara and Segal, 1991; Aston-Jones, Chiang, and Alexinsky, 1991; Rajkowski, Kubiak, and Aston-Jones, 1994) cell firing rates, what is needed is an understanding of the influence of these neuromodulators on the representations in hippocampus and the other structures discussed in this book. There has been some progress in this issue for acetylcholine (Hasselmo and Bower, 1993; Hasselmo and Schnell, 1994; Fox et al., 1997), but further work is still needed.

Navigation and the hippocampus is a particularly useful domain in which to study the role of neuromodulators because we have a good understanding of the representation and general function of the structures. This means that if a neuromodulator modifies a representation or specific function, we may be able to identify the informational change and better understand the role of that neuromodulator than we could with the (important but limited) biophysical methods often used.

In animals with cholinergic deficits, do cells with fields in multiple reference frames should pull their neighbors from one frame into the other?

This intriguing prediction comes from an interaction between the interference and reference frame theories. Imagine that two place cells, a and b, have place fields near each other in one environment but that only cell b has a field in another environment. According to this prediction, as the animal gains experience with the two environments, cell a will begin to show a place field adjacent to cell b in the second environment.

The key point made by the interference hypothesis is that representations should blend together along connections made by shared neurons. The reference frame hypothesis requires cells with overlapping place fields in one reference frame to have strong connections. Therefore we can predict which cells will be drawn into a reference frame. Simultaneous recordings of multiple cells made under low ACh conditions should show this effect.

Notes

INTRODUCTION

1. The subtaxonomy of *declarative memory* is still under extensive debate (see, for example Tulving, 1983; Squire, 1992; Cohen and Eichenbaum, 1993; Nadel and Moscovitch, 1997). Some authors include *semantic memory* (facts, lexical information, etc.) as an additional subcomponent of declarative memory (Squire, 1992) and differentiate it from episodic memory (Tulving, 1983; Nadel and Moscovitch, 1997). For our purposes, it will be sufficient to differentiate episodic memory from procedural memory. The subtaxonomy of declarative memory is beyond the scope of this book. I will therefore refer to "episodic memory" when I need to discuss specifics, even though I will continue to refer to "declarative memory" when comparing it to procedural memory. For some reason, a subtaxonomy of procedural memory does not seem to be currently in vogue.

CHAPTER 1

1. When the presynaptic neuron fires spikes (action potentials) and the postsynaptic neuron is depolarized, there is an increase in the synaptic weight between the two neurons. LTP has been suggested as the neural correlate of learning (for reviews, see McNaughton and Morris, 1987; Bliss and Lynch, 1988; McNaughton, 1993; Eichenbaum, 1996b).

CHAPTER 2

1. I only refer to spatial internal cues (such as motor efferent copy or vestibular signals). Spatial internal cues are sometimes called

idiothetic cues (Mittelstaedt and Mittelstaedt, 1980; Mittelstaedt and Glasauer, 1991).

2. Taxon strategies typically require only simple spatial parameters such as egocentric bearing, not complex spatial parameters such as distance and allocentric bearing. Egocentric bearing is the angle between some aspect of the animal's body (such as its midline) and the cue, while allocentric bearing is the angle between the landmark and an external reference direction.

3. Actually, Barnes et al. (1997) used corrected integrative path length. The details of the measurement are not important here.

CHAPTER 3

1. There are two alternative hypotheses explaining crescent-shaped place fields (see chapter 8).

CHAPTER 4

1. *Kybernetic models* are computational models consisting of a network of computational processes (such as addition or multiplication) that detail how sensory and internal variables must be manipulated in order to calculate behaviorally observed variables. They were very popular in Europe over the last half century. (See Schöne, 1984, for examples.) We will encounter them again in the discussion of path integration (chapter 6). In general, no connection is made between representations in kybernetic models and neurophysiological structures, although associations have been made in the oculomotor domain between nodes in kybernetic models and specific brainstem and subcortical structures (e.g., Robinson, 1973).

2. Similar but not identical to hippocampal lesions, fornix lesions disrupt the subcortical input and output from the hippocampus, but leave the cortical connections and the hippocampus itself intact. (See appendix B for more detail.)

3. Amphetamine injected into a structure after training can enhance certain memories by affecting the consolidation of those

memories (McGaugh, 1966, 1989). See chapter 12 for a discussion of consolidation and related issues.

CHAPTER 5

1. Both Blair and Sharp (1995) and Taube and Muller (1995) report an optimal correlation of ATN activity with future head direction and PoS activity with current head direction, but both have recently revised their estimates (Taube et al., 1996; Blair, Lipscomb, and Sharp, 1997), suggesting that although ATN activity still anticipates future head directions (by 25 ms), PoS activity may lag the current head direction (by 15 ms).

2. A coherent representation is one in which the firing rates of all component cells are consistent with each other (i.e., only cells representing similar directions are firing at high rates).

CHAPTER 6

1. This description of Jander (1957) is a paraphrasing of the review of Maurer and Seguinot (1995).

2. Although head direction is generally correlated with direction of motion, animals can obviously travel in directions they are not facing. It is not clear how the path integration system handles motion in a direction different from the animal's heading (McNaughton et al., 1996; Touretzky and Redish, 1996; Redish and Touretzky, 1997a; Samsonovich and McNaughton, 1997). One possibility is that there is an override mechanism that updates the path integrator correctly; alternatively, the path integrator might produce incorrect results. A third possibility (B. McNaughton, personal communication) is that some head direction cells are actually tuned to direction of motion and that when the animal moves in a direction it is not facing, these cells will fire relative to the direction of motion, not the direction the animal is facing. Experiments have not yet been done to distinguish between these three possibilities.

3. Gaussian representations covering a space are sometimes called *radial basis function* representations and are used in many neural networks (Hertz, Krogh, and Palmer, 1991).

4. Alyan et al. (1997) only describe paths that lead to the center, which would imply that the task could be solved using angular integration. The actual experiment, however, included paths to other points in the environment (S. Alyan, B. McNaughton, personal communication), which implies that the task does indeed require both linear and angular integration and can be considered a true path integration task.

CHAPTER 7

1. As discussed in previous chapters, although the head direction and path integrator representations do not have predefined correlates with the external environment, once a direction has been identified with the preferred direction of a head direction cell, the preferred directions of all of the other cells are defined. This means that the head direction representations can be understood as representing the orientation of the animal relative to an arbitrary reference direction. An analogous case can be made for the path integrator representing position relative to an arbitrary reference point. See discussions of head direction (chapter 5), path integration (chapter 6), and reference frames (chapter 10).

2. Some researchers (e.g., Neave et al., 1994) have reported a lack of effect of cytotoxic lesions of posterior cingulate cortex in spatial tasks. These authors suggest that the earlier experiments (such as those by Sutherland and Hoesing, 1993) may have damaged the cingulum bundle which passes through the area and connects the anterior thalamic nuclei and other subcortical structures with the postsubiculum and the rest of the subicular complex (Neave, Nagle, and Aggleton, 1997).

CHAPTER 8

1. Although local view is not strictly continuous because of occlusions, it is at least piecewise continuous. It should be noted

that none of the published models actually model the effect of occlusions.

2. The early models of McNaughton and colleagues (McNaughton, 1989; McNaughton, Leonard, and Chen, 1989; Leonard and McNaughton, 1990; McNaughton, Chen, and Markus, 1991; McNaughton, Knierim, and Wilson, 1994) had some similarities to path integration models in that they included abilities to navigate in the dark by updating place representations from self-motion information. Because they accomplish this by associations between local views and self-motion information, they require exploration before showing path integration abilities. These models are better described as *associative memory models* than *path integration models*.

3. The papers presented prior to Wan, Touretzky, and Redish (1994c) hypothesized that place cells were partially driven by path integrator information, but none of them included explicit simulations.

4. For properties 1, 2, and 4, connections are assumed to be unmodifiable. Data exists suggesting that these connections are modifiable, but the functionality of this modifiability is not yet clear.

CHAPTER 9

1. Place fields change from environment to environment (O'Keefe and Conway, 1978; Kubie and Ranck, 1983; Muller and Kubie, 1987; Thompson and Best, 1989; see review in chapter 10), which means that the mapping from anatomy to space changes from one environment to the next and thus place fields cannot be laid out topologically.

2. Actually, the local excitation component produces synaptic efficacy inversely related to the travel time between two place fields, but correlational LTP will average over different speeds and the inverse relation to travel time should be an acceptable approximation to the inverse relation to distance for nearby place fields. Place fields that are far apart will have zero effective weight anyway.

3. The *multiple-map hypothesis* combines ideas from O'Keefe and Nadel (1978), Muller and Kubie (1987), McNaughton and colleagues (McNaughton et al., 1996; Samsonovich and McNaughton, 1997; Samsonovich, 1997), and Touretzky and Redish (Touretzky and Redish, 1996; Redish and Touretzky, 1997a; Redish, 1997).

4. The EPSP is a measure of the voltage change in a neuron induced by a synapse or a population of synapses, and thus can be used to guage the effectiveness of synaptic transmission.

5. The recall and replay processes, although similar, differ in that the replay process does not include candidate locations in the input. The replay process and its relation to the recall process will be discussed in chapter 11.

6. Actually, self-localization must occur uniquely after a context-switch, because some environments are represented by multiple maps (see chapter 10).

CHAPTER 10

1. Although place cells represent more than place, I will continue to refer to them as "place cells" for historical reasons.

2. What does it mean to say that the path integrator reference point changes? While, as we saw in chapter 6, there is no *center* of the path integrator representation, mathematically, the path integrator represents the position of the animal relative to some point in space. Thus what it means neurophysiologically when the reference point changes is that the path integrator place fields translate or rotate relative to the external world. (Remember that, in this theory, the path integrator place field topology never changes.)

3. *Orthogonalization* is a mathematical property that occurs by projecting a low-dimensional space onto a higher one (Marr, 1969). It is equivalent to the outer product in linear algebra. Each unit in the high-dimensional space fires if and only if all elements of some subset of the low-dimensional space is active. In other words, each unit calculates an *and* function of its inputs. For example, let the low-

dimensional set be of dimension five $(a_1, a_2, a_3, a_4, a_5)$ and the high-dimensional set be of dimension fifteen. Each unit in the high-dimensional set will be the product of two units in the inputs set: $(a_1^2, a_1a_2, a_1a_3, a_1a_4, a_1a_5, a_2^2, a_2a_3, a_2a_4, a_2a_5, a_3^2, a_3a_4, a_3a_5, a_4^2, a_4a_5, a_5^2)$. If we have two inputs $A = (1, 1, 1, 0, 0)$ and $B = (0, 0, 1, 1, 1)$ that overlap by one element ($\frac{1}{5}$ of the input space), the representations A' and B' in the high-dimensional space still only overlap by one element which is $\frac{1}{15}$ of the input space. This has *separated* the input.

CHAPTER 11

1. The hippocampal formation includes the hippocampus and its surrounding cortices (i.e. entorhinal cortex, the subicular complex, the perirhinal and parahippocampal cortices). Whether the hippocampus itself is the critical component for consolidation will be discussed in chapter 12.

CHAPTER 13

1. *Spontaneous alternation* is a behavior in which animals alternate choices in a two-choice paradigm (Dember and Richman, 1989). It is a specific example of win-shift behavior and is one reason why the delayed nonmatch-to-sample (Mishkin, 1978) and eight-arm maze (Olton and Samuelson, 1976) are so easily trained.
2. Wilson and McNaughton (1994) only showed that the cognitive graph exists after exploration. Whether it also exists prior to exploration, as suggested by McNaughton et al. (1996), or is learned through exploration, as suggested by Muller, Kubie, and Saypoff (1991), is still an open question.

CHAPTER 14

1. Some axons, called *fibers of passage*, pass through without synapsing on local neurons.
2. Patients with Korsakoff's syndrome show anterograde and retrograde amnesias similar but not identical to patients with

ischemia-caused and other hippocampal lesions (for reviews, see Luria, 1973; Squire, 1987, 1992).

APPENDIX B

1. Te2 is a ventral visual area (Zilles, 1990).
2. Humans also make similar errors. Hermer and Spelke (1994) did an equivalent experiment on young children and on adults. A toy was hidden (in the children's presence) in one of two differently colored boxes in two corners of a rectangular room. The children were then spun and asked to find the toy. They chose the wrong box 50 percent of the time. But if the boxes were moved out of the corners of the room (so the children could no longer use spatial strategies), they always chose the correct box. While normal adults did not show any problems, even when spun, if they were given a distractor task that interfered with linguistic memory, they showed these same errors.
3. This percentage range must be taken as a rough estimate only; determining the exact proportions is a complex experiment requiring issues of rescaling, multiple reference frames within a single environment, and so on.

APPENDIX C

1. Two triangles are *geometrically similar* if each pair of corresponding angles is the same, that is, if one triangle is a rescaled, rotated, or translated version of the other.

References

Abbott, L. F. and K. I. Blum (1996). Functional significance of long-term potentiation for sequence learning and prediction. *Cerebral Cortex* 6(3): 406–416.

Abraham, L. and M. Potegal (1979). Caudate nucleus involvement in spatial cognition. *Society for Neuroscience Abstracts* 5: 67.

Abraham, L., M. Potegal, and S. Miller (1983). Evidence for caudate nucleus involvement in an egocentric spatial task: Return from passive transport. *Physiological Psychology* 11(1): 11–17.

Afifi, A. K. (1994). Basal ganglia: Functional anatomy and physiology. Part 1. *Journal of Child Neurology* 9: 249–260.

Aggleton, J. P. (1993). The contribution of the amygdala to normal and abnormal emotional states. *Trends in Neurosciences* 16(8): 328–333.

Aldridge, J. W. and K. C. Berridge (1998). Coding of serial order by neostriatal neurons: A "natural action" approach to movement sequence. *Journal of Neuroscience* 18(7): 2777–2787.

Alexander, G. E. and M. D. Crutcher (1990). Functional architecture of basal ganglia circuits: Neural substrates of parallel processing. *Trends in Neurosciences* 13(7): 266–271.

Altman, J., R. L. Brunner, and S. A. Bayer (1973). The hippocampus and behavioral maturation. *Behavioral Biology* 8: 557–596.

Alvarado, M. C. and J. W. Rudy (1995a). rats with damage to the hippocampal-formation are impaired on the transverse-patterning problem but not on elemental discriminations. *Behavioral Neuroscience* 109(2): 204–211.

Alvarado, M. C. and J. W. Rudy (1995b). a comparison of kainic acid plus colchicine and ibotenic acid-induced hippocampal formation damage on four configural tasks in rats. *Behavioral Neuroscience* 109(6): 1052–1062.

Alvarez, P. and L. R. Squire (1994). Memory consolidation and the medial temporal lobe: A simple network model. *Proceedings of the National Academy of Sciences, USA* 91: 7041–7045.

Alyan, S. H. and R. Jander (1994). Short-range homing in the house mouse *mus musculus:* Stages in the learning of directions. *Animal Behavior* 48(2): 285–298.

Alyan, S. H., B. M. Paul, E. Ellsworth, R. D. White, and B. L. McNaughton (1997). Is the hippocampus required for path integration? *Society for Neuroscience Abstracts* 23: 504.

Alyan, S. H., D. S. Touretzky, and J. S. Taube (1995). The involvement of passive path integration in learning the Morris water maze. *Society for Neuroscience Abstracts* 21: 1939.

Amari, S.-I. (1977). Dynamics of pattern formation in lateral-inhibition type neural fields. *Biological Cybernetics* 27: 77–87.

American Heritage (1969). *The American Heritage Dictionary of the English Language.* American Heritage and Houghton Mifflin, New York.

Andersen, R. (1988). The neurobiological basis of spatial cognition: Role of the parietal lobe. In Stiles-Davis, J., M. Kritchevsky, and U. Bellugi, editors, *Spatial Cognition: Brain Bases and Development.* Erlbaum, Hillsdale NJ.

Andersen, R. A., G. K. Essick, and R. M. Siegel (1985). Encoding of spatial location by posterior parietal neurons. *Science* 230: 456–458.

Andersen, R. A., L. H. Snyder, C. S. Li, and B. Stricanne (1993). Coordinate transformations in the representation of spatial information. *Current Opinion in Neurobiology* 3: 171–176.

Annett, L. E., A. McGregor, and T. W. Robbins (1989). The effects of ibotenic acid lesions of the nucleus accumbens on spatial learning and extinction in the rat. *Behavioral Brain Research* 31(3): 231–242.

Arai, K., E. L. Keller, and J. A. Edelman (1994). Two-dimensional neural network model of the primate saccadic system. *Neural Networks* 7(6/7): 1115–1135.

Archer, J. and L. Birke, editors (1983). *Exploration in Animals and Humans*. Van Nostrand Reinhold, Cambridge.

Arolfo, M. P., L. Nerad, F. Schenk, and J. Bures (1994). Absence of snapshot memory of the target view interferes with place navigation learning by rats in the water maze. *Behavioral Neuroscience* 108(2): 308–316.

Aston-Jones, G., C. Chiang, and T. Alexinsky (1991). Discharge of noradrenergic locus coeruleus neurons in behaving rats and monkeys suggests a role in vigilance. *Progress in Brain Research* 88: 501–520.

Austin, K. B., W. F. Fortin, and M. L. Shapiro (1990). Place fields are altered by NMDA antagonist MK-801 during spatial learning. *Society for Neuroscience Abstracts* 16: 263.

Austin, K. B., L. H. White, and M. L. Shapiro (1993). Short- and long-term effects of experience on hippocampal place fields. *Society for Neuroscience Abstracts* 19: 797.

Bach, M. E., R. D. Hawkins, M. Osman, E. R. Kandel, and M. Mayford (1995). Impairment of spatial but not contextual memory in CaMKII mutant mice with a selective loss of hippocampal LTP in the range of the theta frequency. *Cell* 81: 905–915.

Bachevalier, J. and M. Meunier (1996). Cerebral ischemia: Are the memory deficits associated with hippocampal cell loss? *Hippocampus* 6: 553–560.

Barlow, J. S. (1964). Inertial navigation as a basis for animal navigation. *Journal of Theoretical Biology* 6: 76–117.

Barnes, C. A. (1979). Memory deficits associated with senscence: A neurophysiological and behavioral study in the rat. *Journal of Comparative and Physiological Psychology* 93: 74–104.

Barnes, C. A. (1988). Spatial learning and memory processes: The search for their neurobiological mechanisms in the rat. *Trends in Neurosciences* 11: 163–169.

Barnes, C. A. (1994). Normal aging: Regionally specific changes in hippocampal synaptic transmission. *Trends in Neurosciences* 17(1): 13–18.

Barnes, C. A. (1998). Memory changes during normal aging: Neurobiological correlates. In Martinez, Jr., J. L. and R. P. Kesner, editors, *Learning and Memory: A Biological View*, pp. 247–273. Academic Press, New York.

Barnes, C. A., B. L. McNaughton, S. J. Y. Mizumori, B. W. Leonard, and L. H. Lin (1990). Comparison of spatial and temporal characteristics of neuronal activity in sequential stages of hippocampal processing. *Progress in Brain Research* 83: 287–300.

Barnes, C. A., B. L. McNaughton, and J. O'Keefe (1983). Loss of place specificity in hippocampal complex spike cells of senescent rat. *Neurobiology of Aging* 4: 113–119.

Barnes, C. A., L. Nadel, and W. K. Honig (1980). Spatial memory deficit in senescent rats. *Canadian Journal of Psychology* 34(1): 29–39.

Barnes, C. A., G. Rao, and B. L. McNaughton (1996). Functional integrity of NMDA-dependent LTP induction mechanisms across the lifespan of F-344 rats. *Learning and Memory* 3: 124–137.

Barnes, C. A., M. S. Suster, J. Shen, and B. L. McNaughton (1997). Multistability of cognitive maps in the hippocampus of old rats. *Nature* 388(6639): 272–275.

Barto, A. G. (1995). Adaptive critics and the basal ganglia. In Houk, J. C., J. L. Davis, and D. G. Beiser, editors, *Models of Information Processing in the Basal Ganglia*, pp. 215–232. MIT Press, Cambridge MA.

Bear, M. F. and A. Kirkwood (1993). Neocortical long-term potentiation. *Current Opinion in Neurobiology* 3(2): 197–202.

Beiser, D. G., S. E. Hua, and J. C. Houk (1997). Network models of the basal ganglia. *Current opinion in neurobiology* 7(2): 185–190.

Bellman, R. (1958). On a routing problem. *Quarterly Journal of Applied Mathematics* 16(1): 87–90.

Benhamou, S., P. Bovet, and B. Poucet (1995). A model for place navigation in mammals. *Journal of Theoretical Biology* 173: 163–178.

Benhamou, S., J. P. Sauve, and P. Bovet (1990). Spatial memory in large-scale movements: Efficiency and limitation of the egocentric coding process. *Journal of Theoretical Biology* 145: 1–12.

Bentivoglio, M., K. Kultas-Ilinsky, and I. Illinsky (1993). Limbic thalamus: Structure, intrinsic organization, and connections. In Vogt, B. A. and M. Gabriel, editors, *Neurobiology of Cingulate Cortex and Limbic Thalamus: A Comprehensive Handbook*, pp. 71–122. Birkhäuser, Boston.

Beritashvili, I. S. (1965). *Neural Mechanisms of Higher Vertebrate Behavior*. Little, Brown, Boston.

Berridge, K. C. and I. Q. Whishaw (1992). Cortex, striatum and cerebellum: Control of serial order in a grooming sequence. *Experimental Brain Research* 90(2): 275–290.

Biegler, R. and R. G. M. Morris (1993). Landmark stability is a prerequisite for spatial but not discrimination learning. *Nature* 361: 631–633.

Biegler, R. and R. G. M. Morris (1996). Landmark stability: Studies exploring whether the perceived stability of the environment influences spatial representation. *Journal of Experimental Biology* 199(1): 187–193.

Birke, L. I. A. (1983). Some issues and problems in the study of animal exploration. In Archer, J. and Birke, editors, *Exploration in Animals and Humans*, pp. 1–21. Van Nostrand Reinhold, Cambridge.

Bisiach, E. and G. Vallar (1988). Hemineglect in humans. In Boller, F. and J. Grafman, editors, *Handbook of Neuropsychology*, Vol. 1, pp. 195–222. Elsevier, New York.

Bizzi, E., F. A. Mussa-Ivaldi, and S. Giszter (1991). Computations underlying the execution of movement: A biological perspective. *Science* 253: 287–291.

Bjorklund, A., O. G. Nilsson, and P. Kalen (1990). Reafferentation of the subcortically denervated hippocampus as a model for transplant-induced functional recovery in the CNS. *Progress in Brain Research* 83: 411–426.

Blair, H. T. (1996). A thalamocortical circuit for computing directional heading in the rat. In Touretzky, D. S., M. C. Mozer, and M. E. Hasselmo, editors, *Advances in Neural Information Processing Systems 8*, pp. 152–158, Cambridge, MA. MIT Press.

Blair, H. T., B. W. Lipscomb, and P. E. Sharp (1997). Anticipatory time intervals of head-direction cells in the anterior thalamus of the rat, implications for path integration in the head-direction circuit. *Journal of Neurophysiology* 78(1): 145–159.

Blair, H. T. and P. E. Sharp (1995). Anticipatory head direction signals in anterior thalamus: Evidence for a thalamocortical circuit that integrates angular head motion to compute head direction. *Journal of Neuroscience* 15(9): 6260–6270.

Bliss, T. V. P. and M. A. Lynch (1988). Long-term potentiation of synaptic transmission in the hippocampus: Properties and mechanisms. In Landfield, P. W. and S. A. Deadwyler, editors, *Long-Term Potentiation: From Biophysics to Behavior*, pp. 3–72. Liss, New York.

Blodget, H. C. (1921). The effect of the introduction of reward upon the maze performance of rats. *University of California Publications in Psychology* 4(8): 113–134.

Blum, K. I. and L. F. Abbott (1996). A model of spatial map formation in the hippocampus of the rat. *Neural Computation* 8(1): 85–93.

Bohbot, V. (1997). The medial temporal lobes and human memory. Ph.D. diss., University of Arizona.

Bohbot, V., Z. Liu, S. L. Thurm, L. Nadel, and J. Bures (1996). Spatial memory? Never without a hippocampus. *Society for Neuroscience Abstracts* 22: 1873.

Bolhuis, J. J., C. A. Stewart, and E. M. Forrest (1994). Retrograde amnesia and memory reactivation in rats with ibotenate lesions to the hippocampus or subiculum. *Quarterly Journal of Experimental Psychology* 47B(2): 129–150.

Bondy, J. A. and U. S. R. Murty (1976). *Graph Theory with Applications*. Elsevier, New York.

Bostock, E., R. U. Muller, and J. L. Kubie (1991). Experience-dependent modifications of hippocampal place cell firing. *Hippocampus* 1(2): 193–206.

Bragin, A., G. Jando, Z. Nadasdy, J. Hetke, K. Wise, and G. Buzsáki (1995). Gamma (40–100 Hz) oscillation in the hippocampus of the behaving rat. *Journal of Neuroscience* 15(1): 47–60.

Brooks, V. B. (1986). *The Neural Basis of Motor Control*. Oxford University Press, New York.

Brown, M. A. and P. E. Sharp (1995). Simulation of spatial learning in the Morris water maze by a neural network model of the hippocampal formation and nucleus accumbens. *Hippocampus* 5(3): 171–188.

Brown, M. W. (1982). Effect of context on the response of single units recorded from the hippocampal region of behaviourally trained monkeys. In Marsan, C. A. and H. Matthies, editors, *Neuronal Plasticity and Memory Formation*, pp. 557–573. Raven Press, New York.

Brown, T. H., A. M. Zador, Z. F. Mainen, and B. J. Clairborne (1991). Hebbian modifications in hippocampal neurons. In Boudry, M. and J. L. Davis, editors, *Long-Term Potentiation: A Debate of Current Issues*, pp. 357–389. MIT Press, Cambridge MA.

Buhot, M.-C. and S. Naili (1995). Changes in exploratory activity following stimulation of hippocampal 5-HT1A and 5-HT1B receptors in the rat. *Hippocampus* 5(3): 198–208.

Bunsey, M. and H. Eichenbaum (1995). Selective damage to the hippocampal region blocks long-term retention of a natural and nonspatial stimulus-stimulus association. *Hippocampus* 5(6): 546–556.

Bures, J. (1996). Paradigms for examination of the role played by hippocampal place cells in different forms of place navigation. In Ono, T., B. L. McNaughton, S. Molotchnikoff, E. T. Rolls, and H. Nishijo, editors, *Perception, Memory and Emotion: Frontiers in Neuroscience*, pp. 291–303. Pergamon Press, New York.

Buresova, O., J. J. Bolhuis, and J. Bures (1986). Differential effects of cholinergic blockade on performance of rats in the water tank navigation task and in a radial water task. *Behavioral Neurology* 100: 476–482.

Burgess, N. and J. O'Keefe (1996). Neuronal computations underlying the firing of place cells and their role in navigation. *Hippocampus* 7: 749–762.

Burgess, N., J. O'Keefe, and M. Recce (1993). Using hippocampal 'place cells' for navigation, exploiting phase coding. In Hanson, S., J. Cowan, and L. Giles, editors, *Advances in Neural Information Processing Systems 5*, pp. 929–936. Morgan Kaufmann, San Mateo, CA.

Burgess, N., M. Recce, and J. O'Keefe (1994). A model of hippocampal function. *Neural Networks* 7(6/7): 1065–1081.

Burnham, W. H. (1903). Retroactive amnesia: Illustrative cases and a tentative explanation. *American Journal of Psychology* 14: 382–396.

Burwell, R. D. and D. G. Amaral (1998). Perirhinal and postrhinal cortices of the rat: Interconnectivity and connections with the entorhinal cortex. *Journal of Comparative Neurology* 391(3): 293–321.

Burwell, R. D. and H. Eichenbaum (1997). Perirhinal cortex neurons do not exhibit spatial firing patterns. *Society for Neuroscience abstracts* 23: 503.

Burwell, R. D., M. P. Witter, and D. G. Amaral (1995). Perirhinal and postrhinal cortices of the rat: A review of the neuroanatomical literature and comparison with findings from the monkey brain. *Hippocampus* 5(5): 309–408.

Bussey, T. J., B. J. Everitt, and T. W. Robbins (1997). Dissociable effects of cingulate and medial frontal cortex lesions on stimulus-reward learning using a novel Pavlovian autoshaping procedure for the rat: Implications for the neurobiology of emotion. *Behavioral Neuroscience* 111(5): 908–919.

Bussey, T. J., J. L. Muir, B. J. Everitt, and T. W. Robbins (1997). Triple dissociation of anterior cingulate, posterior cingulate, and medial frontal cortices on visual discrimination tasks using a touchscreen testing procedure for the rat. *Behavioral Neuroscience* 111(5): 920–936.

Buxton, R. B. and L. R. Frank (1997). A model for the coupling between cerebral blood flow and oxygen metabolism during neural stimulation. *Journal of Cerebral Blood Flow and Metabolism* 17: 64–72.

Buzsáki, G. (1989). Two-stage model of memory trace formation: A role for "noisy" brain states. *Neuroscience* 31(3): 551–570.

Carr, H. (1917). Maze studies with the white rat. *Journal of Animal Behavior* 7: 259–306.

Carr, H. and J. B. Watson (1908). Orientation in the white rat. *Journal of Comparative Neurology and Psychology* 18: 27–44.

Cassaday, H. J. and J. N. P. Rawlins (1995). Fornix-fimbria section and working memory deficits in rats: Stimulus complexity and stimulus size. *Behavioral Neuroscience* 109(4): 594–606.

Cassaday, H. J. and J. N. P. Rawlins (1997). The hippocampus, objects, and their contexts. *Behavioral Neuroscience* 111(6): 1228–1244.

Castro, C. A., L. H. Silbert, B. L. McNaughton, and C. A. Barnes (1989). Recovery of spatial learning deficits after decay of electrically induced synaptic enhancement in the hippocampus. *Nature* 342: 545–548.

Chance, M. R. A. and A. P. Mead (1955). Competition between feeding and investigation in the rat. *Behavior* 8: 174–181.

Chandler, H. C., V. King, J. V. Corwin, and R. L. Reep (1992). Thalamocortical connections of rat posterior parietal cortex. *Neuroscience Letters* 143: 237–242.

Chapuis, N. and P. Scardigli (1993). Shortcut ability in hamsters (*mesocricetus auratus*): The role of environmental and kinesthetic information. *Animal Learning and Behavior* 21(3): 255–265.

Chen, L. L. (1989). Spatial representation in the rat posterior parietal cortex. Master's thesis, University of Colorado, Department of Psychology.

Chen, L. L. (1991). Head-directional information processing in the rat posterior cortical areas. Ph.D. diss., University of Colorado.

Chen, L. L., L. H. Lin, E. J. Green, C. A. Barnes, and B. L. McNaughton (1994a). Head-direction cells in the rat posterior cortex: I. Anatomical distribution and behavioral modulation. *Experimental Brain Research* 101: 8–23.

Chen, L. L., L. H. Lin, C. A. Barnes, and B. L. McNaughton (1994b). Head-direction cells in the rat posterior cortex: II. Contributions of visual and ideothetic information to the directional firing. *Experimental Brain Research* 101: 24–34.

Chen, L. L., B. L. McNaughton, C. A. Barnes, and E. R. Ortiz (1990). Head-directional and behavioral correlates of posterior cingulate and medial prestriate cortex neurons in freely-moving rats. *Society for Neuroscience Abstracts* 16: 441.

Cheng, K. (1986). A purely geometric module in the rat's spatial representation. *Cognition* 23: 149–178.

Cho, Y. H., D. Berracochea, and R. Jaffard (1993). Extended temporal gradient for the retrograde and anterograde amnesia produced by ibotenate entorhinal cortex lesions in mice. *Journal of Neuroscience* 13(4): 1759–1766.

Christian, E. P. and S. A. Deadwyler (1986). Behavioral function and hippocampal cell types: Evidence for two non-overlapping populations in the rat. *Journal of Neurophysiology* 55: 331–348.

Chrobak, J. J. and G. Buzáki (1998). Gamma oscillations in the entorhinal cortex of the freely behaving rat. *Journal of Neuroscience* 18(1): 388–398.

Chrobak, J. J. and G. Buzsáki (1994). Selective activation of deep layer (V-VI) retrohippocampal neurons during hippocampal sharp waves in the behaving rat. *Journal of Neuroscience* 14(10): 6160–6170.

Chrobak, J. J. and G. Buzsáki (1996).   High-frequency oscillations in the output networks of the hippocampal-entorhinal axis of the freely behaving rat. *Journal of Neuroscience* 16(9): 3056–3066.

Cohen, N. J. and H. Eichenbaum (1993). *Memory, Amnesia, and the Hippocampal System*. MIT Press, Cambridge, MA.

Cohen, N. J. and L. R. Squire (1980).   Preserved learning and retention of pattern-analyzing skill in amnesia: Dissociation of knowing how and knowing that. *Science* 210: 207–210.

Colby, C. L. and J.-R. Duhamel (1991). Heterogeneity of extrastriate visual areas and multiple parietal areas in the macaque monkey. *Neuropsychologia* 29(6): 517–537.

Colby, C. L., J.-R. Duhamel, and M. E. Goldberg (1993). The analysis of visual space by the lateral intraparietal area of the monkey: The role of extraretinal signals. *Progress in Brain Research* 95: 307–316.

Colby, C. L., J.-R. Duhamel, and M. E. Goldberg (1995).   Occulocentric spatial representation in parietal cortex. *Cerebral Cortex* 5(5): 470–481.

Collett, T. S., B. A. Cartwright, and B. A. Smith (1986). Landmark learning and visuo-spatial memories in gerbils. *Journal of Comparative Physiology* A158: 835–851.

Collinder, P. (1955). *A History of Marine Navigation*. St. Martin's Press, New York. Translated from the Swedish by M. Michael.

Connolly, C. I. and J. B. Burns (1995).   A state space striatal model.   In Houk, J. C., J. L. Davis, and D. G. Beiser, editors, *Models of Information Processing in the Basal Ganglia*, pp. 163–178. MIT Press, Cambridge MA.

Connolly, C. I., J. B. Burns, and R. Weiss (1990). Path planning using Laplace's equation. *Proceedings of the 1990 IEEE International Conference on Robotics and Automation* pp. 2102–2106.

Connolly, C. I. and R. A. Grupen (1992). Applications of harmonic functions to robotics. Technical report COINS-92-12, Computer and Information Science Department, University of Massachusetts.

Cook, D. and R. P. Kesner (1988). Caudate nucleus and memory for egocentric localization. *Behavioral and Neural Biology* 49: 332–343.

Cooper, J. R., F. E. Bloom, and R. H. Roth (1986). *The Biochemical Basis of Neuropharmacology*. Oxford University Press, New York, 5th edition.

Corkin, S. (1968). Acquisition of motor skill after bilateral medial temporal-lobe excision. *Neuropsychologia* 6: 255–265.

Cormen, T. H., C. E. Leiserson, and R. L. Rivest (1990). *Introduction to Algorithms*. MIT Press and McGraw-Hill, Cambridge MA and New York NY.

Corodimas, K. P. and J. E. LeDoux (1995). Disruptive effects of posttraining perirhinal cortex lesions on conditioned fear: Contributions of contextual cues. *Behavioral Neuroscience* 4: 613–619.

Cotter, C. H. (1968). *A History of Nautical Astronomy*. American Elsevier, New York.

Cressant, A., R. U. Muller, and B. Poucet (1997). Failure of centrally placed objects to control firing fields of hippocampal place cells. *Journal of Neuroscience* 17(7): 2531–2542.

Cromwell, H. C. and K. C. Berridge (1996). Implementation of action sequences by a neostriatal site: A lesion mapping study of grooming syntax. *Journal of Neuroscience* 16(10): 3444–3458.

Darwin, C. A. (1873a). Perception in the lower animals. *Nature* 7: 360.

Darwin, C. A. (1873b). Origin of certain instincts. *Nature* 7: 417–418.

Dassonville, P., J. Boline, and A. P. Georgopoulos (1993). A dynamic representation of hand in space for 3D tactile localization. *Society for Neuroscience Abstracts* 19: 147.

Dassonville, P., J. Schlag, and M. Schlag-Rey (1994). Directional constancy in the oculomotor system. *Current Directions in Psychological Science* 2(5): 143–147.

Davidson, T. L., M. G. McKernan, and L. E. Jarrard (1993). Hippocampal lesions do not impair negative patterning: A challenge to configural association theory. *Behavioral Neuroscience* 107(2): 227–234.

Davis, M., D. Rainnie, and M. Cassell (1994). Neurotransmission in the rat amygdala related to fear and anxiety. *Trends in Neurosciences* 17(5): 208–214.

Davis, S., S. P. Butcher, and R. G. Morris (1992). The NMDA receptor antagonist D-2-amino-5-phosphonopentanoate (D-AP5) impairs spatial learning and LTP in vivo at intracerebral concentrations comparable to those that block LTP in vitro. *Journal of Neuroscience* 12(1): 21–34.

Day, L. B. and T. Schallert (1996). Anticholinergic effects on acquisition of place learning in the Morris water task: Spatial mapping deficit or inability to inhibit non-place strategies. *Behavioral Neuroscience* 110(5): 998–1005.

Dayan, P. (1991). Navigating through temporal difference. In Lippmann, R. P., J. E. Moody, and D. S. Touretzky, editors, *Advances in Neural Information Processing Systems 3*, pp. 464–470. Morgan Kauffman, San Mateo CA.

Dean, P. (1990). Sensory cortex: Visual perception functions. In Kolb, B. and R. C. Tees, editors, *The Cerebral Cortex of the Rat*, pp. 275–308. MIT Press, Cambridge MA.

Dean, P. and P. Redgrave (1984a). The superior colliculus and visual neglect in rat and hamster: I. Behavioural evidence. *Brain Research Reviews* 8: 129–141.

Dean, P. and P. Redgrave (1984b). The superior colliculus and visual neglect in rat and hamster: II. Possible mechanisms. *Brain Research Reviews* 8: 141–153.

Dean, P. and P. Redgrave (1984c). The superior colliculus and visual neglect in rat and hamster: III. Functional implications. *Brain Research Reviews* 8: 155–163.

Dean, P., P. Redgrave, and G. W. M. Westby (1989). Event or emergency? Two response systems in the mammalian superior colliculus. *Trends in Neurosciences* 12(4): 137–147.

Decker, M. W. and J. L. McGaugh (1991). The role of interactions between the cholinergic system and other neuromodulatory systems in learning and memory. *Synapse* 7: 151–168.

Dember, W. N. and C. L. Richman, editors (1989). *Spontaneous Alternation Behavior*. Springer, New York.

Dennis, W. (1932). Multiple visual discrimination in the block elevated maze. *Journal of Comparitive and Physiological Psychology* 13: 391–396.

Desimone, R., S. J. Schein, J. Moran, and L. G. Ungerleider (1985). Contour, color, and shape analysis beyond the striate cortex. *Vision Research* 25(3): 444–452.

DeVietti, T. L., S. M. Pellis, V. C. Pellis, and P. Teitelbaum (1985). Previous experience disrupts atropine-induced stereotyped "trapping" in rats. *Behavioral Neuroscience* 99(6): 1128–1141.

Dijkstra, E. W. (1959). A note on two problems in connexion with graphs. *Numerische Mathematik* 1: 269–271.

DiMattia, B. V. D. and R. P. Kesner (1988). Spatial cognitive maps: Differential role of parietal cortex and hippocampal formation. *Behavioral Neuroscience* 102(4): 471–480.

Douglas, R. J. (1967). The hippocampus and behavior. *Psychological Bulletin* 67(6): 416–442.

Douglas, R. J. (1975). The development of hippocampal function: Implications for theory and for therapy. In Isaacson, R. L. and K. H. Pribram, editors, *The Hippocampus*, Vol. 2, pp. 327–361. Plenum Press, New York.

Douglas, R. J. (1989). Spontaneous alternation behavior and the brain. In Dember, W. N. and C. L. Richman, editors, *Spontaneous Alternation Behavior*, pp. 73–108. Springer, New York.

Drager, U. C. and D. H. Hubel (1975). Responses to visual stimulation and relationship between visual, auditory, and somatosensory inputs in mouse superior colliculus. *Journal of Neurophysiology* 38: 690–713.

Drager, U. C. and D. H. Hubel (1976). Topography of visual and somatosensory projections to mouse superior colliculus. *Journal of Neurophysiology* 39: 91–101.

Droulez, J. and A. Berthoz (1991). A neural network model of sensoritopic maps with predictive short-term memory properties. *Proceedings of the National Academy of Sciences, USA* 88: 9653–9657.

Dudchenko, P. A. and J. S. Taube (1997). Correlation between head direction cell activity and spatial behavior on a radial arm maze. *Behavioral Neuroscience* 111(1): 3–19.

Eckerman, D. A., W. A. Gordon, J. D. Edwards, R. C. MacPhail, and M. I. Gage (1980). Effects of scopolomine, pentobarbitol, and amphetamine on radial arm maze performance in the rat. *Pharmacology Biochemistry and Behavior* 12: 595–602.

Efron, B. (1982). *The Jackknife, the Bootstrap, and Other Resampling Plans*, Vol. 38 of *Regional Conference Series in Applied Mathematics*. Society for Industrial and Applied Mathematics, Philadelphia PA.

Eichenbaum, H. (1996a). Is the rodent hippocampus just for "place"? *Current Opinion in Neurobiology* 6: 187–195.

Eichenbaum, H. (1996b). Learning from LTP: A comment on recent attempts to identify cellular and molecular mechanisms of memory. *Learning and Memory* 3(2/3): 61–73.

Eichenbaum, H. and N. J. Cohen (1988). Representation in the hippocampus: What do hippocampal neurons code? *Trends in Neurosciences* 11(6): 244–248.

Eichenbaum, H., M. Kuperstein, A. Fagan, and J. Nagode (1987). Cue-sampling and goal-approach correlates of hippocampal unit activity in rats performing an odor-discrimination task. *Journal of Neuroscience* 7(3): 716–732.

Eichenbaum, H., T. Otto, and N. J. Cohen (1992). The hippocampus – what does it do? *Behavioral and Neural Biology* 57: 2–36.

Eichenbaum, H., T. Otto, and N. J. Cohen (1994). Two functional components of the hippocampal memory system. *Behavioral and Brain Sciences* 17: 449–472. See also commentary and response, pages 472–518.

Eichenbaum, H., C. Stewart, and R. G. M. Morris (1990). Hippocampal representation in place learning. *Journal of Neuroscience* 10(11): 3531–3542.

Eifuku, S., H. Nishijo, T. Kita, and T. Ono (1995). Neuronal activity in the primate hippocampal formation during a conditional association task based on the subject's location. *Journal of Neuroscience* 15(7): 4952–4969.

Eilam, D. and I. Golani (1989). Home base behavior of rats (*rattus norvegicus*) exploring a novel environment. *Behavioral Brian Research* 34: 199–211.

Ellard, C. G. and M. A. Goodale (1988). A functional analysis of the collicular output pathways: A dissociation of deficits following lesions of the dorsal tegmental decussation and the ipsilateral collicular efferent bundle in the Mongolian gerbil. *Experimental Brain Research* 71: 307–319.

Encyclopædia Britannica (1994). *Encyclopædia Britannica*. 15th ed. Chicago.

Ermentrout, B. and J. Cowan (1979). A mathematical theory of visual hallucination patterns. *Biological Cybernetics* 34: 137–150.

Etienne, A. S. (1987). The control of short-distance homing in the golden hamster. In Ellen, P. and C. Thinus-Blanc, editors, *Cognitive Processes and Spatial Orientation in Animals and Man*, Vol. I, *Experimental Animal Psychology and Ethology*, pp. 233–251. Nijhoff, Boston.

Etienne, A. S. (1992). Navigation of a small mammal by dead reckoning and local cues. *Current Directions in Psychological Science* 1(2): 48–52.

Etienne, A. S., R. Maurer, and F. Saucy (1988). Limitations in the assessment of path dependent information. *Behavior* 106: 81–111.

Etienne, A. S., R. Maurer, F. Saucy, and E. Teroni (1986). Short-distance homing in the golden hamster after a passive outward journey. *Animal Behavior* 34: 696–715.

Farrall, L. (1984). *Unwritten Knowledge: Case Study of the Navigators of Micronesia*. Deakin University, Victoria, Australia.

Finch, D. M. (1993). Hippocampal, subicular, and entorhinal afferents and synaptic integration in rodent cingulate cortex. In Vogt, B. A. and M. Gabriel, editors, *Neurobiology of Cingulate Cortex and Limbic Thalamus: A Comprehensive Handbook*, pp. 224–248. Birkhäuser, Boston.

Finch, D. M. (1996). Neurophysiology of converging synaptic inputs from rat prefrontal cortex, amygdala, midline thalamus, and hippocampal formation onto single neurons of the caudate/putamen and nucleus accumbens. *Hippocampus* 6: 495–512.

Fishbein, W. and B. M. Gutwein (1977). Paradoxical sleep and memory storage processes. *Behavioral Biology* 19: 425–464.

Flicker, C. and M. A. Geyer (1982). Behavior during hippocampal microinfusions. I. Norepinephrine and diversive exploration. *Brain Research Reviews* 4: 79–103.

Floresco, S. B., J. K. Seamans, and A. G. Phillips (1997). Selective roles for hippocampal, prefrontal cortical, and ventral striatal circuits in radial-arm maze tasks with or without a delay. *Journal of Neuroscience* 17(5): 1880–1890.

Ford, L. R. and D. R. Fulkerson (1962). *Flows in Networks*. Princeton University Press, Princeton NJ.

Forde, H. (1873). Sense of direction. *Nature* 7: 463–464.

Foster, T. C., C. A. Castro, and B. L. McNaughton (1989). Spatial selectivity of rat hippocampal neurons: Dependence on preparedness for movement. *Science* 244: 1580–1582.

Fox, P. T. and M. E. Raichle (1986). Focal phsyiological uncoupling of cerebral blood flow and oxidative metabolism during somatosensory stimulation in human subjects. *Proceedings of the National Academy of Sciences, USA* 83: 1140–1144.

Fox, S. E., N. Ludvig, J. L. Kubie, R. U. Muller, M. Stead, and A. Fenton (1997). The effects of scopolamine, delivered via intrahippocampal microdialysis, on the firing of local place cells. *Society for Neuroscience Abstracts* 22: 431.

Fraenkel, G. S. and D. L. Gunn (1961). *The Orientation of Animals, Kineses, Taxes, and Compass Reactions*. Dover, New York.

Freud, S. (1899). *The Interpretation of Dreams*. Translated by A. A. Brill. Random House, New York, 1950.

Freud, S. (1923). *The Ego and the Id*, Vol. 19 of *The Standard Edition of the Complete Psychological Works of Sigmund Freud*. Translated and edited by J. Strachey. Hogarth Press, London, 1961.

Freund, T. F. and G. Buzsáki (1996). Interneurons of the hippocampus. *Hippocampus* 6(4): 345–370.

Fried, I., K. A. MacDonald, and C. L. Wilson (1997). Single neuron activity in human hippocampus and amygdala during recognition of faces and objects. *Neuron* 18(5): 753–765.

Fuhs, M., A. D. Redish, and D. S. Touretzky (1998). A visually driven hippocampal model. In Bower, J., editor, *Computational Neuroscience: Trends in Research, 1998*, pp. 379–384. Plenum, New York.

Fujita, N., J. M. Loomis, R. L. Klatzky, and R. G. Golledge (1990). A minimal representation for dead-reckoning navigation: Updating the homing vector. *Geographical Analysis* 22(4): 326–335.

Fuster, J. M. (1997). *The Prefrontal Cortex: Anatomy, Physiology, and Neuropsychology of the Frontal Lobe.* Lippincott-Raven, Third edition.

Gabrieli, J. (1995). Contribution of the basal ganglia to skill learning and working memory in humans. In Houk, J. C., J. L. Davis, and D. G. Beiser, editors, *Models of Information Processing in the Basal Ganglia*, pp. 277–294. MIT Press, Cambridge MA.

Gaffan, D. (1972). Loss of recognition memory in rats with lesions of the fornix. *Neuropsychologia* 10: 327–341.

Gaffan, D. (1974). Recognition impaired and association intact in the memory of monkeys after transection of the fornix. *Journal of Comparative and Physiological Psychology* 86: 1100–1109.

Gaffan, D., R. C. Sanders, E. A. Gaffan, S. Harrison, C. Shields, and M. J. Owen (1984). Effects of fornix transection upon associative memory in monkeys: Role of the hippocampus in learned actions. *Quarterly Journal of Experimental Psychology* 36B: 173–221.

Gallagher, M., R. Burwell, and M. Burchinal (1993). Severity of spatial learning impairment in aging: Development of a learning index for performance in the Morris water maze. *Behavioral Neuroscience* 107(4): 618–626.

Gallagher, M. and R. D. Burwell (1989). Relationship of age-related decline across several behavioral domains. *Neurobiology of Aging* 10: 691–708.

Gallagher, M. and P. J. Colombo (1995). Aging: The cholinergic hypothesis of cognitive decline. *Current Opinion in Neurobiology* 5: 161–168.

Gallagher, M. and P. C. Holland (1992). Preserved configural learning and spatial learning impairment in rats with hippocampal damage. *Hippocampus* 2(1): 81–88.

Gallagher, M., A. H. Nagahara, and R. D. Burwell (1995). Cognition and hippocampal systems in aging: Animal models. In McGaugh, J. L., N. M. Weinberger, and G. Lynch, editors, *Brain and Memory: Modulation and Mediation of Neuroplasticity*, pp. 103–126. Oxford, New York NY.

Gallagher, M. and M. M. Nicole (1993). Animal models of normal aging: Relationship between cognitive decline and markers in hippocampal circuitry. *Behavioral Brain Research* 57: 155–162.

Gallistel, C. R. (1980). *The Organization of Action: A New Synthesis*. Erlbaum, Hillsdale NJ.

Gallistel, C. R. (1990). *The Organization of Learning*. MIT Press, Cambridge, MA.

Gavrilov, V. V., S. I. Wiener, and A. Berthoz (1996). Discharge correlates of hippocampal neurons in rats passively displaced on a mobile robot. *Society for Neuroscience Abstracts* 22: 910.

Georgopoulos, A. P., R. Caminiti, J. F. Kalaska, and J. T. Massey (1983). Spatial coding of movement: A hypothesis concerning the coding of movement direction by motor cortical populations. *Experimental Brain Research* Suppl.(7): 327–336.

Georgopoulos, A. P., R. E. Kettner, and A. B. Schwartz (1988). Primate motor cortex and free arm movements to visual targets in three-dimensional space. II. Coding of the direction of movement by a neuronal population. *Journal of Neuro-science* 8(8): 2928–2937.

Gerstner, W. and L. F. Abbott (1997). Learning navigational maps through potentiation and modulation of hippocampal place cells. *Journal of Computational Neuroscience* 4: 79–94.

Gladwin, T. (1970). *East is a Big Bird*. Harvard University Press, Cambridge MA.

Gluck, M. A. and C. E. Myers (1993). Hippocampal mediation of stimulus representation: A computational theory. *Hippocampus* 3(4): 491–516.

Gluck, M. A. and C. E. Myers (1996). Integrating behavioral and physiological models of hippocampal function. *Hippocampus* 6(6): 643–653.

Golani, I., Y. Benjamini, and D. Eilam (1993). Stopping behavior: Constraints on exploration in rats (*rattus norvegicus*). *Behavioral Brain Research* 53(1-2): 21–33.

Goldman-Rakic, P. S. (1995). Toward a circuit model of working memory and the guidance of voluntary motor action. In Houk, J. C., J. L. Davis, and D. G. Beiser, editors, *Models of Information Processing in the Basal Ganglia*, pp. 131–148. MIT Press, Cambridge MA.

Goldman-Rakic, P. S., S. Funahashi, and C. J. Bruce (1990). Neocortical memory circuits. *Cold Spring Harbor Symposia on Quantitative Biology* LV: 1025–1038.

Goldschmidt, R. B. and O. Steward (1980). Preferential neurotoxicity of colchicine for granule cells of the dentate gyrus of the adult rat. *Proceedings of the National Academy of Sciences, USA* 77(5): 3047–3051.

Golob, E. J. and J. S. Taube (1994). Head direction cells recorded from the postsubiculum in animals with lesions of the lateral dorsal thalamic nucleus. *Society for Neuroscience Abstracts* 20: 805.

Good, M. and R. C. Honey (1991). Conditioning and contextual retrieval in hippocampal rats. *Behavioral Neuroscience* 105: 499–509.

Goodale, M. A. (1983). Neural mechanisms of visual orientation in rodents: Targets vs. places. In Hain, A. and M. Jeannerod, editors, *Spatially Oriented Behavior*, pp. 35–61. Springer-Verlag, New York.

Goodale, M. A. and D. P. Carey (1990). The role of the cerebral cortex in visuomotor control. In Kolb, B. and R. C. Tees, editors, *The Cerebral Cortex of the Rat*, pp. 309–340. MIT Press, Cambridge MA.

Goodale, M. A., N. P. Foreman, and A. D. Milner (1978). Visual orientation in the rat: A dissociation of deficits following cortical and collicular lesions. *Experimental Brain Research* 31: 445–457.

Goodale, M. A., J. P. Meenan, H. H. Bulthoff, D. A. Nicolle, K. J. Murphy, and C. I. Racicot (1994). Separate neural pathways for the visual analysis of object shape in perception and prehension. *Current Biology* 4(7): 604–610.

Goodale, M. A. and R. C. C. Murison (1975). The effects of lesions of the superior colliculus on locomotor orientation and the orienting reflex in the rat. *Brain Research* 88: 243–261.

Goodridge, J. P., P. A. Dudchenko, K. A Worboys, E. J. Golob, and J. S. Taube (1998). Cue control and head direction cells. *Behavioral Neuroscience* 112(4): 749–761.

Goodridge, J. P., A. D. Redish, D. S. Touretzky, H. T. Blair, and P. E. Sharp (1997). Lateral mamillary input explains distortions in tuning curve shapes of anterior thalamic head direction cells. *Society for Neuroscience Abstracts* 23: 503.

Goodridge, J. P. and J. S. Taube (1994). The effect of lesions of the postsubiculum on head direction cell firing in the anterior thalamic nuclei. *Society for Neuroscience Abstracts* 20(1): 805.

Goodridge, J. P. and J. S. Taube (1995). Preferential use of the landmark navigational system by head direction cells in rats. *Behavioral Neuroscience* 109(1): 49–61.

Gothard, K. M., W. E. Skaggs, and B. L. McNaughton (1996). Dynamics of mismatch correction in the hippocampal ensemble code for space: Interaction between path integration and environmental cues. *Journal of Neuroscience* 16(24): 8027–8040.

Gothard, K. M., W. E. Skaggs, K. M. Moore, and B. L. McNaughton (1996). Binding of hippocampal CA1 neural activity to multiple reference frames in a landmark-based navigation task. *Journal of Neuroscience* 16(2): 823–835.

Gray, J. A. (1982a). *The Neuropsychology of Anxiety: An Enquiry into the Functions of the Septo-Hippocampal System*. Oxford University Press, New York.

Gray, J. A. (1982b). Précis of *The Neuropsychology of Anxiety: An Enquiry into the Functions of the Septo-Hippocampal System. Behavioral and Brain Sciences* 5: 469–484. See also commentary and response, pages 484–534.

Graybiel, A. (1990). Neurotransmitters and neuromodulators in the basal ganglia. *Trends in Neurosciences* 13(7): 244–254.

Groves, P. M., M. Garcia-Munoz J. C. Linden, M. S. Markey, M. E. Martone, and S. J. Young (1995). Elements of the intrinsic organization and information processing in the neostriatum. In Houk, J. C., J. L. Davis, and D. G. Beiser, editors, *Models of Information Processing in the Basal Ganglia*, pp. 51–96. MIT Press, Cambridge MA.

Gustafsson, B. and H. Wigström (1990). Basic features of long-term potentiation in the hippocampus. *Seminars in the Neurosciences* 2: 321–333.

Halgren, E., T. L. Babb, and P. H. Crandall (1978). Activity of human hippocampal formation and amygdala neurons during memory testing. *Electroencephalography and Clinical Neurophysiology* 45: 585–601.

Hampson, R. E., C. J. Heyser, and S. A. Deadwyler (1993). Hippocampal cell firing correlates of delayed-match-to-sample performance in the rat. *Behavioral Neuroscience* 107(5): 715–739.

Hasselmo, M. E. (1993). Acetylcholine and learning in a cortical associative memory. *Neural Computation* 5: 32–44.

Hasselmo, M. E. (1995). Neuromodulation and cortical function: Modeling the physiological basis of behavior. *Behavioral and Brain Research* 67(1): 1–27.

Hasselmo, M. E. and J. M. Bower (1993). Acetylcholine and memory. *Trends in Neurosciences* 16(6): 218–222.

Hasselmo, M. E. and E. Schnell (1994). Laminar selectivity of the cholinergic suppression of synaptic transmission in rat hippocampal region CA1: Computational modeling and brain slice physiology. *Journal of Neuroscience* 14(6): 3898–3914.

Hasselmo, M. E., B. P. Wyble, and G. V. Wallenstein (1996). Retrieval of episodic memories: Role of cholinergic and GABAergic modulation in the hippocampus. *Hippocampus* 6(6): 693–708.

Haxby, J. V., L. G. Ungerleider, B. Horowitz, J. M. Maisog, S. I. Rapoport, and C. L. Grady (1996). Face encoding and recognition in the human brain. *Proceedings of the National Academy of Sciences, USA* 93: 922–927.

Hebb, D. O. (1949). *The Organization of Behavior*. Wiley, New York.

Henke, K., A. Buck, B. Weber, and H. G. Wieser (1997). Human hippocampus establishes associations in memory. *Hippocampus* 7: 249–256.

Hennevin, E., B. Hars, C. Maho, and V. Bloch (1995). Processing of learned information in paradoxical sleep: Relevance for memory. *Behavioural Brain Research* 69: 125–135.

Herman, R. M., S. Grillner, P. S. G. Stein, and D. G. Stuart, editors (1975). *Neural Control of Locomotion*. Plenum Press, New York.

Hermer, L. and E. S. Spelke (1994). A geometric process for spatial reorientation in young children. *Nature* 370: 57–59.

Hertz, J., A. Krogh, and R. G. Palmer (1991). *Introduction to the Theory of Neural Computation*. Addison-Wesley, Reading MA.

Hetherington, P. A. and M. L. Shapiro (1993). A simple network model simulates hippocampal place fields: 2. Computing goal-directed trajectories and memory fields. *Behavioral Neuroscience* 107(3): 434–443.

Hill, A. J. (1978). First occurrence of hippocampal spatial firing in a new environment. *Experimental Neurology* 62: 282–297.

Hill, A. J. and P. J. Best (1981). Effects of deafness and blindness on the spatial correlates of hippocampal unit activity in the rat. *Experimental neurology* 74: 204–217.

Hirsh, R. (1974). The hippocampus and contextual retrieval of information from memory: A theory. *Behavioral Biology* 12: 421–444.

Hirsh, R. (1980). The hippocampus, conditional operations, and cognition. *Physiological Psychology* 8(2): 175–182.

Hirsh, R., B. Leber, and K. Gillman (1978). Fornix fibers and motivational states as controllers of behavior: A study stimulated by the contextual retrieval theory. *Behavioral Biology* 22: 463–478.

Hodges, H., Y. Allen, T. Kershaw, P. L. Lantos, J. A. Gray, and J. Sinden (1991a). Effects of cholinergic-rich neural grafts on radial maze performance of rats after excitotoxic lesions of the forebrain cholinergic system — I. Amelioration of cognitive deficits by transplants into cortex and hippocampus but not into basal forebrain. *Neuroscience* 45(3): 587–607.

Hodges, H., Y. Allen, J. Sinden, and J. A. Gray (1991b). Effects of cholinergic-rich neural grafts on radial maze performance of rats after excitotoxic lesions of the forebrain cholinergic system — II. Cholinergic drugs as probes to investigate lesion-induced deficits and transplant-induced functional recovery. *Neuroscience* 45(3): 609–623.

Honey, R. C. and M. Good (1993). Selective hippocampal lesions abolish the contextual specificity of latent inhibition and of conditioning. *Behavioral Neuroscience* 107: 23–33.

Honzik, C. H. (1936). The sensory basis of maze learning in rats. *Comparative Psychology Monographs* 13(4): 1–113.

Houk, J. C., J. L. Adams, and A. G. Barto (1995). A model of how the basal ganglia generate and use neural signals that predict reinforcement. In Houk, J. C., J. L. Davis, and D. G. Beiser, editors, *Models of Information Processing in the Basal Ganglia*, pp. 249–270. MIT Press, Cambridge MA.

Houk, J. C., J. L. Davis, and D. G. Beiser (1995). *Models of Information Processing in the Basal Ganglia*. MIT Press, Cambridge MA.

Huerta, P. T. and J. E. Lisman (1993). Heightened synaptic plasticity of hippocampal CA1 neurons during a cholinergically induced rhythmic state. *Nature* 364: 723–725.

Hull, C. L. (1943). *Principles of behavior*. Appleton-Century-Crofts, New York.

Hull, C. L. (1952). *A Behavior System: An Introduction to Behavior Theory Concerning the Individual Organism*. Yale University Press, New Haven.

Hyvarinen, J. (1982). *The Parietal Cortex of Monkey and Man*. Springer, New York.

Isaacson, R. L. (1974). *The Limbic System*. Plenum Press, New York. See also 2d ed., 1982.

Jacobs, L. F. (1992). Memory for cache locations in Merriam's kangaroo rats. *Animal Behaviour* 43(4): 585–593.

Jacobs, L. F. and E. R. Liman (1991). Grey squirrels remember the locations of buried nuts. *Animal Behavior* 41: 103–110.

James, W. (1890). *The Principles of Psychology*. Reprint, Dover Press, New York, 1960.

Jammer, M. (1969). *Concepts of Space: The History of Theories of Space in Physics*. Harvard University Press, Cambridge MA.

Jander, R. (1957). Die optische Richtungsorientierung der roten Waldameise (*formica rufa* l.). *Zeitschrift für Vergleichende Physiologie*. 40: 162–238. Cited in Maurer and Seguinot (1995).

Jarrard, L. E. (1989). On the use of ibotenic acid to lesion selectively different components of the hippocampal formation. *Journal of Neuroscience Methods* 29: 251–259.

Jarrard, L. E. (1991). Use of ibotenic acid to selectively lesion brain structures. In Conn, P. M., editor, *Lesions and Transplantation*, Vol. 7 of *Methods in Neurosciences*, pp. 58–69. Academic Press, San Diego CA.

Jarrard, L. E. (1993). On the role of the hippocampus in learning and memory in the rat. *Behavioral Neural Biology* 60(1): 9–26.

Jones, D. L. and G. J. Mogenson (1980). Nucleus accumbens to globus pallidus GABA projection subserving ambulatory activity. *American Journal of Physiology* 238: R65–R69.

Jung, M. W. and B. L. McNaughton (1993). Spatial selectivity of unit activity in the hippocampal granular layer. *Hippocampus* 3(2): 165–182.

Jung, M. W., S. I. Wiener, and B. L. McNaughton (1994). Comparison of spatial firing characteristics of the dorsal and ventral hippocampus of the rat. *Journal of Neuroscience* 14(12): 7347–7356.

Kalaska, J. F., D. A. D. Cohen, M. Prud'homme, and M. L. Hyde (1990). Parietal area 5 neuronal activity encodes movement kinematics not movement dynamics. *Experimental Brain Research* 80: 351–364.

Kalaska, J. F. and D. J. Crammond (1992). Cerebral cortical mechansims of reaching movements. *Science* 255: 1517–1523.

Kanno, I., J. Hatazawa, H. Fujita, E. Shimosegawa, M. Murakami, and K. Uemura (1995). Neural activation does not require increase in absolute CBF but normalized CBF: Revisit quantitative PET-CBF during functional activation. *Journal of Cerebral Blood Flow and Metabolism* 15(Suppl. 1): S48.

Karni, A., D. Tanne, B. S. Rubenstein, J. J. Askenasy, and D. Sagi (1994). Dependence on REM sleep of overnight improvement of a perceptual skill. *Science* 265: 697–682.

Keith, J. R. and K. M. McVety (1988). Latent place learning in a novel environment and the influences of prior training in rats. *Psychobiology* 16(2): 146–151.

Kelly, J. B. (1990). Rat auditory cortex. In Kolb, B. and R. C. Tees, editors, *The Cerebral Cortex of the Rat*, pp. 381–405. MIT Press, Cambridge MA.

Kesner, R. P., B. L. Bolland, and M. Dakis (1993). Memory for spatial locations, motor responses, and objects: Triple dissociation among the hippocampus, caudate nucleus, and extrastriate visual cortex. *Experimental Brain Research* 93: 462–470.

Kesner, R. P., G. Farnsworth, and B. V. DiMattia (1989). Double dissociation of egocentric and allocentric space following medial prefrontal and parietal cortex lesions in the rat. *Behavioral Neuroscience* 103(5): 956–961.

Khatib, O. (1986). Real-time obstacle avoidance for manipulators and mobile robots. *International Journal of Robotics Research* 5(1): 90–98.

Kim, J. J. and M. S. Fanselow (1992). Modality-specific retrograde amnesia of fear. *Science* 256: 675–677.

Kimble, D. P. (1968). Hippocampus and internal inhibition. *Psychological Bulletin* 70(5): 285–295.

Kimble, D. P. (1975). Choice behavior in rats with hippocampal lesions. In Isaacson, R. L. and K. H. Pribram, editors, *The Hippocampus*, Vol. 2, pp. 209–236. Plenum Press, New York.

Kishimoto, K. and S. Amari (1979). Existence and stability of local excitations in homogenous neural fields. *Journal of Mathematical Biology* 7(4): 303–318.

Kiyatkin, E. A. and A. Gratton (1994). Electrochemical monitoring of extracellular dopamine in nucleus accumbens of rats lever-pressing for food. *Brain Research* 652: 225–234.

Knierim, J. J., H. S. Kudrimoti, and B. L. McNaughton (1995). Place cells, head direction cells, and the learning of landmark stability. *Journal of Neuroscience* 15: 1648–1659.

Knierim, J. J., H. S. Kudrimoti, and B. L. McNaughton (1998). Interactions between idiothetic cues and external landmarks in the control of place cells and head direction cells. *Journal of Neurophysiology* 80: 425–446.

Knierim, J. J. and B. L. McNaughton (1995). Differential effects of dentate gyrus lesions on pyramidal cell firing in 1- and 2-dimensional spatial tasks. *Society For Neuroscience Abstracts* 21: 940.

Koerner, A., M. J. Thomas, M. P. Weisend, and R. J. Sutherland (1996). Hippocampal-dependent memory consolidation: An evaluation of three hypotheses. *Society for Neuroscience Abstracts* 22: 1118.

Koerner, A., M. J. Thomas, M. P. Weisend, and R. J. Sutherland (1997). Further tests of hippocampal-dependent memory consolidation. *Society for Neuroscience Abstracts* 23: 1603.

Kohler, C. (1986). Intrinsic connections of the retrohippocampal region in the rat brain. II. The medial entorhinal area. *Journal of Comparative Neurology* 246: 149–169.

Kohler, C. (1988). Intrinsic connections of the retrohippocampal region in the rat brain. III. The lateral entorhinal area. *Journal of Comparative Neurology* 271: 208–228.

Kohonen, T. (1977). *Associative Memory: A System-Theoretical Approach*. Springer, New York.

Kohonen, T. (1980). *Content-Addressable Memories*. Springer, New York.

Kohonen, T. (1982). Self-organized formation of topologically correct feature maps. *Biological Cybernetics* 43: 59–69.

Kohonen, T. (1984). *Self-Organization and Associative Memory*. Springer-Verlag, New York.

Kolb, B. (1990a). Posterior parietal and temporal association cortex. In Kolb, B. and R. C. Tees, editors, *The Cerebral Cortex of the Rat*, pp. 459–471. MIT Press, Cambridge MA.

Kolb, B. (1990b). Prefrontal cortex. In Kolb and R. C. Tees, editors, *The Cerebral Cortex of the Rat*, pp. 437–458. MIT Press, Cambridge MA.

Kolb, B., K. Burhmann, R. McDonald, and R. J. Sutherland (1994). Dissociation of the medial prefrontal, posterior parietal, and posterior temporal cortex for spatial navigation and recognition memory in the rat. *Cerebral Cortex* 6: 664–680.

Kolb, B. and J. Walkey (1987). Behavioural and anatomical studies of the posterior parietal cortex in the rat. *Behavioral and Brain Research* 23: 127–145.

Krieg, W. J. S. (1946). Connections of the cerebral cortex. I. The albino rat: A. Topography of the cortical areas. *Journal of Comparative Neurology* 84: 221–275.

Kubie, J. L. and R. U. Muller (1991). Multiple representations in the hippocampus. *Hippocampus* 1(3): 240–242.

Kubie, J. L., R. U. Muller, and E. Bostock (1990). Spatial firing properties of hippocampal theta cells. *Journal of Neuroscience* 10(4): 1110–1123.

Kubie, J. L. and J. B. Ranck, Jr. (1983). Sensory-behavioral correlates in individual hippocampus neurons in three situations: Space and context. In Seifert, W., editor, *Neurobiology of the Hippocampus*, pp. 433–447. Academic Press, New York.

Kuipers, B. J. (1977). Representing knowledge of large-scale space. Ph.D. diss., Massachusetts Institute of Technology.

Kuipers, B. J. (1978). Modeling spatial knowledge. *Cognitive Science* 2: 129–153.

Kuipers, B. J., R. Froom, W.-Y. Lee, and D. Pierce (1993). The semantic hierarchy in robot learning. In Connell, J. H. and S. Mahadevan, editors, *Robot Learning*, pp. 141–170. Kluwer, Boston.

Kuipers, B. J. and T. S. Levitt (1988). Navigation and mapping in large-scale space. *AI Magazine* 9(2): 25–43.

Lanczos, C. (1970). *Space through the Ages: The Evolution of Geometrical Ideas from Pythagoras to Hilbert and Einstein.* Academic Press, New York.

Landfield, P. W. and S. A. Deadwyler, editors (1988). *Long-Term Pontentiation: From Biophysics to Behavior*, Vol. 35 of *Neurology and Neurobiology*. Alan R. Liss, Inc., New York.

Lavoie, A. M. and S. J. Y. Mizumori (1994). Spatial-, movement- and reward-sensitive discharge by medial ventral striatum neurons in rats. *Brain Research* 638: 157–168.

Lefévre, P. and H. L. Galiana (1992). Dynamic feedback to the superior colliculus in a neural network model of the gaze control system. *Neural Networks* 5: 871–890.

Leonard, B. and B. L. McNaughton (1990). Spatial representation in the rat: Conceptual, behavioral, and neurophysiological perspectives. In Kesner, R. P. and D. S. Olton, editors, *Neurobiology of Comparative Cognition*, pp. 363–422. Erlbaum, Hillsdale, NJ.

Leonhard, C. L., R. W. Stackman, and J. S. Taube (1996). Head direction cells recorded from the lateral mammillary nuclei in rats. *Society for Neuroscience Abstracts* 22: 1873.

Levitt, T., D. Lawton, D. Chelberg, and P. Nelson (1987). Qualitative navigation. In *Proceedings of the DARPA Image Understanding Workshop*, pp. 447–465. Kaufmann, Los Altos CA.

Levy, W. B. (1989). A computational approach to hippocampal function. In Hawkins, R. D. and G. H. Bower, editors, *Computational Models of Learning in Simple Neural Systems*, Vol. 23 of *The Psychology of Learning and Motivation*, pp. 243–305. Academic Press, San Diego CA.

Levy, W. B. (1996). A sequence predicting CA3 is a flexible associator that learns and uses context to solve hippocampal-like tasks. *Hippocampus* 6(6): 579–591.

Levy, W. B. and X. Wu (1996). The relationship of local context cues to sequence length memory capacity. *Network: Computation in Neural Systems* 7: 371–384.

Lorento do Nó, R. (1933). Studies on the structure of the cerebral cortex. *J. Psychol. Neurol.* 45: 381–442.

Lorento do Nó, R. (1934). Studies on the structure of the cerebral cortex II. Continuation of the study of the ammonic system. *J. Psychol. Neurol.* 46: 113–177.

Luria, A. R. (1973). *The Working Brain: An Introduction to Neuropsychology*. Basic Books, New York. Translated by B. Haigh.

MacLean, P. D. (1973). *A Triune Concept of the Brain and Behavior*. Ontario Mental Health Foundation and University of Toronto Press, Toronto.

MacLean, P. D. (1990). *The Triune Brain in Evolution*. Plenum Press, New York.

Malenka, R. C. (1995). LTP and LTD: Dynamic and interactive processes of synaptic plasticity. *The Neuroscientist* 1(1): 35–42.

Mardia, K. V. (1972). *Statistics of Directional Data*. Academic Press, New York.

Margules, J. and C. R. Gallistel (1988). Heading in the rat: Determination by environmental shape. *Animal Learning and Behavior* 16(4): 404–410.

Markus, E. J., C. A. Barnes, B. L. McNaughton, V. L. Gladden, and W. E. Skaggs (1994). Spatial information content and reliability of hippocampal CA1 neurons: Effects of visual input. *Hippocampus* 4: 410–421.

Markus, E. J., Y. Qin, B. Leonard, W. E. Skaggs, B. L. McNaughton, and C. A. Barnes (1995). Interactions between location and task affect the spatial and directional firing of hippocampal neurons. *Journal of Neuroscience* 15: 7079–7094.

Marr, D. (1969). A theory of cerebellar cortex. *Journal of Physiology* 202: 437–470. Reprinted in Marr (1991).

Marr, D. (1970). A theory for cerebral neocortex. *Proceedings of the Royal Society* 176: 161–234. Reprinted in Marr (1991).

Marr, D. (1971). Simple memory: A theory of archicortex. *Philosophical Transactions of the Royal Society of London* 262(841): 23 81. Reprinted in Marr (1991).

Marr, D. (1982). *Vision*. W. H. Freeman and Co., New York.

Marr, D. (1991). *From the Retina to the Neocortex: Selected Papers of David Marr*. Edited by L. M. Vaina. Birkhäuser, Boston.

Martin, G. M., C. W. Harley, A. R. Smith, E. S. Hoyles, and C. S. Rideout (1995). How rats are transported to the maze determines success or failure of spatial problem solving: Environmental cues are not sufficient to support spatial learning. *Society for Neuroscience Abstracts* 21: 1939.

Matthews, D. B., A. M. White, E. D. Brush, and P. J. Best (1995). Construction of the spatial cognitive map does not require active exploration of the environment. *Society for Neuroscience Abstracts* 21: 2086.

Maurer, R. and V. Seguinot (1995). What is modelling for? A critical review of the models of path integration. *Journal of Theoretical Biology* 175: 457–475.

McClelland, J. L. and N. H. Goddard (1996). Considerations arising from a complementary learning systems perspective on hippocampus and neocortex. *Hippocampus* 6(6): 654–665.

McClelland, J. L., B. L. McNaughton, and R. C. O'Reilly (1995). Why there are complementary learning systems in the hippocampus and neocortex: Insights from the successes and failures of connectionist models of learning and memory. *Psychological Review* 102(3): 419–457.

McDonald, R. J. and N. M. White (1994). Parallel information processing in the water maze: Evidence for independent memory systems involving dorsal striatum and hippocampus. *Behavioral and Neural Biology* 61: 260–270.

McDonald, R. J. and N.M. White (1993). Parallel information processing by hippocampal and dorsal striatal memory systems in the Morris water maze. *Society for Neuroscience Abstracts* 19(1): 362.

McGaugh, J. L. (1966). Time-dependent processes in memory storage. *Science* 153: 1351–1358.

McGaugh, J. L. (1989). Dissociating learning and performance: Drug and hormone enhancement of memory storage. *Brain Research Bulletin* 23: 339–345.

McGuire, F. A., N. Burgess, J. Donnett, C. D. Frith, and J. O'Keefe (1997). Right hippocampus, left hippocampus and inferior parietal cortex are differentially involved in human spatial navigation. *Society for Neuroscience Abstracts* 23: 2107.

McHugh, T. J., K. I. Blum, J. Z. Tsien, S. Tonegawa, and M. A. Wilson (1996). Impaired hippocampal represntation of space in CA1-specific NMDAR1 knockout mice. *Cell* 87: 1339–1349.

McNaughton, B. L. (1989). Neuronal mechanisms for spatial computation and information storage. In Nadel, L., L. Cooper, P. Culicover, and R. M. Harnish, editors, *Neural Connections, Mental Computation*, pp. 285–350. MIT Press, Cambridge, MA.

McNaughton, B. L. (1993). The mechanism of expression of long-term enhancement of hippocampal synapses: Current issues and theoretical implications. *Annual Review of Physiology* 55: 375–396.

McNaughton, B. L., C. A. Barnes, J. L. Gerrard, K. Gothard, M. W. Jung, J. J. Knierim, H. Kudrimoti, Y. Qin, W. E. Skaggs, M. Suster, and K. L. Weaver (1996). Deciphering the hippocampal polyglot: The hippocampus as a path integration system. *Journal of Experimental Biology* 199(1): 173–186.

McNaughton, B. L., C. A. Barnes, J. Meltzer, and R. J. Sutherland (1989). Hippocampal granule cells are necessary for normal spatial learning but not for spatially-selective pyramidal cell discharge. *Experimental Brain Research* 76: 485–496.

McNaughton, B. L., C. A. Barnes, and J. O'Keefe (1983). The contributions of position, direction, and velocity to single unit activity in the hippocampus of freely-moving rats. *Experimental Brain Research* 52: 41–49.

McNaughton, B. L., C. A. Barnes, G. Rao, J. Baldwin, and M. Rasmussen (1986). Long-term enhancement of hippocampal synaptic transmission and the acquisition of spatial information. *Journal of Neuroscience* 6(2): 563–571.

McNaughton, B. L., L. L. Chen, and E. J. Markus (1991). "Dead reckoning," landmark learning, and the sense of direction: A neurophysiological and computational hypothesis. *Journal of Cognitive Neuroscience* 3(2): 190–202.

McNaughton, B. L., J. J. Knierim, and M. A. Wilson (1994). Vector encoding and the vestibular foundations of spatial cognition: Neurophysiological and computational mechanisms. In Gazzaniga, M., editor, *The Cognitive Neurosciences*, pp. 585–595. MIT Press, Cambridge MA.

McNaughton, B. L., B. Leonard, and L. Chen (1989). Cortical-hippocampal interactions and cognitive mapping: A hypothesis based on reintegration of the parietal and inferotemporal pathways for visual processing. *Psychobiology* 17(3): 230–235.

McNaughton, B. L., S. J. Y. Mizumori, C. A. Barnes, B. J. Leonard, M. Marquis, and E. J. Green (1994). Cortical representation of motion during unrestrained spatial navigation in the rat. *Cerebral Cortex* 4(1): 27–39.

McNaughton, B. L. and R. G. M. Morris (1987). Hippocampal synaptic enhancement and information storage within a distributed memory system. *Trends in Neurosciences* 10(10): 408–415.

McNaughton, B. L. and L. Nadel (1990). Hebb-Marr networks and the neurobiological representation of action in space. In Gluck, M. A. and D. E. Rumelhart, editors, *Neuroscience and Connectionist Theory*, pp. 1–63. Erlbaum, Hillsdale NJ.

McNaughton, B. L., J. O'Keefe, and C. A. Barnes (1983). The stereotrode: A new technique for simultaneous isolation of several single units in the central nervous system from multiple unit records. *Journal of Neuroscience Methods* 8: 391–397.

Mehta, M. R., C. A. Barnes, and B. L. McNaughton (1997). Experience-dependent, asymmetric expansion of hippocampal place fields. *Proceedings of the National Academy of Sciences, USA* 94: 8918–8921.

Meunier, M., J. Bachevalier, M. Mishkin, and E. A. Murray (1993). Effects on visual recognition of combined and separate ablations of the entorhinal and perirhinal cortex in rhesus monkeys. *Journal of Neuroscience* 13(12): 5418–5432.

Meunier, M., W. Hadfield, J. Bachevalier, and E. A. Murray (1996). Effects of rhinal cortex lesions combined with hippocampectomy on visual recognition memory in rhesus monkeys. *Journal of Neurophysiology* 75(3): 1190–1205.

Miller, V. M. and P. J. Best (1980). Spatial correlates of hippocampal unit activity are altered by lesions of the fornix and entorhinal cortex. *Brain Research* 194: 311–323.

Milner, A. D. and C. R. Lines (1983). Stimulus sampling and the use of distal visual cues in rats with lesions of the superior colliculus. *Behavioural Brian Research* 8: 387–401.

Milner, B. (1970). Memory and the medial temporal regions of the brain. In Pribram, K. H. and D. E. Broadbent, editors, *Biology of Memory*, pp. 29–50. Academic Press, New York.

Milner, B., S. Corkin, and H.-L. Teuber (1968). Further analysis of the hippocampal amnesia syndrome: 14-year follow-up study of H. M. *Neuropsychologia* 6: 215–234.

Minai, A. A., G. L. Barrows, and W. B. Levy (1994). Disambiguation of pattern sequences with recurrent networks. *INNS World Congress on Neural Networks* pp. IV–178–181.

Minai, A. A. and W. B. Levy (1993). Sequence learning in a single trial. *INNS World Congress on Neural Networks* pp. I–582–586.

Minsky, M. and S. Papert (1969). *Perceptrons*. MIT Press, Cambridge MA.

Mishkin, M. (1978). Memory in monkeys severly impaired by combined but not separate removal of amygdala and hippocampus. *Nature* 273: 297–298.

Mishkin, M. and T. Appenzeller (1987). The anatomy of memory. *Scientific American* 256(6): 80–89.

Mishkin, M. and E. A. Murray (1994). Stimulus recognition. *Current Opinion in Neurobiology* 4: 200–206.

Mishkin, M., L. G. Ungerleider, and K. A. Macko (1983). Object vision and spatial vision: Two cortical pathways. *Trends in Neurosciences* 6: 414–417.

Mittelstaedt, H. (1962). Control systems of orientation in insects. *Annual Review of Entomology* 7: 177–198. Cited in Maurer and Seguinot (1995).

Mittelstaedt, H. (1983). The role of multimodal convergence in homing by path integration. *Fortschritte der Zoologie* 28: 197–212.

Mittelstaedt, H. and M.-L. Mittelstaedt (1982). Homing by path integration. In Papi, F. and H. G. Wallraff, editors, *Avian Navigation*, pp. 290–297. Springer, New York.

Mittelstaedt, M.-L. and S. Glasauer (1991). Idiothetic navigation in gerbils and humans. *Zoologische Jahrbücher — Abteilung für Zoologie und Physiologie der Tiere* 95: 427–435.

Mittelstaedt, M. L. and H. Mittelstaedt (1980). Homing by path integration in a mammal. *Naturwissenschaften* 67: 566–567.

Mittlestaedt, H. (1985). Analytical cybernetics of spider navigation. In Barth, F., editor, *Neurobiology of Arachnids*. Springer, Berlin. Cited in Maurer and Seguinot (1995).

Miyashita, Y., E. T. Rolls, P. M. B. Cahusac, H. Niki, and J. D. Feigenbaum (1989). Activity of hippocampal formation neurons in the monkey related to a conditional spatial response task. *Journal of Neurophysiology* 61(3): 669–678.

Mizumori, S. J. Y., C. A. Barnes, and B. L. McNaughton (1990). Behavioral correlates of theta-on and theta-off cells recorded from hippocampal formation of mature young and aged rats. *Experimental Brain Research* 80: 365–373.

Mizumori, S. J. Y. and B. G. Cooper (1995). Spatial representations of dorsal caudate neurons of freely-behaving rats. *Society for Neuroscience Abstracts* 21: 1929.

Mizumori, S. J. Y. and A. Kalyani (1997). Age and experience-dependent representational reorganization during spatial learning. *Neurobiology of Aging* 18(6): 651–659.

Mizumori, S. J. Y., A. M. Lavoie, and A. Kalyani (1996). Redistribution of spatial representation in the hippocampus of aged rats performing a spatial memory task. *Behavioral Neuroscience* 110(5): 1006–1016.

Mizumori, S. J. Y., B. L. McNaughton, C. A. Barnes, and K. B. Fox (1989). Preserved spatial coding hippocampus CA1 pyramidal cells during reversible suppression in CA3c output: Evidence for pattern completion in hippocampus. *Journal of Neuroscience* 9(11): 3915–3928.

Mizumori, S. J. Y., D. Y. Miya, and K. E. Ward (1994). Reversible inactivation of the lateral dorsal thalamus disrupts hippocampal place representation and impairs spatial learning. *Brain Research* 644: 168–174.

Mizumori, S. J. Y., K. E. Unick, and B. G. Cooper (1996). Dynamic reward and spatial codes of caudate nucleus neurons. *Society for Neuroscience Abstracts* 22: 630.

Mizumori, S. J. Y., K. E. Ward, and A. M. Lavoie (1992). Medial septal modulation of entorhinal single unit activity in anesthetized and freely moving rats. *Brain Research* 570: 188–197.

Mizumori, S. J. Y. and J. D. Williams (1993). Directionally selective mnemonic properties of neurons in the lateral dorsal nucleus of the thalamus of rats. *Journal of Neuroscience* 13(9): 4015–4028.

Mogenson, G. J. (1984). Limbic-motor integration – with emphasis on intiation of exploratory and goal-directed locamotion. In Bandler, R., editor, *Modulation of Sensorimotor Activity*

During Alterations in Behavioral States, pp. 121–138. Liss, New York.

Mogenson, G. J. and M. Nielsen (1984). Neuropharmacological evidence to suggest that the nucleus accumbens and subpallidal region contribute to exploratory locomotion. *Behavioral and Neural Biology* 42: 52–60.

Moghaddam, M. and J. Bures (1994). The contribution of path integration to place navigation in the Morris water maze. *European Journal of Neuroscience* Suppl. 7: 116.

Moravec, H. P. (1988). Sensor fusion in certainty grids for mobile robots. *AI Magazine* 9(2): 61–74.

Morris, R. G., S. Davis, and S. P. Butcher (1990). Hippocampal synaptic plasticity and NMDA receptors: A role in information storage? *Philosophical Transactions of the Royal Society, London* B329(1253): 187–204.

Morris, R. G. M. (1981). Spatial localization does not require the presence of local cues. *Learning and Motivation* 12: 239–260.

Morris, R. G. M., P. Garrud, J. N. P. Rawlins, and J. O'Keefe (1982). Place navigation impaired in rats with hippocampal lesions. *Nature* 297: 681–683.

Morris, R. G. M., F. Schenk, F. Tweedie, and L. E. Jarrard (1990). Ibotenate lesions of hippocampus and/or subiculum: Dissociating components of allocentric spatial learning. *European Journal of Neuroscience* 2: 1016–1028.

Müller, M. and R. Wehner (1988). Path integration in desert ants, *cataglyphis fortis*. *Proceedings of the National Academy of Sciences USA* 85: 5287–5290.

Muller, R. U., E. Bostock, J. S. Taube, and J. L. Kubie (1994). On the directional firing properties of hippocampal place cells. *Journal of Neuroscience* 14(12): 7235–7251.

Muller, R. U. and J. L. Kubie (1987). The effects of changes in the environment on the spatial firing of hippocampal complex-spike cells. *Journal of Neuroscience* 7: 1951–1968.

Muller, R. U., J. L. Kubie, E. M. Bostock, J. S. Taube, and G. J. Quirk (1991). Spatial firing correlates of neurons in the hippocampal formation of freely moving rats. In Paillard, J., editor, *Brain and Space*, pp. 296–333. Oxford University Press, New York.

Muller, R. U., J. L. Kubie, and J. B. Ranck, Jr. (1987). Spatial firing patterns of hippocampal complex-spike cells in a fixed environment. *Journal of Neuroscience* 7: 1935–1950.

Muller, R. U., J. L. Kubie, and R. Saypoff (1991). The hippocampus as a cognitive graph. *Hippocampus* 1(3): 243–246.

Muller, R. U., M. Stead, and J. Pach (1996). The hippocampus as a cognitive graph. *Journal of General Physiology* 107(6): 663–694.

Mumby, D. G., E. R. Wood, C. A. Duva, T. J. Kornecook, J. P. J. Pinel, and A. G. Phillips (1996). Ischemia-induced object-recognition deficits in rats are attenuated by hippocampal ablation before or soon after ischemia. *Behavioral Neuroscience* 110(2): 266–281.

Munoz, D. P., D. Pélisson, and D. Guitton (1991). Movement of neural activity on the superior colliculus motor map during gaze shifts. *Science* 251: 1358–1360.

Murphy, J. J. (1873). Instinct: A mechanical analogy. *Nature* 7: 483.

Murray, E. A. (1992). Medial temporal lobe structures contributing to recognition memory: The amygdaloid complex versus the rhinal cortex. In Aggleton, J. P., editor, *The Amygdala: Neurobiological Aspects of Emotion, Memory, and Mental Dysfunction*, pp. 453–470. Wiley, New York.

Murray, E. A., D. Gaffan, and M. Mishkin (1993). Neural substrates of visual stimulus-stimulus association in rhesus monkeys. *Journal of Neuroscience* 13(10): 4549–4561.

Murray, E. A. and M. Mishkin (1984). Severe tactual as well as visual memory deficits follow combined removal of the amygdala and hippocampus in monkeys. *Journal of Neuroscience* 4(10): 2565–2580.

Murray, E. A. and M. Mishkin (1996). 40-minute visual recognition memory in rhesus monkeys with hippocampal lesions. *Society for Neuroscience Abstracts* 22: 281.

Murray, J. D. (1989). *Mathematical Biology*, Vol. 19 of *Biomathematics*. Springer-Verlag, New York.

Myrher, T. (1991). Retroactive memory of a visual discrimination task in the rat: Role of temporal-entorhinal cortices and their connections. *Experimental Brain Research* 84: 517–524.

Nadel, L. (1991). The hippocampus and space revisited. *Hippocampus* 1(3): 221–9.

Nadel, L. (1994). Multiple memory systems: What and Why, an update. In Schacter, D. L. and E. Tulving, editors, *Memory Systems 1994*, pp. 39–64. MIT Press, Cambridge MA.

Nadel, L. (1995). The role of the hippocampus in declarative memory: A commentary on Zola-Morgan, Squire, and Ramus, 1994. *Hippocampus* 5: 232–234.

Nadel, L. and M. Moscovitch (1997). Memory consolidation, retrograde amnesia and the hippocampal complex. *Current Opinion in Neurobiology* 7: 217–227.

Nadel, L., J. O'Keefe, and A. Black (1975). Slam on the brakes: A critique of Altman, Brunner, and Bayer's response-inhibition model of hippocampal function. *Behavioral Biology* 14: 151–162.

Nadel, L. and J. Willner (1980). Context and conditioning: A place for space. *Physiological Psychology* 8(2): 218–228.

Nadel, L., J. Willner, and E. M. Kurz (1985). Cognitive maps and environmental context. In Balsam, P. D. and A. Tomie, editors, *Context and Learning*, pp. 385–406. Earlbaum, Hillsdale NJ.

Nagahara, A. H., T. Otto, and M. Gallagher (1995). Entorhinal-perirhinal lesions impair performance of rats on two versions of place learning in the Morris water maze. *Behavioral Neuroscience* 109(1): 3–9.

Nature (1873). Perception and instinct in the lower animals. *Nature* 7:377–378.

Neafsey, E. J., R. R. Terreberry, K. M. Hurley, K. G. Ruit, and R. J. Frysztak (1993). Anterior cingulate cortex in rodents: Connections, visceral control, and implications for emotion. In Vogt, B. A. and M. Gabriel, editors, *Neurobiology of Cingulate Cortex and Limbic Thalamus: A Comprehensive Handbook*, pp. 206–223. Birkhäuser, Boston.

Neave, N., S. Lloyd, A. Sahgal, and J. P. Aggleton (1994). Lack of effect of lesions in the anterior cingulate cortex and retrosplenial cortex on certain tests of spatial memory in the rat. *Behavioural Brain Research* 65: 89–101.

Neave, N., S. Nagle, and J. P. Aggleton (1997). Evidence for the involvement of the mammillary bodies and cingulum bundle in allocentric spatial processing by rats. *European Journal of Neuroscience* 9(5): 941–955.

Nilsson, O. G., M. L. Shapiro, F. H. Gage, D. S. Olton, and A. Bjorklund (1987). Spatial learning and memory following fimbria-fornix transection and grafting of fetal septal neurons to the hippocampus. *Experimental Brain Research* 67: 195–215.

Nyberg, L., A. R. McIntosh, S. Houle, L.-G. Nilsson, and E. Tulving (1996). Activation of medial temporal structures during epiosdic memory retrieval. *Nature* 380: 715–717.

Oatley, K. (1974). Mental maps for navigation. *New Scientist* 10 December: 863–866. Reprinted in Farrall (1984), pages 58–65.

Ogawa, S., D. W. Tank, R. Menon, J. M. Ellermann, S.-G. Kim, H. Merkle, and K. Ugurbil (1992). Intrinsic signal changes accompanying sensory stimulation: Functional brain mapping with magnetic resonance imaging. *Proceedings of the National Academy of Sciences, USA* 89: 5951–5955.

Ohta, H., K. Matsumoto, and H. Watanabe (1993). The interaction between central cholinergic and peripheral beta-adrenergic systems on radial maze performance in rats. *Brain Research* 622(1–2): 353–356.

O'Keefe, J. (1976). Place units in the hippocampus of the freely moving rat. *Experimental Neurology* 51: 78–109.

O'Keefe, J. (1989). Computations the hippocampus might perform. In Nadel, L., L. Cooper, P. Culicover, and R. M. Harnish, editors, *Neural Connections, Mental Computation*, pp. 225–284. MIT Press, Cambridge, MA.

O'Keefe, J. (1991). An allocentric spatial model for the hippocampal cognitive map. *Hippocampus* 1(3): 230–235.

O'Keefe, J. and N. Burgess (1996a). Geometric determinants of the place fields of hippocampal neurons. *Nature* 381: 425–428.

O'Keefe, J. and N. Burgess (1996b). Spatial and temporal determinants of the hippocampal place cell activity. In Ono, T., B. L. McNaughton, S. Molotchnikoff, E. T. Rolls, and H. Nishijo, editors, *Perception, Memory and Emotion: Frontiers in Neuroscience*, pp. 359–373. Pergamon, New York.

O'Keefe, J. and D. H. Conway (1978). Hippocampal place units in the freely moving rat: Why they fire where they fire. *Experimental Brain Research* 31: 573–590.

O'Keefe, J. and J. Dostrovsky (1971). The hippocampus as a spatial map. Preliminary evidence from unit activity in the freely moving rat. *Brain Research* 34: 171–175.

O'Keefe, J. and L. Nadel (1978). *The Hippocampus as a Cognitive Map*. Clarendon Press, Oxford.

O'Keefe, J. and L. Nadel (1979). Précis of O'Keefe and Nadel's *The Hippocampus as a Cognitive Map*. *Behavioral and Brain Sciences* 2: 487–494. See also commentary and response, pages 494–533.

O'Keefe, J. and M. Recce (1993). Phase relationship between hippocampal place units and the EEG theta rhythm. *Hippocampus* 3: 317–330.

O'Keefe, J. and A. Speakman (1987). Single unit activity in the rat hippocampus during a spatial memory task. *Experimental Brain Research* 68: 1–27.

Olton, D. S., J. T. Becker, and G. E. Handelmann (1979). Hippocampus, space, and memory. *Behavioral and Brain Sciences* 2: 313–322. See also commentary and response, pages 323–366.

Olton, D. S., J. T. Becker, and G. E. Handelmann (1980). Hippocampal function: Working memory or cognitive mapping? *Physiological Psychology* 8(2): 239–246.

Olton, D. S., M. Branch, and P. J. Best (1978). Spatial correlates of hippocampal unit activity. *Experimental Neurology* 58: 387–409.

Olton, D. S. and R. J. Samuelson (1976). Remembrance of places passed: Spatial memory in rats. *Journal of Experimental Psychology: Animal Behavior Processes* 2(2): 97–116.

O'Mara, S. M. (1995). Spatially selective firing properties of hippocampal formation neurons in rodents and primates. *Progress in Neurobiology* 45: 253–274.

O'Mara, S. M., E. T. Rolls, A. Berthoz, and R. P. Kesner (1994). Neurons responding to whole body motion in the primate hippocampus. *Journal of Neuroscience* 14(11): 6511–6523.

Ono, T., K. Nakamura, M. Fukuda, and R. Tamura (1991). Place recognition responses of neurons in monkey hippocampus. *Neuroscience Letters* 121: 194–198.

Ono, T., R. Tamura, and K. Nakamura (1991). The hippocampus and space: Are there "place neurons" in the monkey hippocampus. *Hippocampus* 1(3): 253–257.

O'Reilly, R. C. and J. L. McClelland (1994). Hippocampal conjunctive encoding, storage, and recall: Avoiding a trade-off. *Hippocampus* 4(6): 661–682.

Orrison, Jr., W. W., J. D. Levine, J. A. Sanders, and M. F. Hartshorne, editors (1995). *Functional Brian Imaging*, St. Louis MO. Mosby.

Otto, T., C. Ding, G. Cousens, and K. Schiller (1996). Effects of lateral vs. medial entorhinal cortex aspiration on the acquisition of odor-place associations. *Society for Neuroscience Abstracts* 22: 1120.

Otto, T. and H. Eichenbaum (1992a). Complementary roles of the orbital prefrontal cortex and the perirhinal-entorhinal cortices in an odor-guided delayed nonmatching-to-sample task. *Behavioral Neuroscience* 106(5): 762–775.

Otto, T. and H. Eichenbaum (1992b). Neuronal activity in the hippocampus during delayed non-match to sample performance in rats: Evidence for hippocampal processing in recognition memory. *Hippocampus* 2(3): 323–334.

Otto, T., F. Schottler, U. Staubli, H. Eichenbaum, and G. Lynch (1991). Hippocampus and olfactory discrimination learning: Effects of entorhinal cortex lesions on olfactory learning and memory in a successive-cue, go-no-go task. *Behavioral Neuroscience* 105(1): 111–119.

Packard, M. G. (1994). "Place" versus "response" learning debate revisited in the brain. *Society for Neuroscience Abstracts* 20: 1016.

Packard, M. G., R. Hirsh, and N. M. White (1989). Differential effects of fornix and caudate nucleus lesions on two radial maze tasks: Evidence for multiple memory systems. *Journal of Neuroscience* 9(5): 1465–1472.

Packard, M. G. and J. L. McGaugh (1992). Double dissociation of fornix and caudate nucleus lesions on acquisition of two water maze tasks: Further evidence for multiple memory systems. *Behavioral Neuroscience* 106(3): 439–446.

Packard, M. G. and J. L. McGaugh (1996). Inactivation of hippocampus or caudate nucleus with lidocaine differentially affects expression of place and response learning. *Neurobiology of Learning and Memory* 65: 65–72.

Packard, M. G. and N. M. White (1991). Dissociation of hippocampus and caudate nucleus memory systems by posttraining intracerebral injection of dopamine agonists. *Behavioral Neuroscience* 105(2): 295–306.

Papez, J. W. (1937). A proposed mechanism of emotion. *Archives of Neurology and Psychiatry* 38: 728–744.

Parent, A. (1990). Extrinsic connections of the basal ganglia. *Trends in Neurosciences* 13(7): 254–258.

Pavlides, C. and J. Winson (1989). Influences of hippocampal place cell firing in the awake state on the activity of these cells during subsequent sleep episodes. *Journal of Neuroscience* 9(8): 2907–2918.

Pearson, K. (1976). The control of walking. *Scientific American* 235(6): 72–86.

Pellis, S. M., E. Castaneda, M. M. McKenna, L. T. Tran-Nguyen, and I. Q. Whishaw (1993). The role of the striatum in organizing sequences of play fighting in neonatally dopamine-depleted rats. *Neuroscience Letters* 158(1): 13–15.

Phillips, R. G. and J. E. Le Doux (1992). Differential contribution of amygdala and hippocampus to cued and contextual fear conditioning. *Behavioral Neuroscience* 106(2): 274–285.

Phillips, R. G., H. Tanila, and H. Eichenbaum (1996). Differences in the spatial coding patterns of ventral subicular neurons in simple and complex environments. *Society for Neuroscience Abstracts* 22: 679.

Pico, R. M., L. K. Gerbrandt, M. Pondel, and G. Ivy (1985). During stepwise cue deletion, rat place behaviors correlate with place unit responses. *Brain Research* 330: 369–372.

Pinto, D. J., J. C. Brumberg, D. J. Simons, and G. B. Ermentrout (1996). A quantitative population model of whisker barrels: Re-examining the Wilson-Cowan equations. *Journal of Computational Neuroscience* 3(3): 247–264.

Plaznik, A., W. Danysz, and W. Kostowski (1983). Some behavioral effects of microinjections of noradrenaline and serotonin into the hippocampus of the rat. *Physiological Behavior* 31: 625–631.

Potegal, M. (1972). The caudate nucleus egocentric localization system. *Acta Neurobiological Experiments* 32: 479–494.

Potegal, M. (1982). Vestibular and neostriatal contributions to spatial orientation. In Potegal, M., editor, *Spatial Abilities: Development and Physiological Foundations*, pp. 361–387. Academic Press, New York.

Poucet, B. (1993). Spatial cognitive maps in animals: New hypotheses on their structure and neural mechanisms. *Psychological Review* 100(2): 163–182.

Poucet, B., N. Chapuis, M. Durup, and C. Thinus-Blanc (1986). A study of exploratory behavior as an index of spatial knowledge in hamsters. *Animal Learning and Behavior* 14(1): 93–100.

Poucet, B., C. Thinus-Blanc, and R. U. Muller (1994). Place cells in the ventral hippocampus of rats. *NeuroReport* 5(16): 2045–2048.

Pouget, A. and T. J. Sejnowski (1995). Spatial representations in parietal cortex may use basis functions. In Tesauro, G., D. Touretzky, and T. Leen, editors, *Advances in Neural Information Processing Systems 7*, pp. 157–164. MIT Press, Cambridge MA.

Pratt, I. (1991a). An algorithm for planning "sensible" routes. *Engineering Applications of Artificial Intelligence* 4(2): 97–108.

Pratt, I. (1991b). Path finding in free space using sinusoidal transforms. In Frank, A. and D. Mark, editors, *Cognitive and Linguistic Aspects of Geographic Space*, pp. 219–233. Kluwer, Boston.

Qin, Y. L., B. L. McNaughton, W. E. Skaggs, and C. A. Barnes (1997). Memory reprocessing in corticocortical and hippocampocortical neuronal ensembles. *Philosophical Transactions of the Royal Society, London* B352(1360): 1525–1533.

Quirk, G. J., R. U. Muller, and J. L. Kubie (1990). The firing of hippocampal place cells in the dark depends on the rat's recent experience. *Journal of Neuroscience* 10(6): 2008–2017.

Quirk, G. J., R. U. Muller, J. L. Kubie, and J. B. Ranck, Jr. (1992). The positional firing properties of medial entorhinal neurons: Description and comparison with hippocampal place cells. *Journal of Neuroscience* 12(5): 1945–1963.

Racine, R. J., N. W. Milgram, and S. Hafner (1983). Long-term potentiation phenomena in the rat limbic forebrain. *Brain Research* 260: 217–231.

Rajkowski, J., P. Kubiak, and G. Aston-Jones (1994). Locus coeruleus activity in monkey: Phasic and tonic changes are associated with altered vigilance. *Brain Research Bulletin* 35(5–6): 607–616.

Ramón y Cajal, S. (1968). *The Structure of Ammon's Horn.* Translated by L. M. Kraft. Thomas, Springfield IL.

Ranck, Jr., J. B. (1984). Head-direction cells in the deep cell layers of dorsal presubiculum in freely moving rats. *Society for Neuroscience Abstracts* 10: 599.

Rasmussen, M., C. A. Barnes, and B. L. McNaughton (1989). A systematic test of cognitive mapping, working-memory, and temporal discontiguity theories of hippocampal function. *Psychobiology* 17: 335–348.

Rawlins, J. N. P. (1985). Associations across time: The hippocampus as a temporary memory store. *Behavioral and Brain Sciences* 8: 479–496. See also commentary and response, pages 497–528.

Rawlins, J. N. P., G. L. Lyford, A. Seferiades, R. M. J. Deacon, and H. J. Cassaday (1993). Critical determinants of nonspatial working memory deficits in rats with conventional lesions of the hippocampus or fornix. *Behavioral Neuroscience* 107(3): 420–433.

Recce, M. and K. D. Harris (1996). Memory for places: A navigational model in support of Marr's theory of hippocampal function. *Hippocampus* 6: 735–748.

Redish, A. D. (1997). Beyond the cognitive map: Contributions to a computational neuroscience theory of rodent navigation. Ph.D. diss., Carnegie Mellon University.

Redish, A. D., A. N. Elga, and D. S. Touretzky (1996). A coupled attractor model of the rodent head direction system. *Network: Computation in Neural Systems* 7(4): 671–685.

Redish, A. D. and D. S. Touretzky (1994). The reaching task: Evidence for vector arithmetic in the motor system? *Biological Cybernetics* 71: 307–317.

Redish, A. D. and D. S. Touretzky (1996). Modeling interactions of the rat's place and head direction systems. In Touretzky,

D. S., M. C. Mozer, and M. E. Hasselmo, editors, *Advances in Neural Information Processing Systems 8*, pp. 61–71, Cambridge, MA. MIT Press.

Redish, A. D. and D. S. Touretzky (1997a). Cognitive maps beyond the hippocampus. *Hippocampus* 7(1): 15–35.

Redish, A. D. and D. S. Touretzky (1997b). Implications of attractor networks for cue conflict situations. *Society for Neuroscience Abstracts* 23: 1601.

Redish, A. D. and D. S. Touretzky (1997c). Navigating with landmarks: Computing goal locations from place codes. In Ikeuchi, K. and M. Veloso, editors, *Symbolic Visual Learning*, pp. 325–351. Oxford University Press, New York.

Redish, A. D. and D. S. Touretzky (1998a). The role of the hippocampus in solving the Morris water maze. *Neural Computation* 10(1): 73–111.

Redish, A. D. and D. S. Touretzky (1998b). Separating hippocampal maps. In Burgess, N., K. Jeffery, and J. O'Keefe, editors, *Spatial Functions of the Hippocampal Formation and the Parietal Cortex*, pp. 203–219. Oxford University Press, New York.

Rempel-Clower, N. L., S. M. Zola, L. R. Squire, and D. G. Amaral (1996). Three cases of enduring memory impairment after bilateral damage limited to the hippocampal formation. *Journal of Neuroscience* 16: 5233–5255.

Renner, M. J. (1990). Neglected aspects of exploratory and investigatory behavior. *Psychobiology* 18(1): 16–22.

Reymann, K. G. (1993). Mechanisms underlying synaptic long-term potentiation in the hippocampus: Focus on postsynaptic glutamate receptors and protein kinases. *Functional Neurology* 5(Suppl.): 7–32.

Ribot, T. A. (1882). *Diseases of Memory*, Vol. 1 of *Significant Contributions to the History of Psychology, Series C, Medical Psy-*

chology. Edited by D. N. Robinson. University Publications of America, Washington D. C. 1977.

Robinson, D. A. (1973). Models of the saccadic eye movement control system. *Kybernetik* 14: 71–83.

Rolls, E. T. (1989). The representation and storage of information in neuronal networks in the primate cerebral cortex and hippocampus. In Durbin, R., C. Miall, and G. Mitchison, editors, *The Computing Neuron*, pp. 125–159. Addison-Wesley, Reading, MA.

Rolls, E. T. (1996). A theory of hippocampal function in memory. *Hippocampus* 6: 601–620.

Rolls, E. T., Y. Miyashita, P. M. B. Cahusac, R. P. Kesner, H. Niki, J. D. Feigenbaum, and L. Bach (1989). Hippocampal neurons in the monkey with activity related to the place in which a stimulus is shown. *Journal of Neuroscience* 9(6): 1835–1845.

Rolls, E. T. and S. M. O'Mara (1995). View responsive neurons in the primate hippocampal complex. *Hippocampus* 5: 409–424.

Rotenberg, A., M. Mayford, R. D. Hawkins, E. R. Kandel, and R. U. Muller (1996). Mice expressing activated CaMKII lack low frequency LTP and do not form stable place cells in the CA1 region of the hippocampus. *Cell* 87: 1351–1361.

Rumelhart, D. E., G. E. Hinton, and J. L. McClelland (1986). A general framework for parallel distributed processing. In Rumelhart and McClelland, editors, *Parallel Distributed Processing: Explorations in the Microstructure of Cognition*, Vol. 1, pp. 45–76. MIT Press, Cambridge MA.

Rumelhart, D. E., G. E. Hinton, and R. J. Williams (1986). Learning internal representations by error propogation. In Rumelhart and McClelland, editors, *Parallel Distribted Processing: Explorations in the Microstructure of Cognition*, Vol. 1, pp. 318–362. MIT Press, Cambridge MA.

Sacks, O. (1985). Lost mariner. In *The Man who Mistook his Wife for a Hat*, chapter 2, pp. 22–41. Summitt Books, New York.

Saint-Cyr, J. A., A. E. Taylor, and A. E. Lang (1988). Procedural learning and neostriatal dysfunction in man. *Brain* 111: 941–959.

Saksida, L. M., A. D. Redish, C. R. Milberg, S. J. Gaulin, and D. S. Touretzky (1995). Landmark-based navigation in gerbils supports vector voting. *Society for Neuroscience Abstracts* 21: 1939.

Sakurai, Y. (1990a). Cells in the rat auditory system have sensory delay correlates during the performance of an auditory working memory task. *Behavioral Neuroscience* 104(6): 856–868.

Sakurai, Y. (1990b). Hippocampal cells have behavioral correlates during the performance of an auditory working memory task in the rat. *Behavioral Neuroscience* 104(2): 253–263.

Sakurai, Y. (1994). Involvement of auditory cortical and hippocampal neurons in auditory working memory and reference memory in the rat. *Journal of Neuroscience* 14(5): 2606–2623.

Samsonovich, A. V. (1997). Attractor map theory of the hippocampal representation of space. Ph.D. diss., Graduate Interdisciplinary Program in Applied Mathematics, University of Arizona.

Samsonovich, A. V. and B. L. McNaughton (1996). Attractor-map-based path integrator model of the hippocampus reproduces the phase precession phenomenon. *Society for Neuroscience Abstracts* 22: 1872.

Samsonovich, A. V. and B. L. McNaughton (1997). Path integration and cognitive mapping in a continuous attractor neural network model. *Journal of Neuroscience* 17(15): 5900–5920.

Sara, S. J. and M. Segal (1991). Plasticity of sensory responses of locus coeruleus neurons in the behaving rat: Implications for cognition. *Progress in Brain Research* 88: 571–585.

Save, E., A. Cressant, C. Thinus-Blanc, and B. Poucet (1998). Spatial firing of hippocampal place cells in blind rats. *Journal of Neuroscience* 18(5): 1818–1826.

Save, E. and M. Moghaddam (1996). Effects of lesions of the associative parietal cortex on the acquisition and use of spatial memory in egocentric and allocentric navigation tasks in the rat. *Behavioral Neuroscience* 110(1): 74–85.

Schacter, D. L., N. M. Alpert, C. R. Savage, S. L. Rauch, and M. S. Albert (1996). Conscious recollection and the human hippocampal formation: Evidence from positron emission tomography. *Proceedings of the National Academy of Sciences, USA* 93: 321–325.

Schaffer, K. (1892). Beitrag zur histologie der Ammons Horn-formation. *Archiv für Mikroscopische Anatomie* 39(1). Cited in Ramón y Cajal (1968).

Schallert, T., L. B. Day, M. Weisend, and R. J. Sutherland (1996). Spatial learning by hippocampal rats in the Morris water task. *Society for Neuroscience Abstracts* 22: 678.

Schallert, T., M. De Ryck, and P. Teitelbaum (1980). Atropine sterotypy as a behavioral trap: A movement subsystem and electroencephalographic analysis. *Journal of Comparative Physiology and Psychology* 94(1): 1–24.

Schenk, F. and R. G. M. Morris (1985). Dissociation between components of spatial memory in rats after recovery from the effects of retrohippocampal lesions. *Experimental Brain Research* 58: 11–28.

Schmajuk, N. A. and H. T. Blair (1993). Place learning and the dynamics of spatial navigation: A neural network approach. *Adaptive Behavior* 1: 355–387.

Schölkopf, B. and H. A. Mallot (1993). View-based cognitive mapping and path planning. Technical report 7, Max-Plank-Institut für Biologische Kybernetik.

Schöne, H. (1984). *Spatial Orientation*. Princeton University Press, Translated by C. Strausfeld. Princeton NJ.

Schultz, W. (1997). Dopamine neurons and their role in reward mechanisms. *Current Opinion in Neurobiology* 7: 191–197.

Schultz, W., P. Apicella, R. Romo, and E. Scarnati (1995a). Context-dependent activity in primate striatum reflecting past and future behavioral events. In Houk, J. C., J. L. Davis, and D. G. Beiser, editors, *Models of Information Processing in the Basal Ganglia*, pp. 11–27. MIT Press, Cambridge MA.

Schultz, W., R. Romo, T. Ljungberg, J. Mirenowicz, J. R. hollerman, and A. Dickinson (1995b). Reward-related signals carried by dopamine neurons. In Houk, J. C., J. L. Davis, and D. G. Beiser, editors, *Models of Information Processing in the Basal Ganglia*, pp. 233–248. MIT Press, Cambridge MA.

Scoville, W. B. (1968). Amnesia after bilateral medial temporal-lobe excision: Introduction to case H.M. *Neuropsychologia* 6: 211–213.

Scoville, W. B. and B. Milner (1957). Loss of recent memory after bilateral hippocampal lesions. *Journal of Neurology, Neurosurgery, and Psychiatry* 20: 11–21.

Seamans, J. K. and A. G. Phillips (1994). Selective memory impairments produced by transient lidocaine-induced lesions of the nucleus accumbens in rats. *Behavioral Neuroscience* 108(3): 456–468.

Seguinot, V., R. Maurer, and A. S. Etienne (1993). Dead reckoning in a small mammal: The evaluation of distance. *Journal of Comparative Physiology* A173: 103–113.

Seifert, W., editor (1983). *Neurobiology of the Hippocampus*. Academic Press, London.

Selden, N. R., B. J. Everitt, L. E. Jarrard, and T. W. Robbins (1991). Complementary roles for the amygdala and hippocampus in aversive conditioning to explicit and contextual cues. *Neuroscience* 42(2): 335–350.

Sesack, S. R., A. Y. Deutch, R. H. Roth, and B. S. Bunney (1989). Topographical organization of the efferent projections of the medial prefrontal cortex in the rat: An anterograde tract-tracing study with *Phaseolus vulgaris leucoagglutinin*. *Journal of Comparative Neurology* 290(2): 213–242.

Sesack, S. R. and V. M. Pickel (1990). In the rat medial nucleus accumbens, hippocampal and catecholaminergic terminals converge on spiny neurons and are in apposition to each other. *Brain Research* 527(2): 266–279.

Shapiro, M. L. and P. A. Hetherington (1993). A simple network model simulates hippocampal place fields: 1. Parametric analyses and physiological predictions. *Behavioral Neuroscience* 107(1): 34–50.

Shapiro, M. L., D. K. Simon, D. S. Olton, F. H. Gage III, O. Nilsson, and A. Bjorklund (1989). Intrahippocampal grafts of fetal basal forebrain tissue alter place fields in the hippocampus of rats with fimbria-fornix lesions. *Neuroscience* 32(1): 1–18.

Sharp, P. E. (1991). Computer simulation of hippocampal place cells. *Psychobiology* 19(2): 103–115.

Sharp, P. E. (1996). Multiple spatial/behavioral correlates for cells in the rat postsubiculum: Multiple regression analysis and comparison to other hippocampal areas. *Cerebral Cortex* 6(2): 238–259.

Sharp, P. E. (1997). Subicular cells generate similar firing patterns in two geometrically and visually distinctive environments: Comparison with hippocampal place cells. *Behavioral Brain Research* 85(1): 71–92.

Sharp, P. E., H. T. Blair, and M. Brown (1996). Neural network modeling of the hippocampal formation spatial signals and their possible role in navigation: A modular approach. *Hippocampus* 6(6): 735–748.

Sharp, P. E., H. T. Blair, D. Etkin, and D. B. Tzanetos (1995). Influences of vestibular and visual motion information on the spatial firing patterns of hippocampal place cells. *Journal of Neuroscience* 15(1): 173–189.

Sharp, P. E. and C. Green (1994). Spatial correlates of firing patterns of single cells in the subiculum of the freely moving rat. *Journal of Neuroscience* 14(4): 2339–2356.

Sharp, P. E., J. L. Kubie, and R. U. Muller (1990). Firing properties of hippocampal neurons in a visually symmetrical environment: Contributions of multiple sensory cues and mnemonic processes. *Journal of Neuroscience* 10(9): 3093–3105.

Shen, B. and B. L. McNaughton (1996). Modeling the spontaneous reactivation of experience-specific hippocampal cell assembles during sleep. *Hippocampus* 6(6): 685–693.

Shen, J., C. A. Barnes, B. L. McNaughton, W. E. Skaggs, and K. L. Weaver (1997). The effect of aging on experience-dependent plasticity of hippocampal place cells. *Journal of Neuroscience* 17(17): 6769–6782.

Shen, J., C. A. Barnes, G. L. Wenk, and B. L. McNauyghton (1996). Differential effects of selective immunotoxic lesions of medial septal cholinergic cells on spatial working and reference memory. *Behavioral Neuroscience* 110(5): 1181–1186.

Sherry, D. F. and S. J. Duff (1996). Behavioral and neural bases of orientation in food storing birds. *Journal of Experimental Biology* 199(1): 165–172.

Silva, A. J., R. Paylor, J. M. Wehner, and S. Tonegawa (1992). Impaired spatial learning in α-calcium-calmodulin kinase II mutant mice. *Science* 257: 206–211.

Skaggs, W. E. (1995). Relations between the theta rhythm and activity patterns of hippocampal neurons. Ph.D. diss., University of Arizona.

Skaggs, W. E. (1997). Influence of landmarks in a model of the head direction system. *Society for Neuroscience Abstracts* 23: 504.

Skaggs, W. E., J. J. Knierim, H. S. Kudrimoti, and B. L. McNaughton (1995). A model of the neural basis of the rat's sense of direction. In Tesauro, G., D. S. Touretzky, and T. K. Leen, editors, *Advances in Neural Information Processing Systems 7*, pp. 173–180, Cambridge MA. MIT Press.

Skaggs, W. E. and B. L. McNaughton (1996). Replay of neuronal firing sequences in rat hippocampus during sleep following spatial experience. *Science* 271: 1870–1873.

Skaggs, W. E., B. L. McNaughton, M. A. Wilson, and C. A. Barnes (1996). Theta phase precession in hippocampal neuronal populations and the compression of temporal sequences. *Hippocampus* 6(2): 149–173.

Smith, A. D. and J. P. Bolam (1990). The neural network of the basal ganglia as revealed by the study of synaptic connections of identified neurones. *Trends in Neurosciences* 13(7): 259–265.

Smith, C. (1995). Sleep states and memory processes. *Behavioural Brain Research* 69: 137–145.

Smith, M. L. and B. Milner (1989). Right hippocampal impairment in the recall of spatial location: Encoding deficit or rapid forgetting? *Neuropsychologia* 27(1): 71–81.

Sobel, D. (1995). *Longitude: The True Story of a Lone Genius Who Solved the Greatest Scientific Problem of his Time*. Penguin, New York.

Sohal, V. S. and M. E. Hasselmo (1998). GABA$_B$ modulation improves sequence disambiguation in computational models of hippocampal region CA3. *Hippocampus* 8(2): 171–193.

Sparks, D. L. (1986). Translation of sensory signals into commands for control of saccadic eye movements: Role of primate superior colliculus. *Physiological Review* 66(1): 118–171.

Sparks, D. L. and J. S. Nelson (1987). Sensory and motor maps in the mammalian superior colliculus. *Trends in Neurosciences* 10(8): 312–317.

Squire, L. R. (1987). *Memory and Brain*. Oxford University Press, New York.

Squire, L. R. (1992). Memory and the hippocampus: A synthesis from findings with rats, monkeys, and humans. *Psychology Review* 99(2): 195–231.

Squire, L. R. and P. Alvarez (1995). Retrograde amnesia and memory consolidation: A neurobiological perspective. *Current Opinion in Neurobiology* 5: 169–177.

Squire, L. R., N. J. Cohen, and L. Nadel (1984). The medial temporal region and memory consolidation: A new hypothesis. In Weingartner, H. and E. S. Parker, editors, *Memory Consolidation: Psychobiology of Cognition*. Erlbaum, Hillsdale NJ.

Squire, L. R. and B. J. Knowlton (1995). Learning about categories in the absense of memory. *Proceedings of the National Academy of Sciences, USA* 92: 12470–12474.

Squire, L. R. and S. Zola-Morgan (1988). Memory: Brain systems and behavior. *Trends in Neurosciences* 11(4): 170–175.

Squire, L. R. and S. M. Zola-Morgan (1991). The medial temporal lobe memory system. *Science* 253: 1380–1386.

Sripanidkulchai, K. and J. M. Wyss (1986). Thalamic projections to retrosplenial cortex in the rat. *Journal of Comparative Neurology* 254: 143–165.

Stackman, R. W. and J. S. Taube (1997). Firing properties of head direction cells in the rat anterior thalamic nucleus: Dependence upon vestibular input. *Journal of Neuroscience* 17(11): 4349–4358.

Staubli, U., G. Ivy, and G. Lynch (1984). Hippocampal denervation causes rapid forgetting of olfactory information in rats. *Proceedings of the National Academy of Sciences, USA* 81: 5885–5887.

Stein, B. E. and M. A. Meredith (1993). *The Merging of the Senses*. MIT Press, Cambridge MA.

Stein, J. F. (1991). Space and the parietal areas. In Paillard, J., editor, *Brain and Space*, pp. 185–222. Oxford University Press, New York.

Stein, J. F. (1992). The representation of egocentric space in the posterior parietal cortex. *Brain and Behavioral Sciences* 15: 691–700.

Stewart, M. and S. E. Fox (1990). Do septal neurons pace the hippocampal theta rhythm? *Trends in Neurosciences* 13(5): 163–168.

Stricanne, B., R. A. Andersen, and P. Mazzoni (1996). Eye-centered, head-centered, and intermediate coding of remembered sound locations in area LIP. *Journal of Neurophysiology* 76(3): 2071–2076.

Sutherland, R. J. and K. A. Arnold (1987). Temporally-graded loss of place memory after hippocampal damage. *Neuroscience* Suppl.: 175.

Sutherland, R. J., G. L. Chew, J. C. Baker, and R. C. Linggard (1987). Some limitations on the use of distal cues in place navigation by rats. *Psychobiology* 15(1): 48–57.

Sutherland, R. J. and J. M. Hoesing (1993). Posterior cingulate cortex and spatial memory: A microlimnology analysis. In Vogt, B. A. and M. Gabriel, editors, *Neurobiology of Cingulate Cortex and Limbic Thalamus: A Comprehensive Handbook*, pp. 461–477. Birkhäuser, Boston.

Sutherland, R. J. and A. J. Rodriguez (1990). The role of the fornix/fimbria and some related subcortical structures in place learning and memory. *Behavioral and Brain Research* 32: 265–277.

Sutherland, R. J. and J. W. Rudy (1989). Configural association theory: The role of the hippocampal formation in learning, memory, and amnesia. *Psychobiology* 17(2): 129–144.

Sutherland, R. J., I. Q. Whishaw, and B. Kolb (1983). A behavioral analysis of spatial localization following electrolytic, kainate-, or colchicine-induced damage to the hippocampal formation in the rat. *Behavioral Brain Research* 7: 133–153.

Sutherland, R. J., I. Q. Whishaw, and B. Kolb (1988). Contributions of cingulate cortex to two forms of spatial learning and memory. *Journal of Neuroscience* 8(6): 1863–1872.

Sutherland, R. J., I. Q. Whishaw, and J. C. Regehr (1982). Cholinergic receptor blockade impairs spatial localization by use of distal cues in the rat. *Journal of Comparative and Physiological Psychology* 96(4): 563–573.

Suzuki, S., G. Augerinos, and A. H. Black (1980). Stimulus control of spatial behavior on the eight-arm maze in rats. *Learning and Motivation* 11: 1–18.

Suzuki, W. A. (1996). The anatomy, physiology, and functions of the perirhinal cortex. *Current Opinion in Neurobiology* 6: 179–186.

Tamura, R., T. Ono, M. Fukuda, and K. Nakamura (1990). Recognition of egocentric and allocentric visual and auditory space by neurons in the hippocampus of monkeys. *Neuroscience Letters* 109: 293–298.

Tamura, R., T. Ono, M. Fukuda, and K. Nakamura (1992a). Spatial responsiveness of monkey hippocampal neurons to various visual and auditory stimuli. *Hippocampus* 2(3): 307–322.

Tamura, R., T. Ono, M. Fukuda, and H. Nishijo (1992b). Monkey hippocampal neuron responses to complex sensory stimulation during object discrimination. *Hippocampus* 2(3): 287–306.

Tanaka, K., H. Saito, Y. Fukada, and M. Moriya (1991). Coding visual images of objects in the inferotemporal cortex of the macaque monkey. *Journal of Neurophysiology* 66(1): 170–189.

Tanila, H., M. Shaprio, M. Gallagher, and H. Eichenbaum (1997a). Brain aging: Changes in the nature of information coding by the hippocampus. *Journal of Neuroscience* 17(13): 5155–5166.

Tanila, H., P. Sipilä, M. Shapiro, and H. Eichenbaum (1997b). Brain aging: Impaired coding of novel environmental cues. *Journal of Neuroscience* 17(13): 5167–5174.

Tarassenko, L. and A. Blake (1991). Analogue computation of collision-free paths. In *Proceedings of the 1991 IEEE International Conference on Robotics and Automation*, pp. 540–545.

Taube, J. S. (1995a). Head direction cells recorded in the anterior thalamic nuclei of freely moving rats. *Journal of Neuroscience* 15(1): 1953–1971.

Taube, J. S. (1995b). Place cells recorded in the parasubiculum of freely moving rats. *Hippocampus* 5(6): 569–583.

Taube, J. S. and H. L. Burton (1995). Head direction cell activity monitored in a novel environment and during a cue conflict situation. *Journal of Neurophysiology* 74(5): 1953–1971.

Taube, J. S., J. P. Goodridge, E. J. Golob, P. A. Dudchenko, and R. W. Stackman (1996). Processing the head direction cell signal: A review and commentary. *Brain Research Bulletin* 40(5/6): 477–486.

Taube, J. S., J. P. Klesslak, and C. W. Cotman (1992). Lesions of the rat postsubiculum impair performance on spatial tasks. *Behavioral and Neural Biology* 5: 131–143.

Taube, J. S., R. I. Muller, and J. B. Ranck, Jr. (1990a). Head direction cells recorded from the postsubiculum in freely moving rats. I. Description and quantitative analysis. *Journal of Neuroscience* 10: 420–435.

Taube, J. S., R. I. Muller, and J. B. Ranck, Jr. (1990b). Head direction cells recorded from the postsubiculum in freely moving rats. II. Effects of environmental manipulations. *Journal of Neuroscience* 10: 436–447.

Taube, J. S. and R. U. Muller (1995). Head direction cell activity in the anterior thalamic nuclei, but not the postsubiculum, predicts the animal's future directional heading. *Society for Neuroscience Abtracts* 21: 946.

Terrazas, A., K. M. Gothard, K. C. Kung, C. A. Barnes, and B. L. McNaughton (1997). All aboard! What train-driving rats can tell us about the neural mechanisms of spatial navigation. *Society for Neuroscience Abstracts* 23: 506.

Teyler, T. J. and P. DiScenna (1985). The role of hippocampus in memory: A hypothesis. *Neuroscience and Biobehavioral Reviews* 9: 377–389.

Teyler, T. J. and P. DiScenna (1986). The hippocampal memory indexing theory. *Behavioral Neuroscience* 100(2): 147–154.

Thinus-Blanc, C., L. Bouzouba, K. Chaix, N. Chapuis, M. Durup, and B. Poucet (1987). A study of spatial parameters encoded during exploration in hamsters. *Journal of Experimental Psychology* 13(4): 418–427.

Thinus-Blanc, C., M. Durup, and B. Poucet (1992). The spatial parameters encoded by hamsters during exploration: A further study. *Behavioural Processes* 26: 43–57.

Thinus-Blanc, C., E. Save, M.-C. Buhot, and B. Poucet (1991). The hippocampus, exploratory activity, and spatial memory. In Paillard, J., editor, *Brain and Space*, pp. 334–352. Oxford University Press, New York.

Thompson, L. T. and P. J. Best (1989). Place cells and silent cells in the hippocampus of freely-behaving rats. *Journal of Neuroscience* 9(7): 2382–2390.

Thompson, L. T. and P. J. Best (1990). Long-term stability of the place-field activity of single units recorded from the dorsal hippocampus of freely behaving rats. *Brain Research* 509(2): 299–308.

Tinbergen, N. (1969). *The Study of Instinct*. Clarendon Press, Oxford.

Tolman, E. C. (1948). Cognitive maps in rats and men. *Psychological Review* 55: 189–208.

Tolman, E. C., B. F. Ritchie, and D. Kalish (1946a). Studies in spatial learning. I. Orientation and the short-cut. *Journal of Experimental Psychology* 36: 13–24.

Tolman, E. C., B. F. Ritchie, and D. Kalish (1946b). Studies in spatial learning. II. Place learning versus response learning. *Journal of Experimental Psychology* 36: 221–229.

Touretzky, D. S., S. J. C. Gaulin, and A. D. Redish (1996). Gerbils regularly return to their entry point when exploring a novel environment. *Society for Neuroscience Abstracts* 22: 449.

Touretzky, D. S. and A. D. Redish (1996). A theory of rodent navigation based on interacting representations of space. *Hippocampus* 6(3): 247–270.

Touretzky, D. S., A. D. Redish, and H. S. Wan (1993). Neural representation of space using sinusoidal arrays. *Neural Computation* 5(6): 869–884.

Treves, A., O. Miglino, and D. Parisi (1992). Rats, nets, maps, and the emergence of place cells. *Psychobiology* 20(1): 1–8.

Trullier, O., S. I. Wiener, A. Berthoz, and J. A. Meyer (1997). Biologically based artificial navigation systems: Review and prospects. *Progress in Neurobiology* 51(5): 483–544.

Tsien, J. Z., D. F. Chen, D. Gerber, C. Tom, E. H. Mercer, D. J. Anderson, M. Mayford, and E. R. Kandel (1996). Subregion- and cell type-restricted gene knockout in mouse brain. *Cell* 87: 1317–1326.

Tsien, J. Z., P. T. Huerta, and S. Tonegawa (1996). The essential role of hippocampal CA1 NMDA receptor dependent synaptic plasticity in spatial memory. *Cell* 87: 1327–1338.

Tsodyks, M. and T. Sejnowski (1995). Associative memory and hippocampal place cells. *International Journal of Neural Systems* 6(Suppl.): 81–86.

Tsodyks, M. V., W. E. Skaggs, T. J. Sejnowski, and B. L. McNaughton (1996). Population dynamics and theta rhythm phase precession of hippocampal place cell firing: A spiking neuron model. *Hippocampus* 6(3): 271–280.

Tulving, E. (1983). *Elements of Episodic Memory*. Oxford University Press, New York.

Tulving, E. and H. J. Markowitsch (1997). Memory beyond the hippocampus. *Current Opinion in Neurobiology* 7: 209–216.

Ungerleider, L. G. and J. V. Haxby (1994). 'What' and 'where' in the human brain. *Current Opinion in Neurobiology* 4: 157–165.

Valentine, D. E., R. Iannucci, and C. F. Moss (1994). Sensorimotor integration of spatial information in the superior colliculus of the echolocating bat. *Society for Neuroscience Abstracts* 20: 168.

Valentine, D. E. and C. F. Moss (1997). Spatially selective auditory responses in the superior colliculus of the echolocating bat. *Journal of Neuroscience* 17(5): 1720–1733.

van Groen, T., B. A. Vogt, and J. M. Wyss (1993). Interconnections between the thalamus and retrosplenial cortex in the rodent brain. In Vogt and M. Gabriel, editors, *Neurobiology of Cingulate Cortex and Limbic Thalamus: A Comprehensive Handbook*, pp. 123–150. Birkhäuser, Boston.

van Groen, T. and J. M. Wyss (1990). The postsubicular cortex in the rat: Characterization of the fourth region of the subicular cortex and its connections. *Brain Research* 529: 165–177.

Van Hoesen, G. W. (1982). The parahippocampal gyrus: New observations regarding its cortical connections in the monkey. *Trends in Neurosciences* 5: 345–350.

van Opstal, A. J. and H. Kappen (1993). A two-dimensional ensemble coding model for spatial-temporal transformation of saccades in monkey superior colliculus. *Network: Computation in Neural Systems* 4: 19–38.

Vander Wall, S. B. (1990). *Food Hoarding in Animals*. University of Chicago Press, Chicago.

Vanderwolf, C. H. (1971). Limbic-diencephalic mechanisms of voluntary movement. *Psychological Review* 78(2): 83–113.

Vanderwolf, C. H. (1990). An introduction to the electrical activity of the cerebral cortex: Relations to behavior and control by subcortical inputs. In Kolb, B. and R. C. Tees, editors, *The Cerebral Cortex of the Rat*, pp. 151–189. MIT Press, Cambridge MA.

Vanderwolf, C. H. (1995). Does a history of convulsions increase the amnestic effect of temporal region brain lesions? *Physiology and Behavior* 57(1): 193–197.

Vanderwolf, C. H. and L.-W. S. Leung (1983). Hippocampal rhythmical slow activity: A brief history and the effects of entorhinal lesions and phencyclidine. In Seifert, W., editor, *Neurobiology of the Hippocampus*, pp. 275–302. Academic Press, New York.

Vitte, E., C. Derosier, Y. Caritu, A. Berthoz, D. Hasboun, and D. Soulié (1996). Activiation of the hippocampal formation by vestibular stimulation: A functional magnetic resonance imaging study. *Experimental Brain Research* 112: 523–526.

Vogt, B. A. (1985). Cingulate cortex. In Peters, A. and E.G. Jones, editors, *Association and Auditory Cortices*, Vol. 4 of *Cerebral Cortex*, pp. 89–150. Plenum Press, New York.

Vogt, B. A., R. W. Sikes, and L. J. Vogt (1993). Anterior cingulate cortex and the medial pain system. In Vogt and M. Gabriel, editors, *Neurobiology of Cingulate Cortex and Limbic Thalamus: A Comprehensive Handbook*, pp. 313–344. Birkhauser, Boston.

von Saint Paul, U. (1982). Do geese use path integration for walking home? In Papi, F. and H. G. Wallraff, editors, *Avian Navigation*, pp. 298–307. Springer, New York.

Wallace, A. R. (1873a). Inherited feeling. *Nature* 7: 303.

Wallace, A. R. (1873b). Perception and instinct in the lower animals. *Nature* 8: 65–66.

Wan, H. S., D. S. Touretzky, and A. D. Redish (1994a). Computing goal locations from place codes. In *Proceedings of the Sixteenth Annual Conference of the Cognitive Science Society*, pp. 922–927. Erlbaum, Hillsdale NJ.

Wan, H. S., D. S. Touretzky, and A. D. Redish (1994b). A rodent navigation model that combines place code, head direction, and path integration information. *Society for Neuroscience Abstracts* 20: 1205.

Wan, H. S., D. S. Touretzky, and A. D. Redish (1994c). Towards a computational theory of rat navigation. In Mozer, M., P. Smolensky, D. Touretzky, J. Elman, and A. Weigend, editors, *Proceedings of the 1993 Connectionist Models Summer School*, pp. 11–19. Erlbaum, Hillsdale NJ.

Watanabe, T. and H. Niki (1985). Hippocampal unit activity and delayed response in the monkey. *Brain Research* 325: 241–254.

Watson, J. B. (1907). Kinaesthetic and organic sensations: Their role in the reactions of the white rat to the maze. *Psychological Review* 8(2): 43–100.

Weaver, K. L., J. Shen, B. L. McNaughton, C. A. Barnes, W. E. Skaggs, M. S. Suster, and J. L. Gerrard (1996). Theta phase precession in hippocampal pyramidal cells does not depend on visual input. *Society for Neuroscience Abstracts* 22: 1871.

Wehner, R. and M. V. Srinivasan (1981). Searching behavior of desert ants, genus *Cataglyphis* (Formicidae, Hymenera). *Journal of Comparative Physiology A* 142: 315–338.

Weingartner, H. and E. S. Parker, editors (1984). *Memory Consolidation: Psychobiology of Cognition*, Hillsdale NJ. Erlbaum.

Weisend, M. P., R. S. Astur, and R. J. Sutherland (1996). The specificity and temporal characteristics of retrograde amnesia after hippocampal lesions. *Society for Neuroscience Abstracts* 22: 1118.

West, M. O., R. M. Carelli, M. Pomerantz, S. M. Cohen, J. P. Gardner, J. K. Chapin, and D. J. Woodward (1990). A region in the dorsolateral striatum of the rat exhibiting single-unit correlations with specific locomotor limb movements. *Journal of Neurophysiology* 64(4): 1233–1246.

Whishaw, I. Q. (1985). Cholinergic receptor blockade in the rat impairs locale but not taxon strategies for place navigation in a swimming pool. *Behavioral Neuroscience* 99(5): 979–1005.

Whishaw, I. Q. (1992). What are voluntary movements made of? *Behavioral and Brain Sciences* 15(2): 290–291.

Whishaw, I. Q., J-C. Cassel, and L. E. Jarrard (1995). Rats with fimbria-fornix lesions display a place response in a swimming pool: A dissociation between getting there and knowing where. *Journal of Neuroscience* 15(8): 5779–5788.

Whishaw, I. Q. and L. E. Jarrard (1996). Evidence for extrahippocampal involvement in place learning and hippocampal involvement in path integration. *Hippocampus* 6: 513–524.

Whishaw, I. Q. and H. Maaswinkel (1997). Absence of dead reckoning in hippocampal rats. *Society for Neuroscience Abstracts* 23: 1839.

Whishaw, I. Q. and G. Mittleman (1986). Visits to starts, routes, and places by rats (*Rattus norvegicus*). *Journal of Comparative Psychology* 100(4): 422–431.

Whishaw, I. Q. and G. Mittleman (1991). Hippocampal modulation of nucleus accumbens: Behavioral evidence from amphetamine-induced activity profiles. *Behavioral and Neural Biology* 55: 289–306.

Whishaw, I. Q. and J. A. Tomie (1991). Acquisition and retention by hippocampal rats of simple, conditional, and configural tasks using tactile and olfactory cues: Implications for hippocampal function. *Behavioral Neuroscience* 105(6): 787–797.

Whishaw, I. Q. and J. A. Tomie (1995). Rats with fimbria-fornix lesions can acquire and retain a visual-tactile transwitching (configural) task. *Behavioral Neuroscience* 109(4): 607–612.

White, N. M. (1989). A functional hypothesis concerning the striatal matrix and patches: Mediation of S-R memory and reward. *Life Sciences* 45: 1943–1957.

White, N. M. (1997). Mnemonic functions of the basal ganglia. *Current Opinion in Neurobiology* 7: 164–169.

White, N. M. and N. Hiroi (1998). Preferential localization of self-stimulation sites in striosomes/patches in the rat striatum. *Proceedings of the National Academy of Sciences, USA* 95: 6486–6491.

Whiting, P. D. and J. A. Hillier (1960). A method for finding the shortest route through a road network. *Operational Research Quarterly* 11: 37–40.

Wible, C. G., R. L. Findling, M. Shapiro, E. J. Lang, S. Crane, and D. S. Olton (1986). Mnemonic correlates of unit activity in the hippocampus. *Brain Research* 399: 97–110.

Wickens, J. and R. Kotter (1995). Cellular models of reinforcement. In Houk, J. C., J. L. Davis, and D. G. Beiser, editors, *Models of Information Processing in the Basal Ganglia*, pp. 187–214. MIT Press, Cambridge MA.

Wiener, S. I. (1993). Spatial and behavioral correlates of striatal neurons in rats performing a self-initiated navigation task. *Journal of Neuroscience* 13(9): 3802–3817.

Wiener, S. I., C. A. Paul, and H. Eichenbaum (1989). Spatial and behavioral correlates of hippocampal neuronal activity. *Journal of Neuroscience* 9(8): 2737–2783.

Wiig, K. A. and D. K. Bilkey (1994). Perirhinal cortex lesions in rats disrupt performance in a spatial DNMS task. *NeuroReport* 5: 1405–1408.

Wilson, D. M. (1966). Insect walking. *Annual Review of Entomology* 11: 103–122. Reprinted in Gallistel (1980).

Wilson, H. R. and J. D. Cowan (1973). A mathematical theory of the functional dynamics of cortical and thalamic tissue. *Kybernetik* 13: 55–80.

Wilson, M. A. and B. L. McNaughton (1993). Dynamics of the hippocampal ensemble code for space. *Science* 261: 1055–1058.

Wilson, M. A. and B. L. McNaughton (1994). Reactivation of hippocampal ensemble memories during sleep. *Science* 265: 676–679.

Wilson, M. A. and S. Tonegawa (1997). Synaptic plasticity, place cells and spatial memory: Study with second generation knockouts. *Trends in Neurosciences* 20(3): 102–106.

Wilson, R. C. and O. Steward (1978). Polysynaptic activation of the dentate gyrus of the hippocampal formation: An olfactory input via the lateral entorhinal cortex. *Experimental Brain Research* 33: 523–534.

Winocur, G. (1974). Functional dissociation within the caudate nucleus of rats. *Journal of Comparative and Physiological Psychology* 86(3): 432–439.

Winocur, G. (1990). Anterograde and retrograde amnesia in rats with dorsal hippocampal or dorsomedial thalamic lesions. *Behavioural Brain Research* 38: 145–154.

Wirsching, B. A., R. J. Beninger, K. Jhamandas, R. J. Boegman, and S. R. El-Defrawy (1984). Differential effects of scopolomine on working and reference memory of rats in the radial maze. *Pharmacology Biochemistry and Behavior* 20: 659–662.

Witter, M. P., H. J. Groenewegen, F. H. Lopes da Silva, and A. H. M. Lohman (1989). Functional organization of the extrinsic and intrinsic circuitry of the parahippocampal region. *Progress in Neurobiology* 33: 161–253.

Witter, M. P., R. H. Ostendorf, and H. J. Groenwegen (1990). Heterogeneity in the dorsal subiculum of the rat. Distinct neuronal zones project to different cortical and subcortical targets. *European Journal of Neuroscience* 2: 718–725.

Wittmann, T. and H. Schwegler (1995). Path integration — a network model. *Biological Cybernetics* 73(6): 569–575.

Wolske, M., P. P. Rompre, R. A. Wise, and M. O. West (1993). Activation of single neurons in the rat nucleus accumbens during self-stimulation of the ventral tegmental area. *Journal of Neuroscience* 13(1): 1–12.

Worden, R. (1992). Navigation by fragment fitting: A theory of hippocampal function. *Hippocampus* 2(2): 165–87.

Wu, X., R. A. Baxter, and W. B. Levy (1996). Context codes and the effect of noisy learning on a simplified hippocampal CA3 model. *Biological Cybernetics* 74: 159–165.

Wu, X. and W. B. Levy (1995). Controlling performance by controlling activity levels in a model of hippocampal region CA3. I. Overcoming the effect of noise by adjusting network excitability parameters. In *INNS World Congress on Neural Networks*, pp. II–557–581.

Wyss, J. M. and T. van Groen (1992). Connections between the retrosplenial cortex and the hippocampal formation in the rat: A review. *Hippocampus* 2(1): 1–12.

Ylinen, A., A. Bragin, Z. Nadasdy, G. Jando, I Szabo, A. Sik, and G. Buzsáki (1995). Sharp wave-associated high-frequency oscillation (200 Hz) in the intact hippocampus: Network and intracellular mechanisms. *Journal of Neuroscience* 15(1): 30–46.

Young, B. J., G. D. Fox, and H. Eichenbaum (1994). Correlates of hippocampal complex-spike cell activity in rats performing a nonspatial radial maze task. *Journal of Neuroscience* 14(11): 6553–6563.

Young, B. J., T. Otto, G. D. Fox, and H. Eichenbaum (1997). Memory representation within the parahippocampal region. *Journal of Neuroscience* 17(13): 5183–5195.

Zhang, K. (1996). Representation of spatial orientation by the intrinsic dynamics of the head-direction cell ensemble: A theory. *Journal of Neuroscience* 16(6): 2112–2126.

Zilles, K. (1990). Anatomy of the neocortex: Cytoarchitecture and myeloarchitecture. In Kolb, B. and R. C. Tees, editors, *The Cerebral Cortex of the Rat*, pp. 77–112. MIT Press, Cambridge MA.

Zipser, D. (1985). A computational model of hippocampal place fields. *Behavioral Neuroscience* 99(5): 1006–1018.

Zipser, D. (1986). Biologically plausible models of place recognition and goal location. In *Parallel Distribted Processing: Explorations in the Microstructure of Cognition*, Vol. 2, pp. 423–470. MIT Press, Cambridge MA.

Zola-Morgan, S. and L. R. Squire (1990). The primate hippocampal formation: Evidence for a time-limited role in memory storage. *Science* 250: 288–290.

Zola-Morgan, S. and L. R. Squire (1993). Neuroanatomy of memory. *Annual Review of Neuroscience* 16: 547–563.

Zola-Morgan, S., L. R. Squire, and D. G. Amaral (1986). Human amnesia and the medial temporal region: Enduring memory impairment following a bilateral lesion limited to field CA1 of the hippocampus. *Journal of Neuroscience* 6(10): 2950–2967.

Zola-Morgan, S., L. R. Squire, and D. G. Amaral (1989). Lesions of the amygdala that spare adjacent cortical regions do not impair memory or exacerbate the impairment following lesions of the hippocampal formation. *Journal of Neuroscience* 9(8): 1922–1936.

Zola-Morgan, S., L. R. Squire, D. G. Amaral, and W. A. Suzuki (1989). Lesions of perirhinal and parahippocampal cortex that spare the amygdala and hippocampal formation produce severe memory impairment. *Journal of Neuroscience* 9(8): 4355–4370.

Zola-Morgan, S., L. R. Squire, and S. J. Ramus (1994). Severity of memory impairment in monkeys as a function of locus and extent of damage within the medial temporal lobe memory system. *Hippocampus* 4: 483–495.

Zoladek, L. and W. A. Roberts (1978). The sensory basis of spatial memory in the rat. *Animal Learning and Behavior* 6(1): 77–81.

Author Index

Abbott, L. F., 6, 16, 106, 151, 153, 157, 188, 198
Abraham, L., 81, 283
Adams, J. L., 40, 41, 44
Afifi, A. K., 40, 183
Aggleton, J. P., 39, 40, 88, 89, 283, 302
Albert, M. S., 200
Aldridge, J. W., 41, 44
Alexander, G. E., 40, 183, 282
Alexinsky, T., 180, 297
Allen, Y., 110, 111, 247, 251
Alpert, N. M., 200
Altman, J., 178
Alvarado, M. C., 180, 234
Alvarez, P., xi, 3, 151, 167, 169, 191, 192, 202, 206, 216
Alyan, S. H., 14, 17, 69, 72, 75, 81, 83, 100, 156, 182, 188, 189, 198, 210, 258, 286, 302
Amaral, D. G., 32, 33, 140, 173–175, 178, 191, 203, 213, 217, 294
Amari, S., 57, 115, 219
Amari, S.-I., 57, 115, 117, 219
Andersen, R., 31
Andersen, R. A., 31, 32, 36, 210, 212, 281
Anderson, D. J., 240
Annett, L. E., 5, 89, 90, 234, 238
Apicella, P., 41, 44, 91, 283
Appenzeller, T., 8, 41, 44, 282
Arai, K., 57, 76, 219
Archer, J., 9, 126, 258
Arnold, K. A., 170
Arolfo, M. P., 126
Askenasy, J. J., 168
Aston-Jones, G., 180, 297

Subject Index